The Management of Meniscal Pathology

Eric J. Strauss • Laith M. Jazrawi
Editors

The Management of Meniscal Pathology

From Meniscectomy to Repair and Transplantation

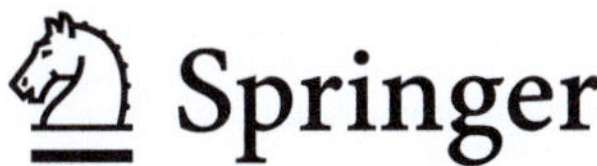

Editors
Eric J. Strauss
Department of Orthopedic Surgery
New York University
New York
USA

Laith M. Jazrawi
Department of Orthopedic Surgery
Sports Medicine Division, NYU Langone
Orthopedic Center
New York
USA

ISBN 978-3-030-49490-2   ISBN 978-3-030-49488-9   (eBook)
https://doi.org/10.1007/978-3-030-49488-9

This Springer imprint is published by the registered company Springer Nature Switzerland AG
The registered company address is: Gewerbestrasse 11, 6330 Cham, Switzerland

Preface

As our understanding of the important role the meniscus plays in normal knee kinematics and function has evolved and numerous advances have been made with respect to surgical techniques and instrumentation, the time is right for a comprehensive text on the management of meniscal pathology. We are extremely thankful to all of the contributing authors for their hard work and to our families for their consistent support, encouragement and love.

New York, NY, USA

Laith M. Jazrawi, MD
Eric J. Strauss, MD

Contents

Contributors

Berkcan Akpinar, MD Department of Orthopedic Surgery, New York University Langone Orthopedic Hospital, New York, NY, USA

Michael Alaia, MD Department of Orthopedic Surgery, Sports Medicine Division, NYU Langone Orthopedic Hospital, New York, NY, USA

Samuel L. Baron, MD NYU Langone Orthopedic Center, New York, NY, USA

Lauren Borowski, MD NYU Langone Orthopedic Center, New York, NY, USA

Dennis Cardone, DO NYU Langone Orthopedic Center, New York, NY, USA

Cordelia Carter, MD Joan H & Preston Robert Tisch Center at Essex Crossing, New York, NY, USA

Jimmy J. Chan, MD Department of Orthopaedic Surgery, Icahn School of Medicine at Mount Sinai, New York, NY, USA

Kevin K. Chen, MD Department of Orthopaedic Surgery, Icahn School of Medicine at Mount Sinai, New York, NY, USA

Philip A. Davidson, MD Davidson Orthopedics, Salt Lake City, UT, USA

Anthony A. Essilfie, MD NYU Langone Orthopedic Center, New York, NY, USA

James N. Gladstone, MD Division of Sports Medicine, Department of Orthopaedic Surgery, Icahn School of Medicine at Mount Sinai, New York, NY, USA

Guillem Gonzalez-Lomas, MD NYU Langone Orthopedic Center, New York, NY, USA

Matthew J. Gotlin, MD Department of Orthopedic Surgery, NYU Langone Orthopedic Hospital, New York, NY, USA

Laith M. Jazrawi, MD Department of Orthopedic Surgery, Sports Medicine Division, NYU Langone Orthopedic Center, New York, NY, USA

Matthew T. Kingery, MD Division of Sports Medicine, Department of Orthopaedic Surgery, NYU Langone Health, New York, NY, USA

David Klein, DO Department of Orthopedic Surgery, Sports Medicine Division, NYU Langone Orthopedic Hospital, New York, NY, USA

Robert Meislin, MD NYU Langone Orthopedic Center, New York, NY, USA

Mehul R. Shah, MD Department of Orthopedic Surgery, NYU Langone Orthopedic Hospital, New York, NY, USA

Eric J. Strauss, MD Division of Sports Medicine, Department of Orthopaedic Surgery, NYU Langone Health, New York, NY, USA

Kamali Thompson, BS, MBA NYU Langone Orthopedic Center, New York, NY, USA

Darryl Whitney, MD NYU Langone Orthopedic Center, New York, NY, USA

Stephen Yu, MD NYU Langone Orthopedic Hospital, New York, NY, USA

Anatomy and Function

1

Samuel L. Baron and Laith M. Jazrawi

Introduction

Once believed to be an unnecessary vestige of human anatomy, the menisci play many critical roles in the biomechanical functioning and long-term health of the knee [1]. The word *meniscus* is derived from the Greek word *mēniskos*, meaning "crescent," which seems appropriately named when viewing its horseshoe-shaped structure.

History in Surgery

Sir Thomas Annandale performed the first documented meniscus surgery in 1885 by suturing together a torn meniscus for a patient with a "locked" knee [2]. Four years later, he introduced and advocated for complete removal of the meniscus instead of repair [3]. In the early twentieth century, and even later throughout, it was commonplace to perform an open total meniscectomy on a patient with symptomatic knee pain or functional impairment secondary to meniscal pathology [4]. In 1942, McMurray advocated for the complete removal of meniscal tissues if there was clinical evidence of posterior meniscus tear, even if the anterior structure was observed to be intact during an open procedure. He even went on to claim insufficient removal of the meniscus was the cause of failed meniscectomy [5].

Although King suggested the amount of degenerative changes seen in the knee was proportional to the amount of meniscus removed during meniscectomy in 1936

S. L. Baron (✉)
NYU Langone Orthopedic Center, New York, NY, USA

L. M. Jazrawi
Department of Orthopedic Surgery, Sports Medicine Division,
NYU Langone Orthopedic Center, New York, NY, USA

© Springer Nature Switzerland AG 2020
E. J. Strauss, L. M. Jazrawi (eds.), *The Management of Meniscal Pathology*,
https://doi.org/10.1007/978-3-030-49488-9_1

[6], it wasn't until 1948 when Fairbank first reported the radiographic evidence of arthropathy following meniscectomy [7]. However, the field was slow to adapt, as open total meniscectomy continued to be the standard approach through the mid-twentieth century.

After its introduction in the 1960s by Ikeuchi [8], arthroscopic meniscectomy replaced its open counterpart as a safer alternative with improved outcomes [9–12]. This change was enhanced by a shift from total to partial meniscectomy, encouraged by reports of decreased contact area and increased contact pressure in the knee following meniscectomy [13, 14]. These practices have evolved into the modern techniques that are used today in an effort to preserve as much of the meniscus and its peripheral rim as possible in order to maintain the biomechanics of the knee joint [15].

Structure and Histology

The meniscus is composed primarily of water (72%) and collagen (22%), with the remaining components being a mixture of cellular tissue, elastins, glycoproteins, and other non-collagenous proteins [16, 17]. The dry-weight composition of a normal human meniscus is roughly 78% collagen, 8% non-collagen proteins, and 1% hexosamine [18]. The noncellular portion, or extracellular matrix (ECM), is produced by hybrid mesenchymal cells called fibrochondrocytes [19, 20]. As implicated by their name, these cells are a phenotypic mixture of fibroblasts and chondrocytes which are critical for the normal function and maintenance of meniscal tissue. Fibrochondrocytes within the meniscus are rich with endoplasmic reticuli and Golgi complexes which aid in the manufacture and transport of extracellular matrix. They typically contain few mitochondria, which suggests their main source of energy is produced via anaerobic glycolysis [17].

Microscopic analysis of meniscal tissue is useful for assessing tissue cellularity and matrix structure. Meniscal tissue may be stained with a traditional hematoxylin and eosin stain to assess cell and tissue morphology; where cell nuclei will stain blueish-purple and cartilage matrix will stain pink or, sometimes, blueish in areas of higher proteoglycan content. Alternatively, Safranin O and Toluidine blue are cationic stains which may be used to better identify glycosaminoglycans and proteoglycans [21].

While the meniscus may appear grossly homogeneous, microscopically its cellular structure varies throughout. Cells in the superficial layer of the meniscus are fusiform, or spindle-shaped, and take on a fibroblastic nature. Conversely, cells of the deep meniscal tissue can be ovoid or polygonal, and are naturally more chondrocytic. While cellular composition changes from superficial to deep portions of the meniscus, cellular morphology does not change in respect to peripheral versus central locations [22, 23].

As cellular composition of the meniscus varies, so too does the makeup of its extracellular matrix. Type I collagen is the predominant collagen fiber type, making up over 90% of extracellular protein. Types II, III, and IV make up the remainder of the collagen content [18, 24]. A study of collagen content in bovine meniscal tissue

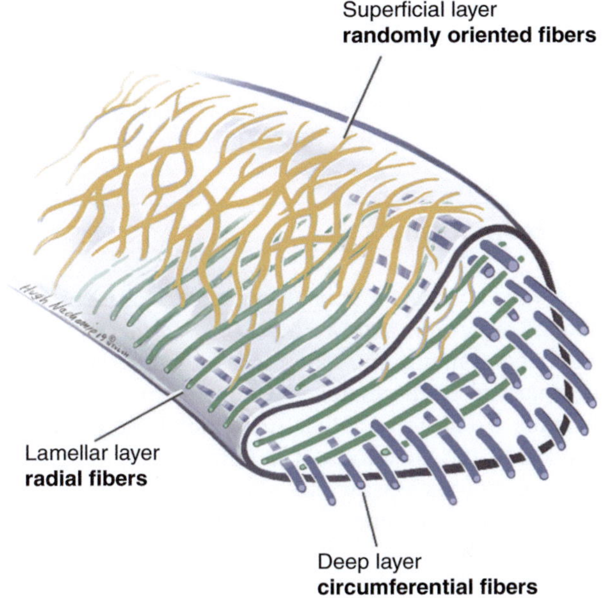

Fig. 1.1 Collagen fiber orientation within the meniscus

found that the outer two-thirds of the meniscus is composed of over 99% type I collagen, while the inner third is a mixture of 60% type II collagen, the major component of articular cartilage, and 40% type I collagen [25].

Collagen fiber orientation changes throughout the cross-sectional surface of the meniscus, depending on the function of each region. Based on fiber orientation, meniscal ultrastructure consists of three distinct layers: a superficial layer, a lamellar layer, and a deep layer (Fig. 1.1). The superficial layer is composed of randomly oriented fibers that provide a smooth and lubricated surface for articulation. The lamellar layer, immediately deep to the superficial layer, is also composed of randomly oriented fibers and interspersed with radially oriented fibers. Lastly, fibers of the deep layer are arranged circumferentially to provide tensile strength, especially in the outer third of meniscal tissue [17, 26–28]. Overall, the majority of fibers are arranged circumferentially, whereas radially oriented fibers can be found more in the inner two-thirds of the meniscus. It is proposed that radial fibers help tie the circumferential fibers together to prevent longitudinal splitting. Additionally, radial fibers of the inner meniscus lay parallel to the articular surface to aid in dispersion of axial loads [29].

Embryology

The paired menisci of the knee obtain their characteristic asymmetrical shape between the 8th and 10th week of gestation. These structures arise from the condensation of intermediate mesenchymal tissue that also forms attachments to the surrounding joint capsule [30, 31]. Early in development, the menisci are highly cellular and vascularized. However, as embryological development progresses, the menisci gradually become peripherally vascularized while cellular density is reduced in exchange for greater collagen content. The collagen, which is initially arranged in a circumferential orientation, is later enhanced by in utero and postnatal joint motion and loading [31, 32].

Gross Anatomy

The knee contains a pair of asymmetrical menisci which are smooth, crescent-shaped structures sandwiched between the femoral condyles and tibial plateau. The medial meniscus, found in the medial compartment of the knee, is larger in comparison to the matched lateral meniscus (Fig. 1.2). Their crescentic shape extends circumferentially, surrounding the periphery of the medial and lateral aspects of the knee joint. The meniscus is wedge-shaped in cross-section along any point on its axis, which allows for the curved femoral condyle to stably and congruently articulate with the tibial plateau. Multiple studies of intra-articular mechanics have shown the menisci occupy roughly 60–70% of the total contact area of the knee joint, thereby alleviating mechanical stress on articular cartilage [33, 34].

Each meniscus is anatomically subdivided into the anterior root, anterior horn, body, posterior horn, and posterior root. Anterior and posterior horns are anchored

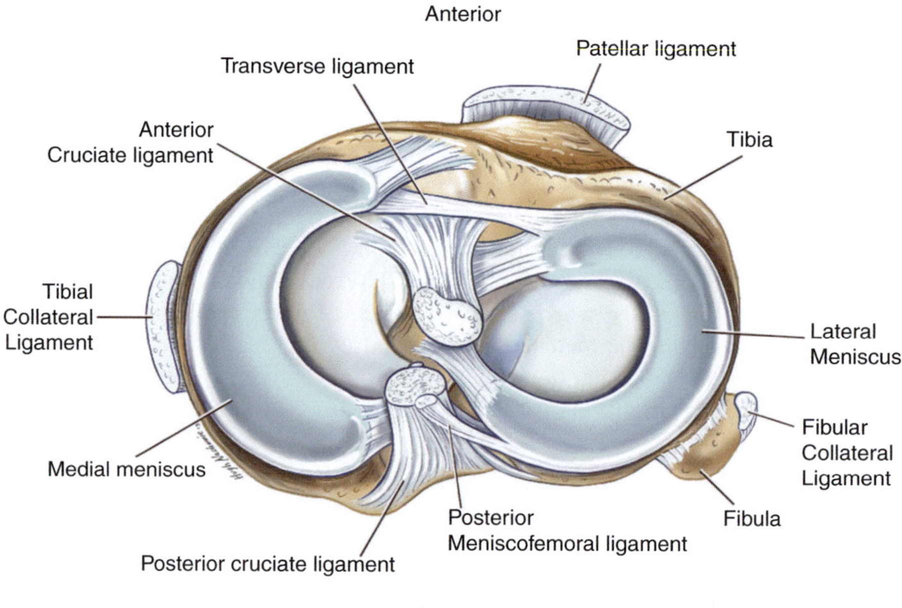

Fig. 1.2 Superior view of the tibial plateau showing menisci and ligaments of the knee

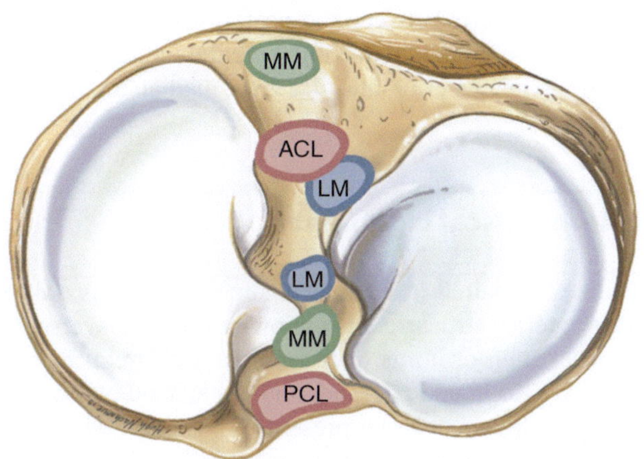

Fig. 1.3 Superior view of the tibial plateau showing footprints of the medial meniscus (MM), lateral meniscus (LM), anterior cruciate ligament (ACL), and posterior cruciate ligament (PCL)

to the tibial plateau by their respective anterior and posterior roots (Fig. 1.3). The body of the meniscus is anchored to the joint capsule throughout its convex peripheral rim via the coronary ligament, with the exception of a segment of the lateral meniscus near the popliteus tendon, which lacks fixation to the capsule. At the midpoint of its body, the medial meniscus is also attached to the deep surface of the medial collateral ligament. The peripheral rim is approximately 110 mm in circumferential length for both the medial and lateral menisci [35].

Tibial Insertion Ligaments

Organized collagen fibers of the meniscus extend from the body to become part of the anterior and posterior insertional ligaments. These ligaments contain transition zones, where increasing stiffness and rigidity toward bony attachments reduce foci of stress during loading. The importance of these ligaments was demonstrated in an animal model, which showed osteochondral changes in the knee equivalent to those of total meniscectomy at 6 and 12 weeks following transection of the anterior or posterior insertional ligaments [36]. While all four ligaments insert onto subchondral bone, each has a distinct footprint and bony landmark.

The fan-shaped anterior insertional ligament of the medial meniscus attaches the anterior horn to the intercondylar fossa roughly 6–7 mm anterior to the attachment site of the anterior cruciate ligament. The anterior insertional ligament of the lateral meniscus also inserts onto the intercondylar fossa, lateral to the anterior cruciate ligament, and somewhat anterior to the lateral intercondylar eminence.

The posterior insertional ligament of the medial meniscus inserts onto the intercondylar fossa between the posterior cruciate ligament and posterior attachment of the lateral meniscus. In an anatomic study, Johannsen et al. described the posterior root attachment of the medial meniscus to be 9.6 mm posterior and 0.7 mm lateral to the apex of the medial tibial eminence [37]. With an insertion less defined than its medial meniscal counterpart, the posterior insertional ligament of the lateral meniscus inserts between the posterior slope of the lateral intercondylar eminence and posterior attachments of the medial meniscus. It was described by Johannsen to be 1.5 mm posterior and 4.2 mm medial to the apex of the lateral tibial eminence [37].

Intermeniscal Ligament

Unlike the paired insertional ligaments, there is only one intermeniscal ligament. This anterior structure, also known as the transverse geniculate ligament, serves to connect anterior horns of the medial and lateral menisci (Fig. 1.2). One cadaveric study by Kohn and Moreno, and another by Nelson and LaPrade, found the intermeniscal ligament to be present in 64% and 94% of knees, respectively [35, 38]. While the presence of the ligament is variable, its functional significance remains unknown.

Nelson and LaPrade went on to describe variations the ligament's attachment pattern. Type I, found in 46% of specimens, was deemed a true anterior intermeniscal ligament and linked the anterior horn of the medial meniscus to the anterior border of the lateral meniscus. Type II intermeniscal ligaments were found in 26% of specimens and passed from the anterior horn of the medial meniscus to the deep surface of the anterior joint capsule. Finally, type III intermeniscal ligaments, which were found in merely 12% of specimens, passed from the anteromedial joint capsule to the anterolateral joint capsule [38].

Meniscofemoral Ligaments

There are two fibrous bands connecting the posterior horn of the lateral meniscus to the lateral portion of the medial condyle within the intercondylar notch of the femur [39]. These structures were first identified by Radoievitch, who coined the term "meniscofemoral ligaments" [40] (Fig. 1.4). The meniscofemoral ligaments were believed to be vestigial structures, however, recent biomechanical studies have discovered they act similarly to the posterior bundle of the PCL, and may also act as secondary resistors to posterior tibial drawer [41, 42].

Each of the two ligaments are named for their positioning with respect to the PCL. The anterior meniscofemoral ligament (aMFL), also known as the ligament of Humphrey, courses anterior to the posterior cruciate ligament and is often confused for the PCL during arthroscopy [43]. The two can be differentiated by pulling on the aMFL, while observing the posterior horn of the lateral meniscus. In a cadaveric study, the ligament of Humphrey was described as being up to one-third the size of the PCL [44]. Another cadaveric study of 92 knees found the aMFL to be present in roughly 50% of specimens [35].

The posterior meniscofemoral ligament (pMFL), also known as the ligament of Wrisberg, runs posterior to the PCL. The insertion of this ligament is in close proximity to that of the PCL at the medial intercondylar notch and, at times, the fibers of

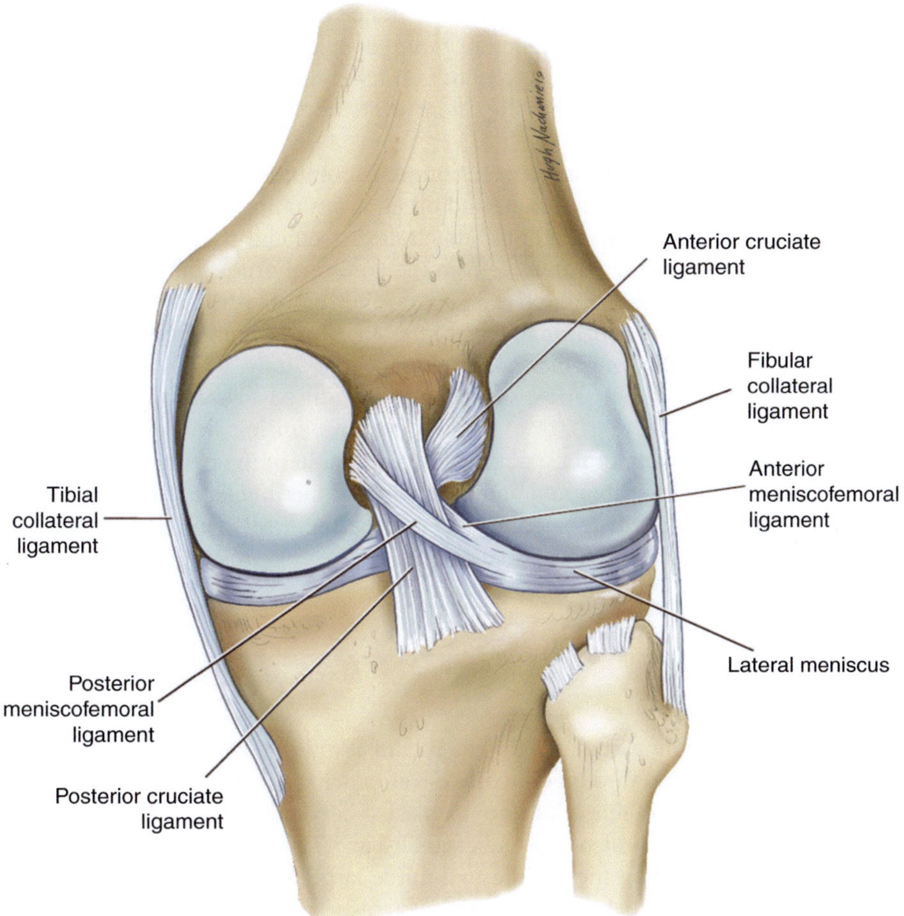

Fig. 1.4 Posterior view of the knee showing anterior and posterior meniscofemoral ligaments

both ligaments may be intermingled [45]. The ligament of Wrisberg is often larger than the ligament of Humphrey, described as being up to half the size of the PCL [44]. Kohn and Moreno found the ligament of Wrisberg to be present in 76% of cadaveric specimens, while Heller and Langman similarly described the pMFL to be present in 71% of 140 knees [35, 44].

The presence of the anterior meniscofemoral ligament is not necessarily associated with presence of the posterior meniscofemoral ligament, and vice versa. Overall, the ligament of Wrisberg is present more often than not, found to be present in 84%, 80%, and 64.4% of cases in three individual MRI-based studies. These same studies found the ligament of Humphrey in 15.8%, 4%, and 11.8% of patients [46–48]. Both ligaments can be found more frequently in males, reported at 67.8% for the aMFL and 74.6% for the pMFL, while females were found to have an aMFL in only 32.3% of cases and a pMFL in

25.4% of cases [48]. Additionally, the prevalence of at least one meniscofemoral ligament is significantly higher in younger knees than in older ones [47, 49]. On imaging, the Wrisberg ligament is thicker and easily identified on coronal sections, while the thinner ligament of Humphrey is best visualized in sagittal sections [46, 48].

In addition to the anterior and posterior meniscofemoral ligaments, structures connecting the menisci to the femur and other surrounding structures have been identified, although they are found much less frequently. The anteromedial meniscofemoral ligament originates from the anterior horn of the medial meniscus and inserts onto the intercondylar area of the femur, while the anterolateral meniscofemoral ligament originates from the anterior horn of the lateral meniscus and inserts onto the same intercondylar area. One study, which reviewed over 2500 arthroscopic knee surgeries, successfully identified an anteromedial meniscofemoral ligament in 13 (0.52%) cases [50]. In addition to these ligaments, fibrous bands from the lateral aspects of the distal pole of the patella insert themselves onto the anterior tibia and anterior horns of the meniscus. These patellomeniscal ligaments (PML), specifically the medial PML, aid in pulling the meniscal horns anteriorly during knee extension, thereby preventing patellar subluxation [51].

Vasculature

The meniscus is highly vascularized in utero and at birth; however, it becomes progressively less perfused throughout child development [31]. By the second year of life, the inner circumference of the meniscus becomes avascular. Vascularity regresses to the outer third of the meniscus by age 10, at which point it reaches vascular maturity, leaving the middle two-thirds largely avascular [52]. This phenomenon is attributed to kinematics and weight-bearing which disrupt vascular structures of the inner two-thirds of the meniscus [31, 32].

Blood supply to the peripheral meniscus originates from the medial, lateral, and middle geniculate arteries [32, 53]. Policard was the first to identify the perimeniscal capillary plexus, which surrounds the peripheral surface of the meniscus and is formed from smaller anastomoses of the popliteal artery [32, 54]. The anterior and posterior horns are most generously supplied with blood via radial branches of the perimeniscal capillary plexus, while the remainder of the periphery is also supplied by radial branches, but less richly so [55]. In fact, merely one-quarter of meniscal periphery receives an adequate blood supply to foster healing, while the remainder relies purely on diffusion of nutrients through the synovial fluid [32]. Of note, the periphery of the adult medial meniscus is slightly more vascularized (10–30%) than the lateral meniscus (10–25%) [53].

The meniscus can be divided into three distinct zones by the extent of their vascularization: a red–red zone in the periphery, an intermediate red–white zone, and a central avascular white–white zone (Fig. 1.5). As one might expect, healing capacity of each zone is directly proportional to its vascular supply. Therefore, injuries

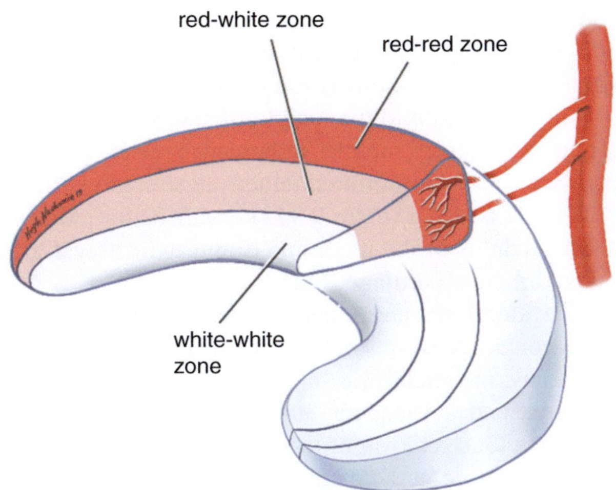

Fig. 1.5 Vascular zones of the meniscus

within the inner white–white zone are far less likely to recover than those of the peripheral red–red zone. Furthermore, the white–white zone is more susceptible to degenerative and posttraumatic lesions [32].

Function

The meniscus is responsible for many functions within the knee joint as it plays critical roles in load-bearing, load transmission, absorption of forces, joint lubrication, and nutrition of articular cartilages [56–58]. When examining meniscal tissue via electron microscopy, Bird and Sweet observed channels running throughout the avascular portions of the deep meniscus and opening to the surface [59]. It is believed that these canals play an important role in fluid transport within the meniscus to carry nutrients from blood and synovial fluid to avascular meniscal tissues [60].

Axial forces are placed on the menisci from the curved femoral condyles and flat tibial plateaus. The meniscus must withstand different types of forces including shear, tension, and compression. As form follows function, its wedge shape allows the meniscus to stabilize the mismatched articular surfaces of the femoral condyles and tibial plateaus [61–63]. This shape, aided by the meniscus' horn-like attachment sites, acts to convert vertical compressive forces into horizontal hoop stress. As they are compressed and deformed radially, fibers within the meniscus must also resist shear forces [34, 63, 64].

Normal human menisci occupy approximately 60% of the contact area within the knee. While the amount of force they transmit is dependent on joint positioning, the menisci transmit over 50% of the axial force applied while in full extension [33, 65]. As the knee is flexed, contact area between the bones of the knee decreases and the menisci transmit a progressively higher amount of the axial load [66]. In full flexion, the lateral meniscus transmits 100% of axial loads in the lateral compartment, while the medial meniscus transmits approximately 50% of medial loads [34]. In compression, the meniscus can withstand axial forces with an aggregate modulus of 100–150 kPa [67]. As a result of ultrastructure and collagen alignment, the tensile strength of the meniscus is roughly tenfold stronger in the circumferential orientation in comparison to the radial orientation. When comparing radially and circumferentially oriented samples of human menisci, Tissakht and Ahmed showed that the meniscus has a circumferential tensile strength with an average elastic modulus of 82.98–111.66 MPa versus 9.94–11.64 MPa for radial specimens [58]. The dynamic shear modulus of the meniscus is approximately 120 kPa, one-fourth to one-sixth that of articular cartilage [68].

The functional and kinematic importance of the meniscus is readily apparent when contact pressures of the knee are examined following varying degrees of meniscectomy. In a cadaveric study, Paletta et al. reported a 50% decrease in total contact area and subsequent 300% increase in peak contact load within the knee following total removal of the lateral meniscus [69]. Similarly, Lee et al. measured contact pressure in the medial compartment following varying degrees of posterior medial meniscectomy. They found reduction of 50% of the radial width of the posterior medial meniscus resulted in significantly higher peak contact stress. These findings were consistent at 0, 30, and 60 degrees of flexion. Furthermore, each serial reduction in meniscal tissue resulted in additional increases in tibiofemoral peak contact pressure [70].

Clinically, removal of meniscal tissue has been associated with cartilage deterioration and progression to osteoarthritis. In the late 1960s, a series of outcomes studies were the first to show that total meniscectomy resulted in a significantly higher incidence of radiographic osteoarthritis (OA) when compared to control groups [71, 72]. Later, a cohort study estimated patients with total meniscectomy were six times more likely to develop OA of the knee [73]. Since partial meniscectomy was shown to result in lower rates of developing OA in comparison to total meniscectomy [74], there has been a general consensus among the orthopedic community that maximum preservation of meniscal tissue is ideal [75]. However, as meniscus tears themselves have also been associated with a greater risk of developing OA, there is controversy surrounding optimal management of meniscal pathology [76]. The risk of OA in the setting of a meniscus tear is likely a result of increased tibiofemoral contact pressure. In a biomechanical model, Lee et al. tested five serial posterior medial meniscectomy conditions. A human cadaveric knee was tested with the medial meniscus intact, 50% radial width, 75% radial width, segmental, and total meniscectomy. All conditions resulted in significantly increased contact pressures compared to the intact meniscus state [77].

Summary

The meniscus is a crescent-shaped, fibrocartilage structure that plays many important roles in the knee. Its anatomic and biomechanical structure are closely related to its function. Deleterious effects of meniscal pathology are often observed in the knee and stress the importance of meniscal tissue conservation in this structure, which has a limited capacity for healing.

References

1. Sutton JB. Nature of ligaments: part II. J Anat Physiol. 1884;19(Pt 1):26 1–50.
2. Annandale T. An operation for displaced semilunar cartilage. Br Med J. 1885;1(1268):779.
3. Annandale T. Excision of the internal semilunar cartilage, resulting in perfect restoration of the joint-movements. Br Med J. 1889;1(1467):291–2.
4. Dandy DJ, Jackson RW. The diagnosis of problems after meniscectomy. J Bone Joint Surg Br. 1975;57(3):349–52.
5. McMurray TP. The semilunar cartilages. Br J Surg. 1942;29:407–14.
6. King D. The function of the semilunar cartilages. J Bone Joint Surg. 1936;18:1069–76.
7. Fairbank TJ. Knee joint changes after meniscectomy. J Bone Joint Surg Br. 1948;30B(4):664–70.
8. Ikeuchi H. Meniscus surgery using the Watanabe arthroscope. Orthop Clin North Am. 1979;10(3):629–42.
9. Benedetto KP, Rangger C. Arthroscopic partial meniscectomy: 5-year follow-up. Knee Surg Sports Traumatol Arthrosc. 1993;1(3-4):235–8.
10. Burks RT, Metcalf MH, Metcalf RW. Fifteen-year follow-up of arthroscopic partial meniscectomy. Arthroscopy. 1997;13(6):673–9.
11. McNicholas MJ, Rowley DI, McGurty D, Adalberth T, Abdon P, Lindstrand A, et al. Total meniscectomy in adolescence. A thirty-year follow-up. J Bone Joint Surg Br. 2000;82(2):217–21.
12. Northmore-Ball MD, Dandy DJ, Jackson RW. Arthroscopic, open partial, and total meniscectomy. A comparative study. J Bone Joint Surg Br. 1983;65(4):400–4.
13. Baratz ME, Fu FH, Mengato R. Meniscal tears: the effect of meniscectomy and of repair on intraarticular contact areas and stress in the human knee. A preliminary report. Am J Sports Med. 1986;14(4):270–5.
14. Krause WR, Pope MH, Johnson RJ, Wilder DG. Mechanical changes in the knee after meniscectomy. J Bone Joint Surg Am. 1976;58(5):599–604.
15. Jeong HJ, Lee SH, Ko CS. Meniscectomy. Knee Surg Relat Res. 2012;24(3):129–36.
16. Herwig J, Egner E, Buddecke E. Chemical changes of human knee joint menisci in various stages of degeneration. Ann Rheum Dis. 1984;43(4):635–40.
17. McDevitt CA, Webber RJ. The ultrastructure and biochemistry of meniscal cartilage. Clin Orthop Relat Res. 1990;252:8–18.
18. Ingman AM, Ghosh P, Taylor TK. Variation of collagenous and non-collagenous proteins of human knee joint menisci with age and degeneration. Gerontologia. 1974;20(4):212–23.
19. McDevitt CA, Miller RR, Sprindler KP. The cells and cell matrix interaction of the meniscus. In: Mow VC, Arnoczky SP, Jackson DW, editors. Knee Meniscus: basic and clinical foundations. New York: Raven Press; 1992. p. 29–36.
20. Webber RJ, Norby DP, Malemud CJ, Goldberg VM, Moskowitz RW. Characterization of newly synthesized pProteoglycans from Rabbit Menisci in organ-culture. Biochem J. 1984;221(3):875–84.
21. Schmitz N, Laverty S, Kraus VB, Aigner T. Basic methods in histopathology of joint tissues. Osteoarthr Cartil. 2010;18(Suppl 3):S113–6.
22. Ghadially FN, Thomas I, Yong N, Lalonde JM. Ultrastructure of rabbit semilunar cartilages. J Anat. 1978;125(Pt 3):499–517.
23. Ghadially FN, Lalonde JM, Wedge JH. Ultrastructure of normal and torn menisci of the human knee joint. J Anat. 1983;136(Pt 4):773–91.
24. Eyre DR, Wu JJ. Collagen of fibrocartilage: a distinctive molecular phenotype in bovine meniscus. FEBS Lett. 1983;158(2):265–70.
25. Cheung HS. Distribution of type I, II, III and V in the pepsin solubilized collagens in bovine menisci. Connect Tissue Res. 1987;16(4):343–56.
26. Rattner JB, Matyas JR, Barclay L, Holowaychuk S, Sciore P, Lo IK, et al. New understanding of the complex structure of knee menisci: implications for injury risk and repair potential for athletes. Scand J Med Sci Sports. 2011;21(4):543–53.

27. Beaupre A, Choukroun R, Guidouin R, Garneau R, Gerardin H, Cardou A. Knee menisci. Correlation between microstructure and biomechanics. Clin Orthop Relat Res. 1986;208:72–5.
28. Bullough PG, Munuera L, Murphy J, Weinstein AM. The strength of the menisci of the knee as it relates to their fine structure. J Bone Joint Surg Br. 1970;52(3):564–7.
29. Skaggs DL, Warden WH, Mow VC. Radial tie fibers influence the tensile properties of the bovine medial meniscus. J Orthop Res. 1994;12(2):176–85.
30. Kaplan EB. The embryology of the menisci of the knee joint. Bull Hosp Joint Dis. 1955;16(2):111–24.
31. Clark CR, Ogden JA. Development of the menisci of the human knee joint. Morphological changes and their potential role in childhood meniscal injury. J Bone Joint Surg Am. 1983;65(4):538–47.
32. Arnoczky SP, Warren RF. Microvasculature of the human meniscus. Am J Sports Med. 1982;10(2):90–5.
33. Fukubayashi T, Kurosawa H. The contact area and pressure distribution pattern of the knee. A study of normal and osteoarthrotic knee joints. Acta Orthop Scand. 1980;51(6):871–9.
34. Walker PS, Erkman MJ. The role of the menisci in force transmission across the knee. Clin Orthop Relat Res. 1975;109:184–92.
35. Kohn D, Moreno B. Meniscus insertion anatomy as a basis for meniscus replacement: a morphological cadaveric study. Arthroscopy. 1995;11(1):96–103.
36. Sommerlath K, Gillquist J. The effect of a meniscal prosthesis on knee biomechanics and cartilage. An experimental study in rabbits. Am J Sports Med. 1992;20(1):73–81.
37. Johannsen AM, Civitarese DM, Padalecki JR, Goldsmith MT, Wijdicks CA, LaPrade RF. Qualitative and quantitative anatomic analysis of the posterior root attachments of the medial and lateral menisci. Am J Sports Med. 2012;40(10):2342–7.
38. Nelson EW, LaPrade RF. The anterior intermeniscal ligament of the knee. An anatomic study. Am J Sports Med. 2000;28(1):74–6.
39. Stoller D, Li A, Anderson L, Cannon W. The knee. 3rd ed. Baltimore: Lippincott Williams & Wilkins; 2007. p. 450.
40. Radoievitch S. Les ligaments des menisques interarticulaires du genous. Ann Anat Path. 1931;8:3–11.
41. Gupte CM, Smith A, Jamieson N, Bull AM, Thomas RD, Amis AA. Meniscofemoral ligaments--structural and material properties. J Biomech. 2002;35(12):1623–9.
42. Gupte CM, Bull AM, Thomas RD, Amis AA. The meniscofemoral ligaments: secondary restraints to the posterior drawer. Analysis of anteroposterior and rotary laxity in the intact and posterior-cruciate-deficient knee. J Bone Joint Surg Br. 2003;85(5):765–73.
43. Standring S. Gray's anatomy, the anatomical basis of clinical practice. 41st ed. Philadelphia, PA: Elsevier Limited; 2016. p. 1383–99.
44. Heller L, Langman J. The Menisco-femoral ligaments of the human knee. J Bone Joint Surg Br. 1964;46:307–13.
45. Amis AA, Gupte CM, Bull AM, Edwards A. Anatomy of the posterior cruciate ligament and the meniscofemoral ligaments. Knee Surg Sports Traumatol Arthrosc. 2006;14(3):257–63.
46. Lee BY, Jee WH, Kim JM, Kim BS, Choi KH. Incidence and significance of demonstrating the meniscofemoral ligament on MRI. Br J Radiol. 2000;73(867):271–4.
47. Cho JM, Suh JS, Na JB, Cho JH, Kim Y, Yoo WK, et al. Variations in meniscofemoral ligaments at anatomical study and MR imaging. Skelet Radiol. 1999;28(4):189–95.
48. Bintoudi A, Natsis K, Tsitouridis I. Anterior and posterior meniscofemoral ligaments: MRI evaluation. Anat Res Int. 2012;2012:839724.
49. Gupte CM, Smith A, McDermott ID, Bull AM, Thomas RD, Amis AA. Meniscofemoral ligaments revisited. Anatomical study, age correlation and clinical implications. J Bone Joint Surg Br. 2002;84(6):846–51.
50. Kim YM, Joo YB. Anteromedial Meniscofemoral ligament of the anterior horn of the medial meniscus: clinical, magnetic resonance imaging, and arthroscopic features. Arthroscopy. 2018;34(5):1590–600.
51. Garth WP Jr, Connor GS, Futch L, Belarmino H. Patellar subluxation at terminal knee extension: isolated deficiency of the medial patellomeniscal ligament. J Bone Joint Surg Am. 2011;93(10):954–62.

52. Petersen W, Tillmann B. Age-related blood and lymph supply of the knee menisci. A cadaver study. Acta Orthop Scand. 1995;66(4):308–12.
53. Danzig L, Resnick D, Gonsalves M, Akeson WH. Blood-supply to the normal and abnormal menisci of the human knee. Clin Orthop Relat Red. 1983;(172):271–6.
54. Policard A. Physiologie générale des articulations à l'état normal et pathologique. Paris: Masson; 1936.
55. Day B, Mackenzie WG, Shim SS, Leung G. The vascular and nerve supply of the human meniscus. Arthroscopy. 1985;1(1):58–62.
56. Proctor CS, Schmidt MB, Whipple RR, Kelly MA, Mow VC. Material properties of the normal medial bovine meniscus. J Orthop Res. 1989;7(6):771–82.
57. Cameron HU, Macnab I. The structure of the meniscus of the human knee joint. Clin Orthop Relat Res. 1972;89:215–9.
58. Tissakht M, Ahmed AM. Tensile stress-strain characteristics of the human meniscal material. J Biomech. 1995;28(4):411–22.
59. Bird MD, Sweet MB. A system of canals in semilunar menisci. Ann Rheum Dis. 1987;46(9):670–3.
60. Bird MD, Sweet MB. Canals in the semilunar meniscus: brief report. J Bone Joint Surg Br. 1988;70(5):839.
61. Radin EL, de Lamotte F, Maquet P. Role of the menisci in the distribution of stress in the knee. Clin Orthop Relat Res. 1984;185:290–4.
62. Hoshino A, Wallace WA. Impact-absorbing properties of the human knee. J Bone Joint Surg Br. 1987;69(5):807–11.
63. Sweigart MA, Athanasiou KA. Toward tissue engineering of the knee meniscus. Tissue Eng. 2001;7(2):111–29.
64. Zhu W, Chern KY, Mow VC. Anisotropic viscoelastic shear properties of bovine meniscus. Clin Orthop Relat Res. 1994;306:34–45.
65. Ahmed AM, Burke DL. In-vitro measurement of static pressure distribution in synovial joints--part I: Tibial surface of the knee. J Biomech Eng. 1983;105(3):216–25.
66. Walker PS, Hajek JV. The load-bearing area in the knee joint. J Biomech. 1972;5(6):581–9.
67. Sweigart MA, Zhu CF, Burt DM, DeHoll PD, Agrawal CM, Clanton TO, et al. Intraspecies and interspecies comparison of the compressive properties of the medial meniscus. Ann Biomed Eng. 2004;32(11):1569–79.
68. Fithian DC, Kelly MA, Mow VC. Material properties and structure-function relationships in the menisci. Clin Orthop Relat Res. 1990;252:19–31.
69. Paletta GA Jr, Manning T, Snell E, Parker R, Bergfeld J. The effect of allograft meniscal replacement on intraarticular contact area and pressures in the human knee. A biomechanical study. Am J Sports Med. 1997;25(5):692–8.
70. Lee SJ, Aadalen KJ, Malaviya P, Lorenz EP, Hayden JK, Farr J, et al. Tibiofemoral contact mechanics after serial medial meniscectomies in the human cadaveric knee. Am J Sports Med. 2006;34(8):1334–44.
71. Jackson JP. Degenerative changes in the knee after meniscectomy. Br Med J. 1968;2(5604):525–7.
72. Tapper EM, Hoover NW. Late results after meniscectomy. J Bone Joint Surg Am. 1969;51(3):517–26 passim.
73. Roos H, Lauren M, Adalberth T, Roos EM, Jonsson K, Lohmander LS. Knee osteoarthritis after meniscectomy: prevalence of radiographic changes after twenty-one years, compared with matched controls. Arthritis Rheum. 1998;41(4):687–93.
74. Englund M, Lohmander LS. Risk factors for symptomatic knee osteoarthritis fifteen to twenty-two years after meniscectomy. Arthritis Rheum. 2004;50(9):2811–9.
75. Lubowitz JH, Poehling GG. Save the meniscus. Arthroscopy. 2011;27(3):301–2.
76. Englund M, Roemer FW, Hayashi D, Crema MD, Guermazi A. Meniscus pathology, osteoarthritis and the treatment controversy. Nat Rev Rheumatol. 2012;8(7):412–9.
77. Lee SJ, Aadalen KJ, Malaviya P, et al. Tibiofemoral contact mechanics after serial medial meniscectomies in the human cadaveric knee. Am J Sports Med. 2006;34(8):1334–44. https://doi.org/10.1177/0363546506286786.

Epidemiology and Classification

2

Guillem Gonzalez-Lomas and Kamali Thompson

Epidemiology

Meniscal injury is the most common intra-articular knee pathology with a prevalence of 60–70 per 100,000 people [1–4], and arthroscopic partial meniscectomy is the most common procedure performed by orthopedic surgeons [5–7]. Several studies have shown one-third of meniscal injuries result from a sports-related activity [8]. Within sports, most meniscus injuries are caused by noncontact injuries, specifically from mechanisms including cutting, decelerating, or landing from a jump [9].

In a 10-year epidemiologic study, Majewski et al. found ski accidents and soccer injuries were responsible for the majority of injury to all knee structures, including the meniscus [3]. Additional high-risk activities for lateral meniscus injury included handball and dance, and for medial meniscus injury included tennis and jogging [3]. Within this study, 84% of patients with meniscal injury required surgical intervention [3].

Gender has been found to be a risk factor for meniscal injury, with males having a 2.5–4 times higher risk than females. This may relate to differential participation in sports and differences in daily activity and occupation [8]. The etiology and classification of meniscal injury are generally specific to age [7, 10, 11]. Most meniscus tears occur between the ages of 20–39 [3, 12–14]. Meniscal injury in children is commonly caused by trauma, discoid meniscus, or meniscal cysts [15]. Traumatic lesions are seen more commonly in younger, more active patients. Degenerative lesions are commonly seen in older patients.

In sports-related internal knee trauma, the medial meniscus is more affected, with a 3:1 ratio of medial to lateral meniscal tears [3]. Anatomically, several differences between lateral and medial menisci may explain the difference in injury occurrence [16]. The medial meniscus is more constrained within the medial

G. Gonzalez-Lomas · K. Thompson (✉)
NYU Langone Orthopedic Center, New York, NY, USA
e-mail: Guillem.Gonzalez-Lomas@nyulangone.org; Kamali.Thompson@nyulangone.org

© Springer Nature Switzerland AG 2020
E. J. Strauss, L. M. Jazrawi (eds.), *The Management of Meniscal Pathology*,
https://doi.org/10.1007/978-3-030-49488-9_2

compartment, whereas the lateral meniscus accommodates motion during knee flexion [15]. The medial meniscus also experiences more force during weight-bearing movements. These characteristics lead to more stress on the medial meniscus during high-impact and torque knee stresses [17, 18]. While medial meniscus tears are more common in an older patient population, lateral meniscus tears are more common in younger patients [16]. Lateral meniscal tears are more frequent in the setting of acute anterior cruciate ligament (ACL) injury, with an incidence ranging from 51% to 72% [19]. This occurs because the lateral meniscus plays an important role in knee stability during the pivot shift mechanism of injury [20].

The peak incidence of traumatic meniscal tears is seen from age 21 to 30 in men and 11 to 19 in women [8, 19, 21, 22]. There may be a correlation between age and injury location. Englund et al. found that 63% of isolated lateral tears were in patients under 20 years old, while 52% of isolated medial tears were in patients above 30 years old. Overall, they identified the prevalence of medial meniscal injury increases with age, present in 50% of adults over 70 years old, suggesting a degenerative etiology [23].

Classification

Meniscus tears are commonly described by orientation: longitudinal/vertical, horizontal, and radial. A combination of tear patterns is often referred to as "complex." Displacement should be noted, as well as specific patterns including bucket handle tears (displaced vertical tears involving a significant amount of meniscus with potential for the torn fragment to flip in and out of the intercondylar notch like a bucket handle) [24]. Orientation is generally linked to etiology (Fig. 2.1), with longitudinal and radial tears resulting from an increased force on a healthy meniscus, and horizontal tears resulting from degeneration [25–27]. Identification of the tear

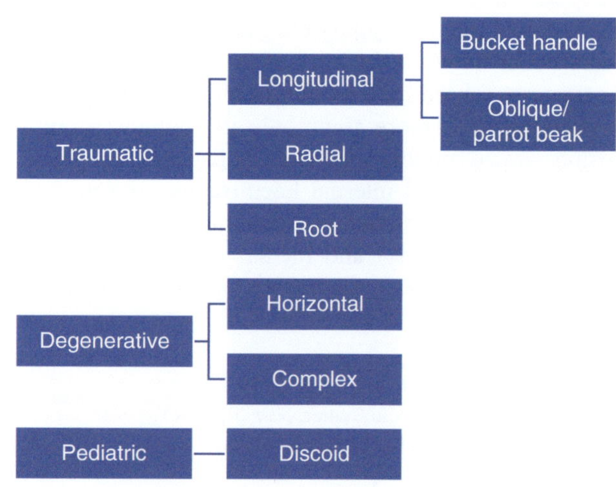

Fig. 2.1 Classification of meniscus tears

pattern impacts operative planning and prognosis [28]. Reparability parameters include the location of the tear with respect to blood supply and healing potential, its orientation, size/length, and chronicity.

Traumatic Tears

During a traumatic event resulting in a tear, the meniscus becomes trapped between the femoral condyle and the tibial plateau while experiencing high forces [29]. Collagen fiber separation ensues either vertically and parallel, creating a longitudinal tear, or vertically and perpendicular, creating a radial tear [29]. Traumatic tears can also be classified as stable or unstable [30].

Longitudinal Tear

Longitudinal tears are perpendicular to the tibial plateau, following the circumference of the meniscus, and separate the meniscus into two portions: central and peripheral [24, 31]. Unlike horizontal and radial tears, these tears do not involve the free edge of the meniscus [24]. However, longitudinal tears may have fluid present, or an irregular outline on the peripheral posterior edge [32]. Usually, longitudinal tears include the peripheral third of the meniscus and posterior horn of the medial or lateral meniscus [24]. The medial meniscus is the most common site, with 75% of longitudinal tears occurring in the posterior horn of the medial meniscus [33].

Tears less than 1 cm and incomplete tears in the peripheral vascularized area have the ability to heal spontaneously [34]. Surgery is not indicated for asymptomatic patients or patients who are not physically active [34]. As meniscal repair is preferred for healthy tissue in vascularized zones, tears in the vascular periphery are repaired, not resected [34].

Radial Tear

Radial tears are perpendicular to the tibial plateau and long axis of the meniscus (Fig. 2.2) [24]. These tears divide the meniscal circumferential fibers [24]. Unlike longitudinal and horizontal tears, radial tears disrupt meniscal hoop strength, resulting in substantial loss of function and potential meniscal extrusion [24]. Meniscal extrusion occurs when the peripheral margin of the meniscus extends 3 mm or more beyond the edge of the tibial plateau [24]. Extrusion exposes the articular surfaces to increased contact stress as the femoral condyles and tibial plateaus interact with each other to higher degree throughout knee flexion and extension [35]. Excessive contact can lead to overload and further damage to the articular cartilage, worsening degeneration [35].

Radial tears represent 15% of meniscus tears, with 79% of tears occurring in the posterior horns [35–37]. Radial tears are frequently located at the junction of the posterior and middle thirds of the medial meniscus or near the posterior attachment of the lateral meniscus [21]. Small radial tears may be subtle and missed. Radial tear extension to the peripheral zone can make the meniscus incompetent [30]. Repair of

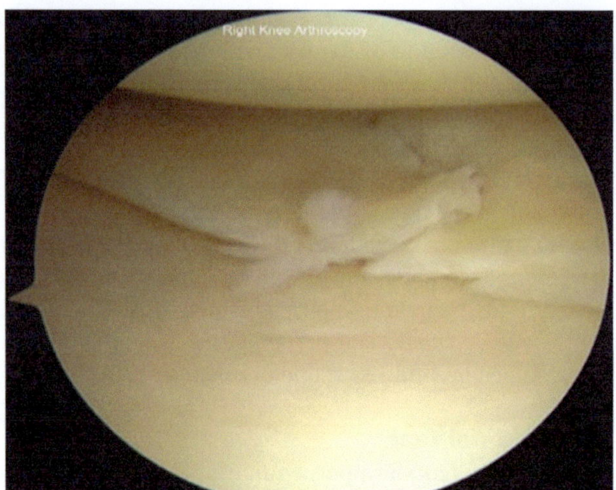

Fig. 2.2 Arthroscopic view of a radial tear

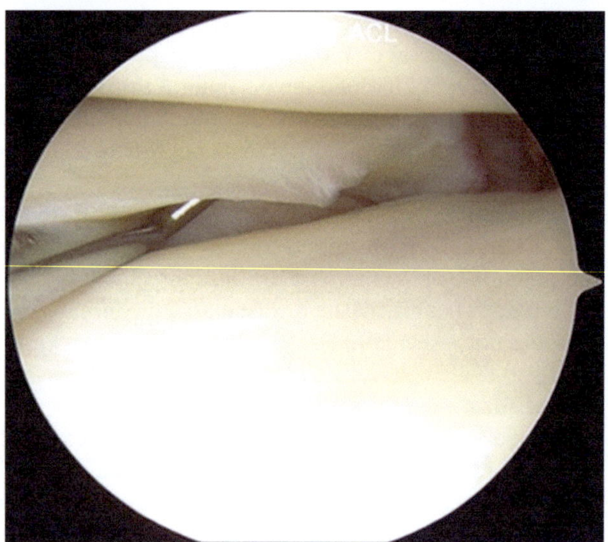

Fig. 2.3 Arthroscopic view of a meniscus root tear

this tear pattern can restore hoop strength and function [34]. However, the typical avascular white–white zone location of these tears may preclude repair and necessitate a partial meniscectomy [24, 34].

Root Tear

Meniscus root tears are radial tears, specifically bony or soft tissue root avulsions injuries, located within 1 cm from the meniscal attachment, and can have either traumatic (e.g., squatting) or degenerative etiologies (Fig. 2.3) [38–44]. Several risk factors have been associated with medial meniscal posterior roots tears, including varus alignment, increased age, high BMI, and female sex [45–48].

Medial root tears are more common and are 5.8 times more likely to have concomitant chondral defects [49]. However, lateral root tears are 10.3 times more likely to occur with an acute ACL injury than medial tears [49]. Root tears, especially medial tears, have a close association with extrusion [39, 50]. Repair should be attempted to prevent further damage [43]. Conservative treatment is reserved for elderly patients or patients with mild to moderate osteoarthritis [43]. Patients with advanced osteoarthritis, who have failed conservativce management, and who complain of persistent mechanical symptoms, may benefit form partial or subtotal meniscectomy [43].

Bucket Handle Tear

Bucket handle tears can either be traumatic or degenerative, but usually present after high velocity accidents [51]. These tears represent 10% of meniscus tears [51]. A bucket handle tear occurs when the longitudinal tear creates fragments and the inner segment fragment migrates centrally while maintaining a connection to the anterior and posterior horns, creating a handle appearance (Fig. 2.4) [24, 52]. Bucket handle tears occur unilaterally, either in the medial or lateral meniscus, rarely in both simultaneously [51]. These tears occur seven times more in the medial meniscus than the lateral meniscus [51].

Degenerative Tears

Degenerative lesions, associated with older age and osteoarthritis, are a result of repeated loads causing microtrauma to the meniscus [53]. Degeneration can lead to horizontal tears, complex tears, and oblique or flap tears [11, 19, 54]. The meniscus experiences various changes after age 40, including a decrease in cellularity and vascularity, as well as an increase in pro-inflammatory cytokines [55–58]. These transformations make the meniscus more susceptible to rupture [56]. Notably,

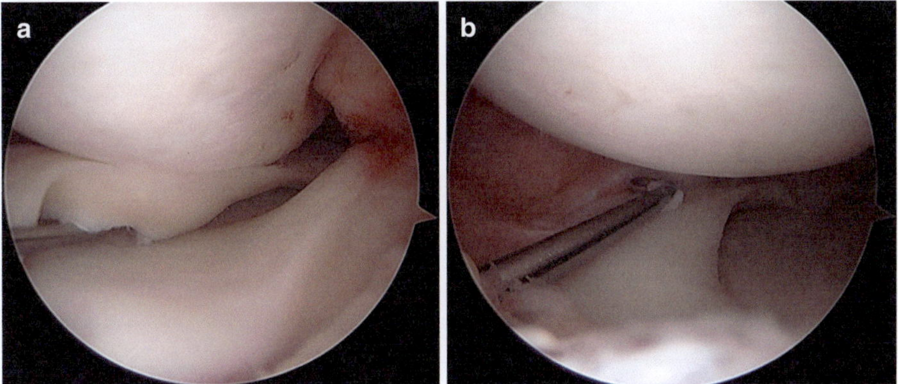

Fig. 2.4 (**a**) Arthroscopic view of meniscus bucket handle tear (**b**) Reduction of bucket handle tear

almost two-thirds of patients with degenerative tears also have an asymptomatic tear in the contralateral knee [59].

Horizontal Tear

A horizontal tear, or cleavage tear, is parallel to the tibial plateau, can involve either the articular surfaces or the central free edge, extend toward the periphery, and separates the meniscus into two fragments: a superior and inferior fragment (Fig. 2.5) [24, 60]. Horizontal fissures are generally stable even with the creation of separate fragments that generally move into surrounding recesses [24, 60, 61]. Complete horizontal tears that extend to the periphery may result in the formation of a parameniscal cyst due to new access to joint space and fluid [62]. The posterior horn of the medial meniscus is the most common location of horizontal cleavages [23].

Horizontal tears represent 32% of meniscus tears [63]. Due to the overall stability of this tear configuration, 60% of patients do not experience mechanical dysfunction and remain asymptomatic [30]. Horizontal tears typically extended into the avascular zone, affecting prognosis and ability to heal [64]. Repair can be considered in patients younger than 50 with no signs of arthritis [65]. Patients who are not appropriate candidates or patients with multiplanar tears with avascular flaps are treated with partial meniscectomy [65].

Complex Tears

Complex tears are seen in conjunction with degenerative joint changes [15]. A complex tear consists of two or more of the following tears: radial, horizontal, or longitudinal [24]. Complex tears give the meniscus a fragmented appearance and extend into more than one plane, most frequently in the posterior horn and midbody (Fig. 2.6) [21, 24]. Complex tears can be treated with repair or partial meniscectomy.

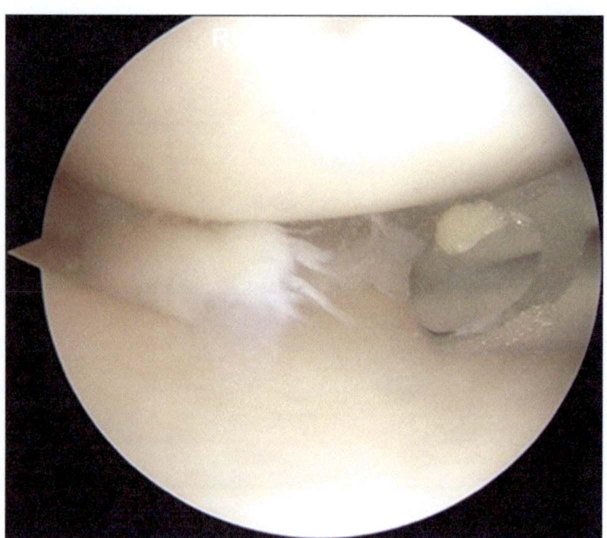

Fig. 2.5 Arthroscopic view of a complex tear

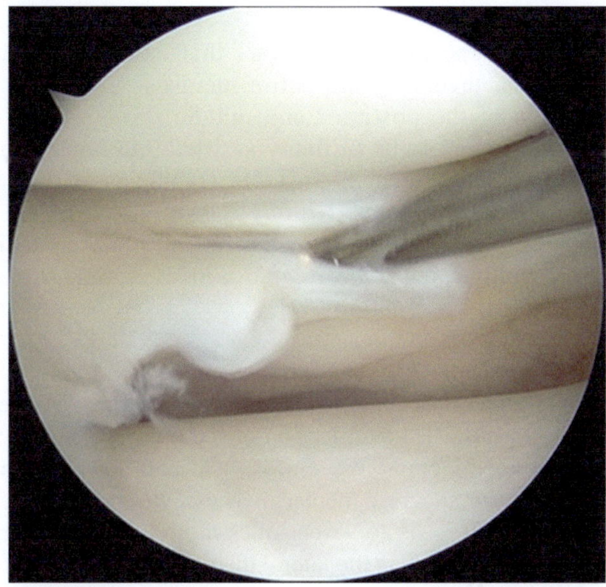

Fig. 2.6 Arthroscopic view of an oblique tear with a horizontal component

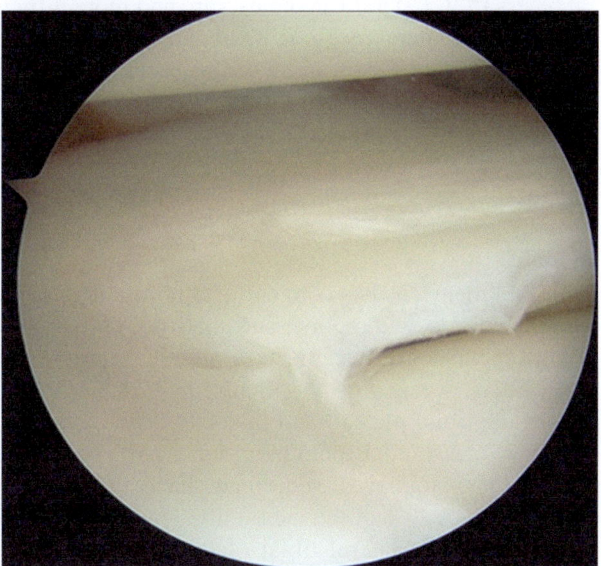

Fig. 2.7 Arthroscopic view of an oblique tear

However, most of these tears form part of the presentation of degenerative joint disease, and isolated management of the meniscus will not alleviate arthritic symptoms [66].

Oblique

Oblique tears are vertical tears that extend toward the anterior horn of the meniscus, involving the entire meniscus. They are frequently located at the junction of the posterior and middle thirds of the meniscus (Fig. 2.7) [21]. Oblique tears can be further classified into flap or parrot beak tears. Flap tears are partially detached, unstable fragments of horizontal tears that produce mechanical symptoms [67, 68]. Parrot beak tears are radial tears with partially detached fragments, connected in one plane and displaced in another plane [68]. Oblique tears are treated with resection to regain stability and reduce mechanical dysfunction [67].

Displaced

Displaced tears occur when a portion of the meniscus separates and becomes a flap or fragment [52]. Identification of the flaps or fragments are vital as retention can lead to knee locking, discomfort, and pain [24]. Fragments are most likely to be found in the superior meniscal recess, inferior meniscal recess, or intercondylar notch [52]. It is six to seven times more likely for fragments to displace from the medial meniscus than the lateral meniscus [69]. Medial fragments are more likely to migrate to the posterior aspect of the intercondylar notch and the medial parameniscal recess [52]. Lateral fragments, rare and more difficult to diagnosis, are likely to migrate to the lateral recess or intercondylar notch [19, 52, 70]. Repair of fragments can be performed if they are in the healing zone. Resection is performed for irreparable fragments [51].

Pediatric Tears

Discoid

A discoid meniscus is a congenital abnormality, creating a hypertrophic, unstable lateral meniscus with poor tissue quality [71]. In comparison to normal meniscus, discoid menisci are thicker, have less vascularity, and decreased number of collagen fibers, weakening the meniscus [72]. Discoid menisci also cover a larger area of the tibial plateau and in some cases cover the entire lateral plateau [71]. Watanabe classified discoid meniscus into Type I, Type II, and Type III [73]. Type I discoid menisci have a semilunar shape and a normal posterior attachment that cover less than 80% of the lateral tibial plateau [73]. Type II discoid menisci completely cover the lateral tibial plateau and have a normal posterior attachment

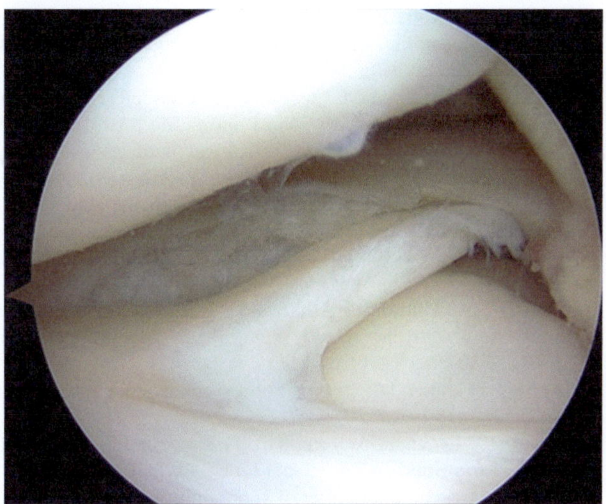

Fig. 2.8 Incomplete discoid lateral meniscus with parrot beak tear

[73]. Type III discoid menisci, Wrisberg menisci, lack the posterior meniscotibial attachment to the tibia [73].

Discoid menisci can cause pain and mechanical symptoms in younger children and present as a tear in older children [71, 74]. Children requiring operative treatment undergo arthroscopic partial central saucerization to revert the meniscus to a normal structure (Fig. 2.8) [74–78].

Conclusion

Meniscus tears are commonly seen on advanced imaging. It is critical to accurately classify the tear in order to develop a treatment plan. The decision between meniscus repair versus debridement is determined based on a constellation of factors including age, chronicity, size, location, and orientation.

References

1. Clayton RA, Court-Brown CM. The epidemiology of musculoskeletal tendinous and ligamentous injuries. Injury. 2008;39(12):1338–44.
2. Hede A, Jensen DB, Blyme P, Sonne-Holm S. Epidemiology of meniscal lesions in the knee. 1,215 open operations in Copenhagen 1982–84. Acta Orthop Scand. 1990;61(5):435–7.
3. Majewski M, Susanne H, Klaus S. Epidemiology of athletic knee injuries: a 10-year study. Knee. 2006;13(3):184–8.
4. Nielsen AB, Yde J. Epidemiology of acute knee injuries: a prospective hospital investigation. J Trauma. 1991;31(12):1644–8.

5. Englund M, Roos EM, Roos HP, Lohmander LS. Patient-relevant outcomes fourteen years after meniscectomy: influence of type of meniscal tear and size of resection. Rheumatology (Oxford). 2001;40(6):631–9.
6. Morgan CD, Wojtys EM, Casscells CD, Casscells SW. Arthroscopic meniscal repair evaluated by second-look arthroscopy. Am J Sports Med. 1991;19(6):632–7; discussion 637–638.
7. Salata MJ, Gibbs AE, Sekiya JK. A systematic review of clinical outcomes in patients undergoing meniscectomy. Am J Sports Med. 2010;38(9):1907–16.
8. Drosos GI, Pozo JL. The causes and mechanisms of meniscal injuries in the sporting and non-sporting environment in an unselected population. Knee. 2004;11(2):143–9.
9. Rath E, Richmond JC. The menisci: basic science and advances in treatment. Br J Sports Med. 2000;34(4):252–7.
10. Makris EA, Hadidi P, Athanasiou KA. The knee meniscus: structure-function, pathophysiology, current repair techniques, and prospects for regeneration. Biomaterials. 2011;32(30):7411–31.
11. Noble J, Hamblen DL. The pathology of the degenerate meniscus lesion. J Bone Joint Surg Br. 1975;57(2):180–6.
12. Baker BE, Peckham AC, Pupparo F, Sanborn JC. Review of meniscal injury and associated sports. Am J Sports Med. 1985;13(1):1–4.
13. Steinbruck K. Epidemiology of sports injuries. A 15 year analysis of sports orthopedic ambulatory care. Sportverletz Sportschaden. 1987;1(1):2–12.
14. Steinbruck K. Epidemiology of sports injuries--25-year-analysis of sports orthopedic-traumatologic ambulatory care. Sportverletz Sportschaden. 1999;13(2):38–52.
15. Fox AJ, Wanivenhaus F, Burge AJ, Warren RF, Rodeo SA. The human meniscus: a review of anatomy, function, injury, and advances in treatment. Clin Anat. 2015;28(2):269–87.
16. Ridley TJ, McCarthy MA, Bollier MJ, Wolf BR, Amendola A. Age differences in the prevalence of isolated medial and lateral meniscal tears in surgically treated patients. Iowa Orthop J. 2017;37:91–4.
17. Costa CR, Morrison WB, Carrino JA. Medial meniscus extrusion on knee MRI: is extent associated with severity of degeneration or type of tear? AJR Am J Roentgenol. 2004;183(1):17–23.
18. Vedi V, Williams A, Tennant SJ, Spouse E, Hunt DM, Gedroyc WM. Meniscal movement. An in-vivo study using dynamic MRI. J Bone Joint Surg Br. 1999;81(1):37–41.
19. Poehling GG, Ruch DS, Chabon SJ. The landscape of meniscal injuries. Clin Sports Med. 1990;9(3):539–49.
20. Musahl V, Citak M, O'Loughlin PF, Choi D, Bedi A, Pearle AD. The effect of medial versus lateral meniscectomy on the stability of the anterior cruciate ligament-deficient knee. Am J Sports Med. 2010;38(8):1591–7. https://doi.org/10.1177/0363546510364402.
21. Greis PE, Bardana DD, Holmstrom MC, Burks RT. Meniscal injury: I. Basic science and evaluation. J Am Acad Orthop Surg. 2002;10(3):168–76.
22. Maher SA, Rodeo SA, Potter HG, Bonassar LJ, Wright TM, Warren RF. A pre-clinical test platform for the functional evaluation of scaffolds for musculoskeletal defects: the meniscus. HSS J. 2011;7(2):157–63.
23. Englund M, Guermazi A, Gale D, et al. Incidental meniscal findings on knee MRI in middle-aged and elderly persons. N Engl J Med. 2008;359(11):1108–15.
24. Nguyen JC, De Smet AA, Graf BK, Rosas HG. MR imaging-based diagnosis and classification of meniscal tears. Radiographics. 2014;34(4):981–99.
25. Fox MG. MR imaging of the meniscus: review, current trends, and clinical implications. Magn Reson Imaging Clin N Am. 2007;15(1):103–23.
26. Hough AJ Jr, Webber RJ. Pathology of the meniscus. Clin Orthop Relat Res. 1990;252:32–40.
27. Jee WH, McCauley TR, Kim JM, et al. Meniscal tear configurations: categorization with MR imaging. AJR Am J Roentgenol. 2003;180(1):93–7.
28. De Smet AA, Tuite MJ, Norris MA, Swan JS. MR diagnosis of meniscal tears: analysis of causes of errors. AJR Am J Roentgenol. 1994;163(6):1419–23.
29. Englund M, Guermazi A, Lohmander SL. The role of the meniscus in knee osteoarthritis: a cause or consequence? Radiol Clin N Am. 2009;47(4):703–12.

30. Beaufils P, Becker R, Kopf S, Matthieu O, Pujol N. The knee meniscus: management of traumatic tears and degenerative lesions. EFORT Open Rev. 2017;2(5):195–203.
31. Rubin DA. MR imaging of the knee menisci. Radiol Clin N Am. 1997;35(1):21–44.
32. De Maeseneer M, Shahabpour M, Vanderdood K, Van Roy F, Osteaux M. Medial meniscocapsular separation: MR imaging criteria and diagnostic pitfalls. Eur J Radiol. 2002;41(3):242–52.
33. Smith JP 3rd, Barrett GR. Medial and lateral meniscal tear patterns in anterior cruciate ligament-deficient knees. A prospective analysis of 575 tears. Am J Sports Med. 2001;29(4):415–9.
34. Vaquero J, Forriol F. Meniscus tear surgery and meniscus replacement. Muscles Ligaments Tendons J. 2016;6(1):71–89.
35. Harper KW, Helms CA, Lambert HS 3rd, Higgins LD. Radial meniscal tears: significance, incidence, and MR appearance. AJR Am J Roentgenol. 2005;185(6):1429–34.
36. Helms CA. The meniscus: recent advances in MR imaging of the knee. AJR Am J Roentgenol. 2002;179(5):1115–22.
37. Magee T, Shapiro M, Williams D. MR accuracy and arthroscopic incidence of meniscal radial tears. Skelet Radiol. 2002;31(12):686–9.
38. Bhatia S, LaPrade CM, Ellman MB, LaPrade RF. Meniscal root tears: significance, diagnosis, and treatment. Am J Sports Med. 2014;42(12):3016–30.
39. Choi CJ, Choi YJ, Lee JJ, Choi CH. Magnetic resonance imaging evidence of meniscal extrusion in medial meniscus posterior root tear. Arthroscopy. 2010;26(12):1602–6.
40. Kim YJ, Kim JG, Chang SH, Shim JC, Kim SB, Lee MY. Posterior root tear of the medial meniscus in multiple knee ligament injuries. Knee. 2010;17(5):324–8.
41. LaPrade CM, Jansson KS, Dornan G, Smith SD, Wijdicks CA, LaPrade RF. Altered tibiofemoral contact mechanics due to lateral meniscus posterior horn root avulsions and radial tears can be restored with in situ pull-out suture repairs. J Bone Joint Surg Am. 2014;96(6):471–9.
42. Marzo JM, Gurske-DePerio J. Effects of medial meniscus posterior horn avulsion and repair on tibiofemoral contact area and peak contact pressure with clinical implications. Am J Sports Med. 2009;37(1):124–9.
43. Pache S, Aman ZS, Kennedy M, et al. Meniscal root tears: current concepts review. Arch Bone Joint Surg. 2018;6(4):250–9.
44. Padalecki JR, Jansson KS, Smith SD, et al. Biomechanical consequences of a complete radial tear adjacent to the medial meniscus posterior root attachment site: in situ pull-out repair restores derangement of joint mechanics. Am J Sports Med. 2014;42(3):699–707.
45. Bin SI, Kim JM, Shin SJ. Radial tears of the posterior horn of the medial meniscus. Arthroscopy. 2004;20(4):373–8.
46. Hwang BY, Kim SJ, Lee SW, et al. Risk factors for medial meniscus posterior root tear. Am J Sports Med. 2012;40(7):1606–10.
47. LaPrade CM, Ellman MB, Rasmussen MT, et al. Anatomy of the anterior root attachments of the medial and lateral menisci: a quantitative analysis. Am J Sports Med. 2014;42(10):2386–92.
48. Ozkoc G, Circi E, Gonc U, Irgit K, Pourbagher A, Tandogan RN. Radial tears in the root of the posterior horn of the medial meniscus. Knee Surg Sports Traumatol Arthrosc. 2008;16(9):849–54.
49. Matheny LM, Ockuly AC, Steadman JR, LaPrade RF. Posterior meniscus root tears: associated pathologies to assist as diagnostic tools. Knee Surg Sports Traumatol Arthrosc. 2015;23(10):3127–31.
50. Brody JM, Lin HM, Hulstyn MJ, Tung GA. Lateral meniscus root tear and meniscus extrusion with anterior cruciate ligament tear. Radiology. 2006;239(3):805–10.
51. Shakespeare DT, Rigby HS. The bucket-handle tear of the meniscus. A clinical and arthrographic study. J Bone Joint Surg Br. 1983;65(4):383–7.
52. Lecouvet F, Van Haver T, Acid S, et al. Magnetic resonance imaging (MRI) of the knee: identification of difficult-to-diagnose meniscal lesions. Diagn Interv Imaging. 2018;99(2):55–64.
53. Vaquero-Picado A, Rodriguez-Merchan EC. Arthroscopic repair of the meniscus: surgical management and clinical outcomes. EFORT Open Rev. 2018;3(11):584–94.
54. Noble J. Lesions of the menisci. Autopsy incidence in adults less than fifty-five years old. J Bone Joint Surg Am. 1977;59(4):480–3.
55. Coppe JP, Desprez PY, Krtolica A, Campisi J. The senescence-associated secretory phenotype: the dark side of tumor suppression. Annu Rev Pathol. 2010;5:99–118.

56. Tsujii A, Nakamura N, Horibe S. Age-related changes in the knee meniscus. Knee. 2017;24(6):1262–70.
57. van Roon JA, Lafeber FP. Role of interleukin-7 in degenerative and inflammatory joint diseases. Arthritis Res Ther. 2008;10(2):107.
58. Zhu Y, Armstrong JL, Tchkonia T, Kirkland JL. Cellular senescence and the senescent secretory phenotype in age-related chronic diseases. Curr Opin Clin Nutr Metab Care. 2014;17(4):324–8.
59. Zanetti M, Pfirrmann CW, Schmid MR, Romero J, Seifert B, Hodler J. Patients with suspected meniscal tears: prevalence of abnormalities seen on MRI of 100 symptomatic and 100 contralateral asymptomatic knees. AJR Am J Roentgenol. 2003;181(3):635–41.
60. Faruch-Bilfeld M, Lapegue F, Chiavassa H, Sans N. Imaging of meniscus and ligament injuries of the knee. Diagn Interv Imaging. 2016;97(7-8):749–65.
61. Lecas LK, Helms CA, Kosarek FJ, Garret WE. Inferiorly displaced flap tears of the medial meniscus: MR appearance and clinical significance. AJR Am J Roentgenol. 2000;174(1):161–4.
62. Ferrer-Roca O, Vilalta C. Lesions of the meniscus. Part II: horizontal cleavages and lateral cysts. Clin Orthop Relat Res. 1980;146:301–7.
63. Metcalf MH, Barrett GR. Prospective evaluation of 1485 meniscal tear patterns in patients with stable knees. Am J Sports Med. 2004;32(3):675–80.
64. Arnoczky SP, Warren RF. Microvasculature of the human meniscus. Am J Sports Med. 1982;10(2):90–5.
65. Woodmass JM, Johnson JD, Wu IT, Saris DBF, Stuart MJ, Krych AJ. Horizontal cleavage meniscus tear treated with all-inside circumferential compression stitches. Arthrosc Tech. 2017;6(4):e1329–33.
66. Rubman MH, Noyes FR, Barber-Westin SD. Arthroscopic repair of meniscal tears that extend into the avascular zone. A review of 198 single and complex tears. Am J Sports Med. 1998;26(1):87–95.
67. Mordecai SC, Al-Hadithy N, Ware HE, Gupte CM. Treatment of meniscal tears: an evidence-based approach. World J Orthop. 2014;5(3):233–41.
68. Raj MA, Bubnis MA. Knee meniscal tears. Treasure Island: StatPearls; 2018.
69. Vande Berg BC, Malghem J, Poilvache P, Maldague B, Lecouvet FE. Meniscal tears with fragments displaced in notch and recesses of knee: MR imaging with arthroscopic comparison. Radiology. 2005;234(3):842–50.
70. McKnight A, Southgate J, Price A, Ostlere S. Meniscal tears with displaced fragments: common patterns on magnetic resonance imaging. Skelet Radiol. 2010;39(3):279–83.
71. Kocher MS, Logan CA, Kramer DE. Discoid lateral meniscus in children: diagnosis, management, and outcomes. J Am Acad Orthop Surg. 2017;25(11):736–43.
72. Atay OA, Pekmezci M, Doral MN, Sargon MF, Ayvaz M, Johnson DL. Discoid meniscus: an ultrastructural study with transmission electron microscopy. Am J Sports Med. 2007;35(3):475–8.
73. Kim JG, Han SW, Lee DH. Diagnosis and treatment of discoid meniscus. Knee Surg Relat Res. 2016;28(4):255–62.
74. Kocher MS, Klingele K, Rassman SO. Meniscal disorders: normal, discoid, and cysts. Orthop Clin North Am. 2003;34(3):329–40.
75. Adachi N, Ochi M, Uchio Y, Kuriwaka M, Shinomiya R. Torn discoid lateral meniscus treated using partial central meniscectomy and suture of the peripheral tear. Arthroscopy. 2004;20(5):536–42.
76. Hart ES, Kalra KP, Grottkau BE, Albright M, Shannon EG. Discoid lateral meniscus in children. Orthop Nurs. 2008;27(3):174–9; quiz 180–171.
77. Ikeuchi H. Arthroscopic treatment of the discoid lateral meniscus. Technique and long-term results. Clin Orthop Relat Res. 1982;167:19–28.
78. Youm T, Chen AL. Discoid lateral meniscus: evaluation and treatment. Am J Orthop (Belle Mead NJ). 2004;33(5):234–8.

Meniscal Pathology: Presentation and Diagnosis

Matthew J. Gotlin and Mehul R. Shah

Clinical Presentation

Meniscus pathology can present in many different ways, depending on the patients' age and mechanism of injury. Tears of the meniscus are common, can represent up to 11% of all acute knee disorders, and may represent up to 31% of all chronic knee disorders [1]. Symptomatic meniscal tears are a leading cause of visits to a healthcare provider [2, 3].

In younger adult patients there is frequently a traumatic etiology, usually caused by a twisting mechanism. There is immediate onset of knee pain, commonly at the joint line, with associated knee effusion. The knee effusion is usually mild to moderate and may take 12–24 hours to declare itself. If a patient develops a large effusion immediately after the injury, one must be concerned about a concomitant anterior cruciate ligament (ACL) rupture. Acute rupture of the ACL is associated with meniscal tears in up to 73% of patients and usually involves the lateral meniscus, while chronic ACL tears are usually associated with medial meniscal tears [4]. Range of motion of the knee may also be limited after a meniscal tear. It is important to distinguish loss of motion due to pain and hemarthrosis versus a mechanical block. If a patient presents with grossly reduced range of motion, a knee aspiration can be performed to help with diagnosis. If range of motion of the knee does not improve after evacuation of the hemarthrosis, then a flipped bucket-handle meniscus tear may be suspected and warrants immediate attention and further work up.

Mechanical symptoms are common in meniscal tears, specifically longitudinal or buckle-handle medial meniscal tears. Mechanical symptoms include catching, popping, and locking. The traditional emphasis on the value of mechanical symptoms in the diagnosis of symptomatic meniscal tears may have limited utility in middle-aged and older patients with knee pain [3]. In this patient population,

M. J. Gotlin · M. R. Shah (✉)
Department of Orthopedic Surgery, NYU Langone Orthopedic Hospital, New York, NY, USA
e-mail: Matthew.gotlin@nyulangone.org; Mehul.shah@nyulangone.org

© Springer Nature Switzerland AG 2020
E. J. Strauss, L. M. Jazrawi (eds.), *The Management of Meniscal Pathology*,
https://doi.org/10.1007/978-3-030-49488-9_3

Table 3.1 Types of meniscal tears

	Acute	Degenerative
Age	20–45 years old	>45 years old
Etiology	Trauma, twisting injury	"Wear-and-tear," remote trauma
Pain	Immediate onset	Intermittent, gradual onset
Swelling	Mild to moderate	Intermittent, activity dependent
Mechanical symptoms	+	+/−
Associate injuries	ACL ruptures, chondral injury	Knee osteoarthritis, chronic ACL tears

localized knee pain lasting <1 year favored the diagnosis of meniscal tear. It is important to note that locking is not pathognomonic of bucket-handle tears but they should raise your suspicion. Locking can also occur secondary to loose bodies, patella maltracking, and articular cartilage defects.

Patients over the age of 45 usually have meniscal tears that are degenerative in nature [5]. Degenerative meniscal tears present differently than acute tears (Table 3.1). These patients may have a remote history of a twisting injury or trauma, but often they are unable to recall an inciting event. They usually have pain with activities in their daily life and may have intermittent swelling and pain. These episodic effusions, which usually improve with rest, ice, and anti-inflammatories, can however progress to cause significant disability. It is often difficult to distinguish pain related to meniscal tears versus degenerative joint disease in this patient population. Patients with meniscal tears usually have faster progression of symptoms, more localized pain, and they may have mechanical symptoms.

Meniscal Root Tears

Meniscal root tears can be challenging to diagnose because they don't typically present with the same signs of symptoms of a meniscal body tear. Patients with posterior root tears may report posterior knee pain, but mechanical symptoms such as locking, catching, or giving way are less likely to be present [6]. They may also experience pain during knee flexion, specifically squatting. Meniscus root injuries are not typically associated with a traumatic event, but some patients report minor trauma. Meniscal root tears are commonly seen in patients with degenerative arthritis.

Children and Adolescents

The incidence of meniscal tears in children and adolescents is growing, likely secondary to increased participation in sports. Diagnosing meniscal pathology in this age group can be challenging. In general, these injuries can occur be divided into two categories: discoid meniscus tears and nondiscoid meniscus tears.

The torn nondiscoid meniscus usually occurs secondary to a traumatic twisting injury and results in medial or lateral knee pain. The pain is usually activity related and improves with rest. Swelling, mechanical symptoms, and giving way may also be present. Medial meniscus tears are more common in this age group. Meniscal tears have been noted in 47% of preadolescents (aged 7–12 years) and in 45% of adolescents (aged 13–18 years) with acute traumatic hemarthrosis [7]. However, in children, other diagnoses can mimic the presentation of meniscal tears, such as osteochondritis dissecans (OCD), patellofemoral syndrome, unstable Wrisberg variant discoid meniscus, pathologic plica, loose body, and osteochondral injury [8].

A discoid meniscus in children can often lead to Snapping Knee Syndrome. This usually presents in children under 10 years of age, and they complain of intermittent, dramatic popping and snapping within the knee. These episodes can occur spontaneously, usually as the knee moves from flexion to extension and may lead to pain and apprehension. In very young children (aged 3–4 years), the snapping is usually asymptomatic, whereas older children (aged 8–10 years) more commonly experience pain with activity [9]. As they are more common laterally, patients usually have lateral side knee symptoms.

Key Points
- Mechanical symptoms are more common in longitudinal tears or bucket-handle medial meniscal tears.
- Locking is NOT pathognomonic of bucket-handle tears: They can also happen with loose bodies, patella maltracking, or articular cartilage defects.
- Degenerative meniscal tears may not have history of any trauma.

Physical Exam

Evaluation begins with basic physical exam principles of inspection, range of motion, palpation, and strength testing. The physical examination should include the entire affected extremity, including a thorough hip and back exam, as well as a comparative exam of the unaffected contralateral knee.

Inspection

Patients with acute meniscal tears often present with an effusion, although the absence of an effusion does not rule out a meniscal tear. One must be suspicious about a concomitant intra-articular ligamentous injury if the hemarthrosis is very large. In contrast, degenerative and meniscal body tears usually do not cause hemarthrosis. Repeat displacement of a pedunculated or extruded meniscus can cause recurrent synovial irritation and lead to chronic synovitis. If a patient presents with a large effusion preventing further examination, an aspiration is indicated.

Range of Motion

Range of motion of the knee is often limited in the setting of an acute meniscal tear, but normal in the setting of degenerative tears. Flexion may be limited secondary to pain or posterior horn tears. Lack of full extension can be due to anterior horn tears, bucket-handle tears, or can be secondary to hemorrhage in the posterior capsule or a collateral ligament with associated hamstring spasm. Aspiration and brief observation may distinguish reduced range of motion secondary to hemarthrosis from real mechanical locking. Always compare the range of motion of the contralateral knee to detect subtle differences.

Palpation

Palpation should include bilateral joint lines and posterior knee structures. Joint line tenderness is the most sensitive test for meniscal tears and is most commonly caused by reactive synovitis and an inflamed capsule. Joint line tenderness has high sensitivity, but lower specificity [10]. Abdon et al. found that joint-line tenderness and mechanical locking were predictive of meniscal tear [11].

Associated Injuries

It is important to assess the knee for concomitant ligamentous injuries. Therefore, one should also complete a thorough ligamentous exam, testing the integrity of the cruciate and collateral ligaments. This should include Lachman testing, anterior/posterior drawer, and testing for varus and valgus instability both at 0° and 30° of flexion.

Special Tests

There are also many special tests reported to diagnose meniscal tears. It is important to know that multiple studies document no single meniscus test that provides adequate diagnostic utility in isolation [10]. It is the combination of symptoms, signs, and physical exam findings that help predict the presence of meniscal pathology.

Thessaly Test

Patients with suspected meniscal tears experience medial or lateral joint-line discomfort and may have a sense of locking or catching during the Thessaly test (Fig. 3.1). The Thessaly test at 20° demonstrated the highest sensitivity and specificity of all special tests (sensitivity: 89% for the medial meniscus, 92% for the lateral meniscus; specificity: 97% for the medial meniscus, 96% for the lateral meniscus) [12].

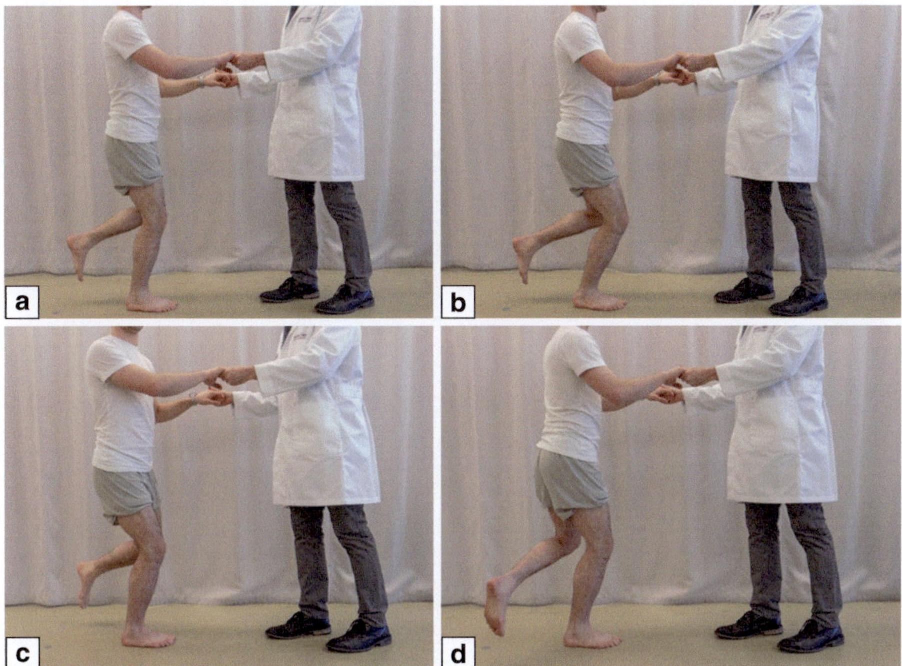

Fig. 3.1 Thessaly test: The examiner supports the patient by holding his or her outstretched hands while the patient stands flatfooted on the affected leg. The patient then rotates his or her knee and body, internally and externally, three times, keeping the knee in 5° of flexion (**a**). Then the same procedure is carried out with the knee flexed at 20° (**b**). (**c**: external, **d**: internal)

McMurray Test

The exam is described in Fig. 3.2. Internal rotation is meant to test the lateral meniscus, while external rotation is meant to test the medial meniscus. The test is positive if the patient feels pain and hears a "pop" from the knee or if the examiner feels a "thud" at the joint line. The McMurray test has low sensitivity but high specificity. Of note, ACL-deficiency decreases the value of the McMurray test.

Apley Test

The patient is in the prone position, the hip is extended, and the knee flexed 90°. The examiner applies axial pressure onto the foot and rotates the tibia (Fig. 3.3). The resulting knee joint pain is regarded as a positive test [13].

Steinmann Part 1 Test

Pain in the medial joint cavity in forced external rotation suggests damage to the medial meniscus; pain in the lateral joint compartment in internal rotation suggests damage to the lateral meniscus [14] (Fig. 3.4).

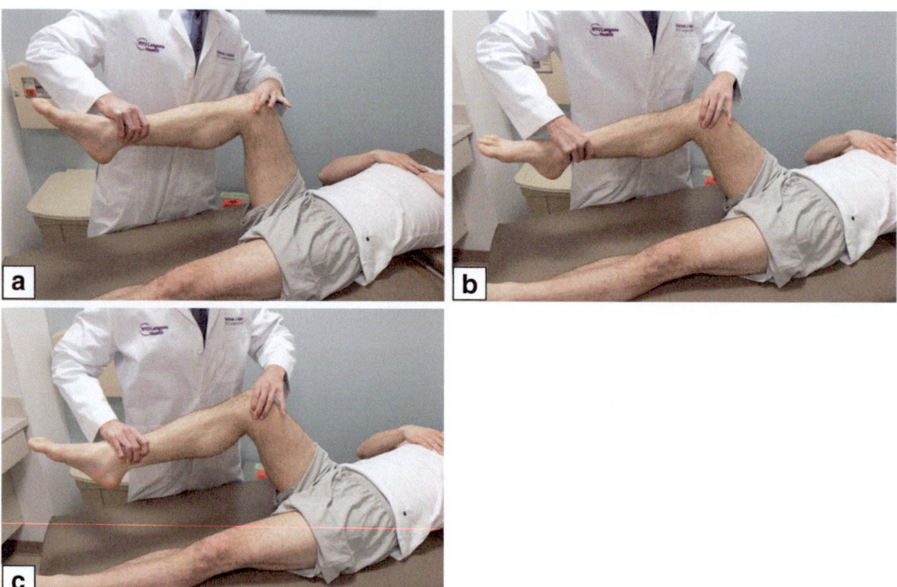

Fig. 3.2 McMurray test: The patient lies supine on the bed while bending the knee and hip. With the knee in full flexion, the examiner holds the knee joint with one hand by placing his index finger and thumbs along the joint line (**a**) and then uses the other hand to extend and twist the leg in internal rotation (**b**) and finally external rotation (**c**)

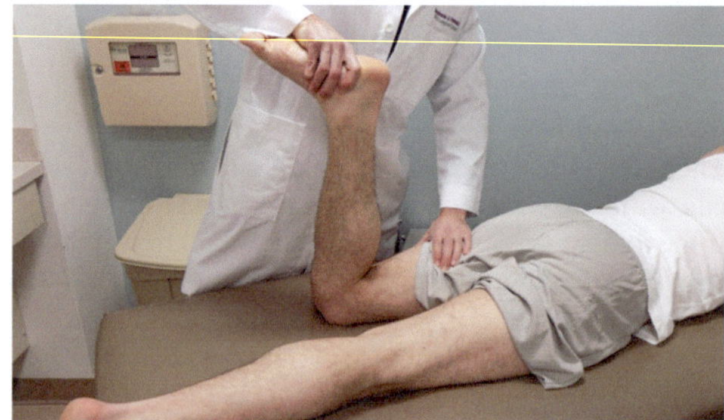

Fig. 3.3 Apley test: The patient is in the prone position, the hip is extended, and the knee flexed at 90°. The examiner applies axial pressure onto the foot and rotates the tibia

Payr's Test

Knees are flexed beyond 90°, and legs crossed. Downward force on the knee leads to pain the medial knee compartment because of compression (Fig. 3.5). A positive test is associated with a lesion of the medial posterior horn [14].

Squat Test (Childress Sign)

The patient squats and walks like a duck (Fig. 3.6). With a positive test, the patient will feel pain, cannot squat all the way down, and will feel a snap or click from the knee joint [15].

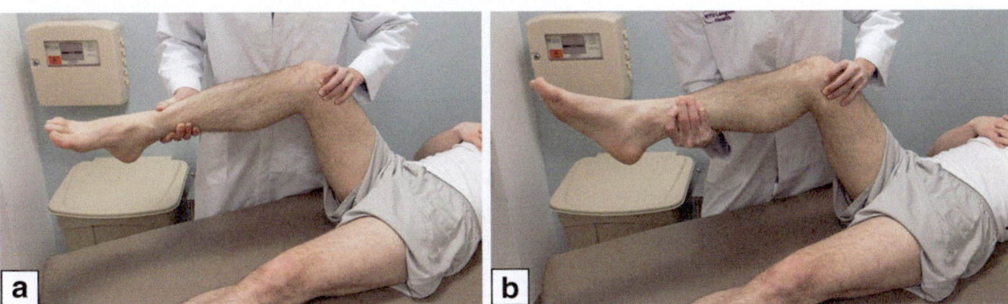

Fig. 3.4 Steinmann part 1 test: The patient is supine. The examiner immobilizes the patient's flexed knee at 90° with one hand and grasps the lower leg with the other hand. The examiner then forcefully rotates the lower leg in internal (**a**) and external rotation (**b**)

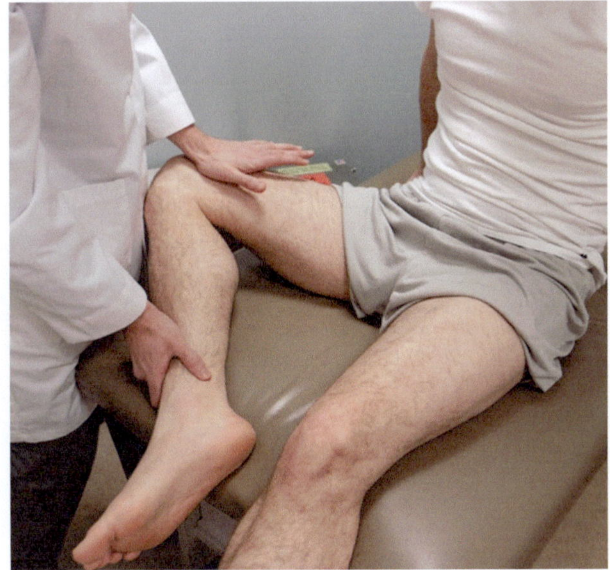

Fig. 3.5 Payr's test is illustrated here. Knees are flexed beyond 90° and legs crossed. Downward force on the knee leads to pain the medial knee compartment because of compression

Ege's Test

The test is positive when pain and/or a click are felt by the patient (sometimes audible to the physician) at the related site of the joint line [16] (Fig. 3.7).

Key Points

- Main physical exam findings include effusion, joint line tenderness, and reproducible click with manual maneuvers. Efforts should be made to reproduce these clicks and to locate them anatomically.
- Always check the contralateral knee.
- An injured locked knee that is not relieved with aspiration of hemarthrosis may need surgical intervention.
- The hip and back should be thoroughly examined.

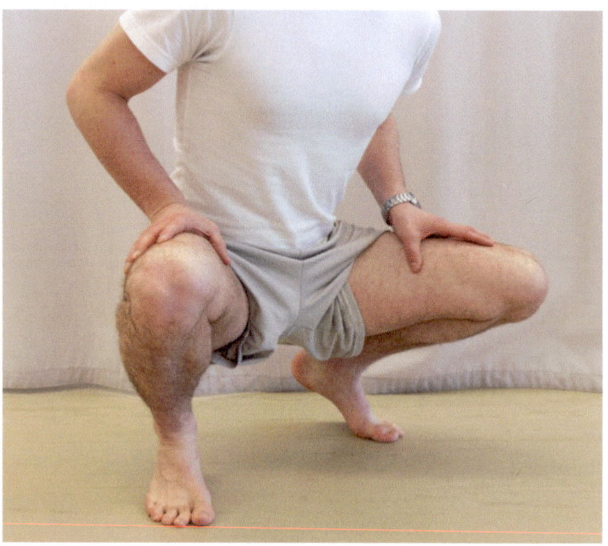

Fig. 3.6 The squat test. The patient gets into a squatting position and walks like a duck

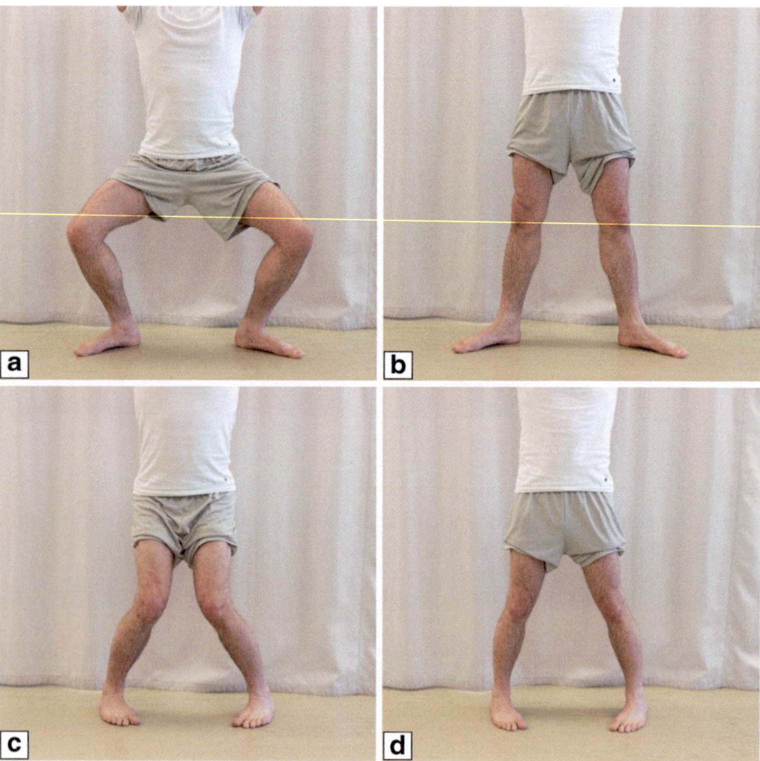

Fig. 3.7 Ege's test: The test is performed with the patient in a standing position. The knees are in extension, and the feet are held 30–40 cm away from each other at the beginning of the test. To detect a medial meniscal tear, the patient squats with both lower legs in maximum external rotation and then stands up slowly (**a** and **b**, respectively). For lateral meniscal tears, both lower extremities are held in maximum internal rotation while the patient squats and stands up (**c** and **d**, respectively)

Imaging

Obtaining imaging is important in the evaluation of a patient with a painful knee and a suspected meniscal injury. Imaging has been shown to improve diagnostic accuracy. Advanced imaging, such as a magnetic resonance imaging (MRI), is not always indicated to evaluate meniscal pathology but it is helpful in the evaluation of associated injuries when a meniscal tear is suspected. The different types of imaging modalities will be reviewed in this section.

Radiographs

Although standard radiographs are not conclusive in diagnosing meniscal injury, they are indicated to confirm or obtain a differential diagnosis. Every patient should get standard X-rays, which includes anterior–posterior (AP), 45° flexion posterior–anterior (PA), lateral, and patellofemoral views (Fig. 3.8). X-rays are used to rule out any other causes of knee pain such as osteoarthritis, chondrocalcinosis, loose bodies, bony pathology, findings consistent with associated injuries such as a Segond sign (ACL tears), or osteochondritis dissecans. Full-length standing lower extremity films can also be obtained to assess the alignment of the lower limb, which may help in decision-making toward treatment.

CT Arthrography

Arthrography was the established way to diagnose meniscal tears in the 1970s and 1980s. It has a reliability between 83% and 94% in the diagnosis of meniscal tears [17]. Arthrography was largely given up in the 2000s with the advent of MRI. However, combined with CT, CT arthrography has a sensitivity and specificity between 86% and 100% for identifying meniscal pathology [18]. CT arthrography is a viable option for patients who are too large for MRI machines, suffer from claustrophobia, or have contraindication for MRIs (pacemakers, etc.). The advent of open MRIs has allowed patients with claustrophobia to obtain MR imaging. The disadvantages of CT arthrography include need for intravenous and intraarticular contrast, joint manipulation, and exposure to ionizing radiation.

Ultrasound

Ultrasound is not used routinely to diagnose meniscal pathology. Dynamic ultrasound has been shown to have a sensitivity of 82% for the detection of meniscal degeneration [19]. Parameniscal cysts, however, are easily diagnosed with ultrasound. It has a sensitivity of 97%, a specificity of 86%, and accuracy of 94% in the setting of meniscal cysts. Practitioners may also choose to puncture and aspirate cysts via ultrasound guidance. Ultrasound is operator dependent, and its accuracy is contingent on the radiologist's and technician's experience.

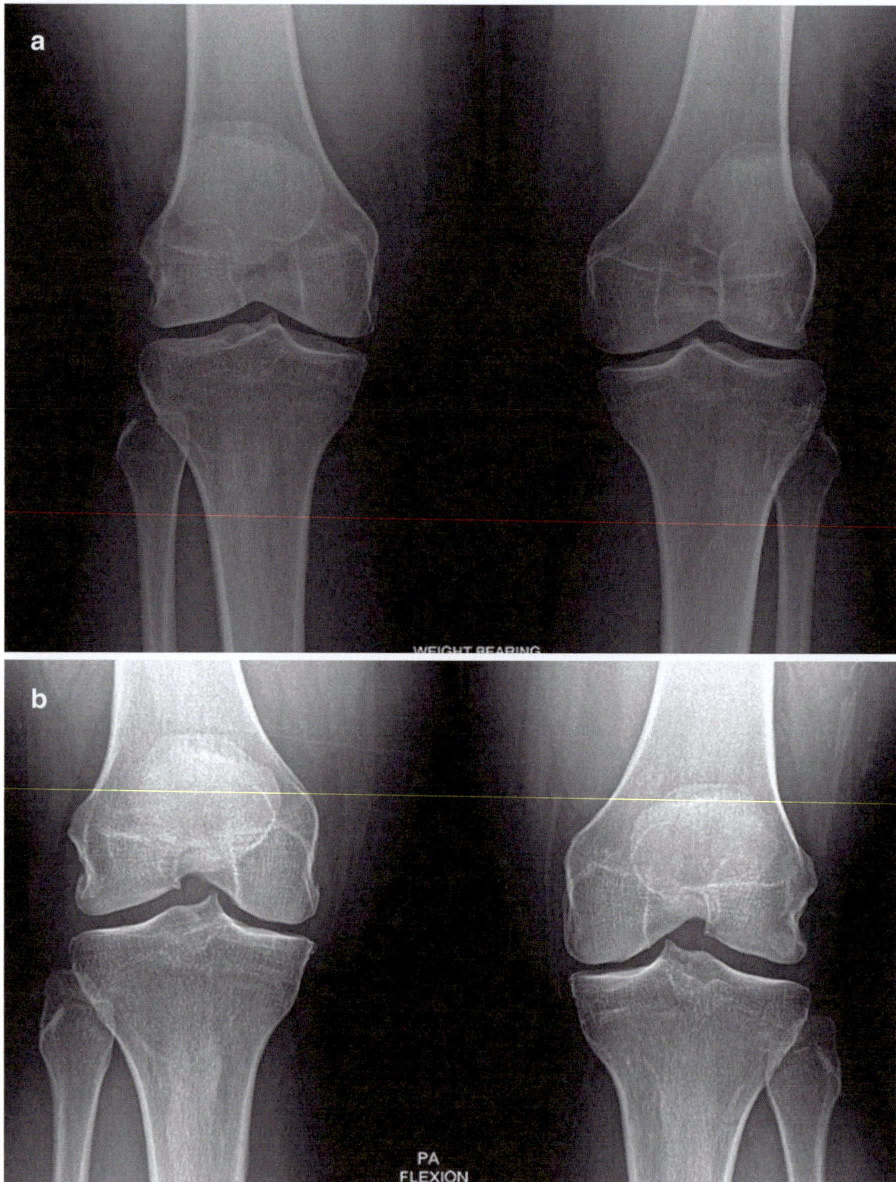

Fig. 3.8 (**a**) Weight-bearing anterior–posterior (AP), (**b**) posterior–anterior (PA) 45° flexion, (**c**) lateral, and (**d**) patellofemoral view radiographs

Fig. 3.8 (continued)

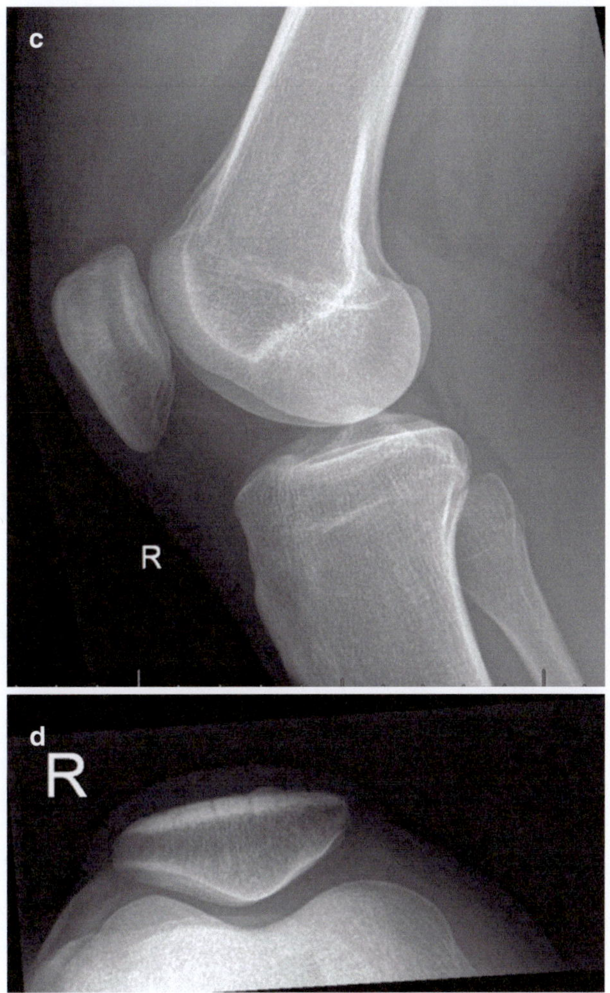

Magnetic Resonance Imaging (MRI)

For detecting meniscal tears, MRI has become the "gold standard" imaging modality. It has many advantages over other imaging techniques (Table 3.2). It is more precise than physical examination and has high correlation with arthroscopic findings [20]. It allows you to analyze the meniscus in all spatial planes, has high-quality resolution, and allows one to thoroughly examine other structures such has articular cartilage, subchondral bone, and cruciate/collateral ligaments. MRI has been shown to have a sensitivity as high as 96% and specificity of 97% [21]. The sensitivity is higher for medial meniscal tears while the specificity is higher for lateral meniscal tears [22]. MRIs using a 1.5 tesla machines have shown similar results to 3.0 tesla machines in terms of diagnostic ability in meniscal pathology [23].

MRI sequences used to detect meniscal tears include T-1-weighted (less sensitive), T-2-weighted, STIR or T-2-weighted fast spin echo with specific fat suppression, and proton density–weighted (FSE) images. Newer 3D isotropic turbo spin echo MRIs have helped improve the diagnosis of meniscal tears [24]. Intravenous or intra-articular gadolinium contrast is rarely needed. Evaluating the meniscus is challenging because scar tissue may cause abnormal signal in standard MRIs. MR arthrograms or gadolinium-enhanced MRIs are useful in evaluating knees with prior meniscectomies or meniscal repair [25].

A classification system has been developed for meniscal degeneration detected on MRI (Table 3.3). This three-stage classification created by Stoller and Crues has been shown to be reliable (88–95%), sensitive (87–97%), and specific (89–98%) [26]. To diagnose a meniscus tear two criteria need to be met:

- *Criteria 1*: Abnormal signal in the meniscus suggesting a tear found on at least two consecutive images.
- *Criteria 2*: Visualization of a meniscal tear in two planes (sagittal and coronal).

If both these clinical criteria are met, the diagnostic accuracy is greater than 90% [27].

Table 3.2 Advantages and disadvantages of MRI

Advantages	Disadvantages
No ionizing radiation	Claustrophobia
No need for intravenous or intra-articular contrast	Contraindicated in some patients (pacemakers, intracranial aneurysm clips, metallic foreign objects in the eye, recent metal stents)
Allows characterization of meniscal lesions	Obese patient may not fit in machine
Allows assessment of other structures (ligaments, tendons, cartilage, subchondral bone)	Resolution hampered by artifact created by nearby orthopedic implants
Useful for diagnosis of residual meniscus lesions following meniscus surgery	

Table 3.3 MRI classification of meniscal tears

	Description	Comment
Grade 1	Small focal area of increased signal, not extending to the joint surface	Early meniscal degeneration Myxoid/hyaline degeneration
Grade 2	Linear area of increased signal that extends to inferior surface of the meniscus, not extending to the joint surface	A progression of a grade 1 lesion No tear or cleavage
Grade 3	Linear area of increased signal extending to the joint surface	Cannot be diagnosed on routine arthroscopy if surface extension is not identified preoperatively

It is important to note incidental meniscal findings on MRI of the knee are common in the general population and increase with increasing age [2]. In patients with knee radiographic osteoarthritis, the prevalence of a meniscus tear is 63% in symptomatic patients, and 60% in asymptomatic patients [2].

Normal Meniscus

On MRI, the normal meniscus appears as a low-signal intensity structure on both T1- and T2-weighed sequences (Fig. 3.9). In the sagittal plane they appear as opposing triangles centrally, sometimes referred to as "bow-ties." In the coronal place, they appear either triangular at the body segment or wedge-shaped at the horns. Surrounding structures that can be identified on MRI include the transverse meniscal ligament, meniscofemoral ligaments (Humphrey and Wrisberg), popliteomeniscal fascicles, and meniscomeniscal ligament.

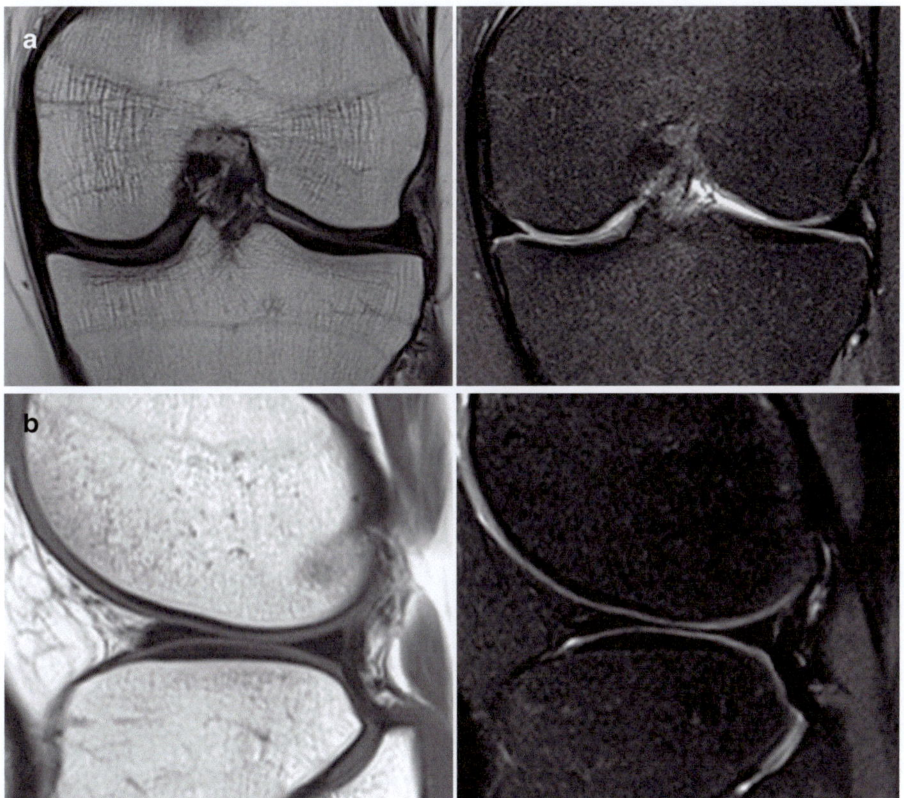

Fig. 3.9 Normal MRI appearance of the menisci – PD-weighted (left) and T2-weighted MR images (right). (**a**) Normal meniscus – coronal. (**b**) Lateral meniscus – sagittal. (**c**) Medial meniscus – sagittal. (**d**) Three-dimensional diagram of a normal meniscus

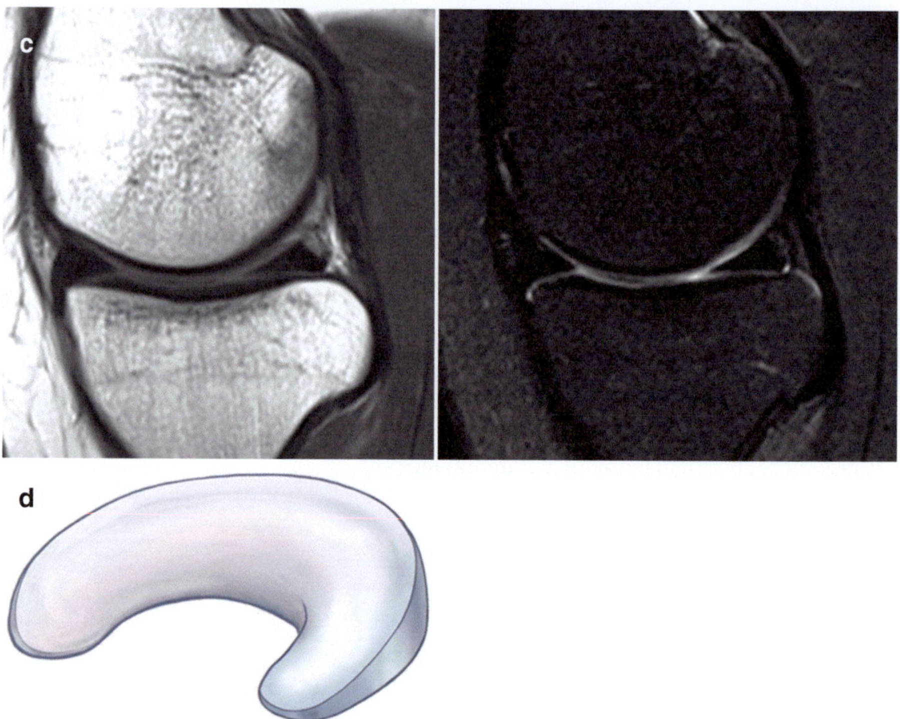

Fig. 3.9 (continued)

Anatomic Variants

Discoid Meniscus

A discoid meniscus is a normal variant seen in 1–5% of knees and is more common in the lateral meniscus than in the medial meniscus [28]. It represents an enlarged meniscus with further central extension onto the tibial plateau (Fig. 3.10). There are three types of discoid menisci: complete, incomplete, and Wrisberg (lacks the normal posterior coronary ligament and capsular attachments). A discoid meniscus is diagnosed on MRI when the body of the meniscus measures 15 mm or more on a midline coronal image or when three or more bowtie shapes are identified on contiguous sagittal (4 mm-thick) images [29]. Tears in discoid menisci are more common with complete discoid variants and often have horizontal or longitudinal tear patterns. Given the increased vascularity of a discoid meniscus, a tear is more difficult to detect on MRI and reliance on morphologic distortion rather than signal changes is often necessary. The sensitivity and specificity of MRI on detecting a tear in a discoid meniscus are highly variable, but if a suspected tear contacts the articular surface in two or more images, then a true tear is likely.

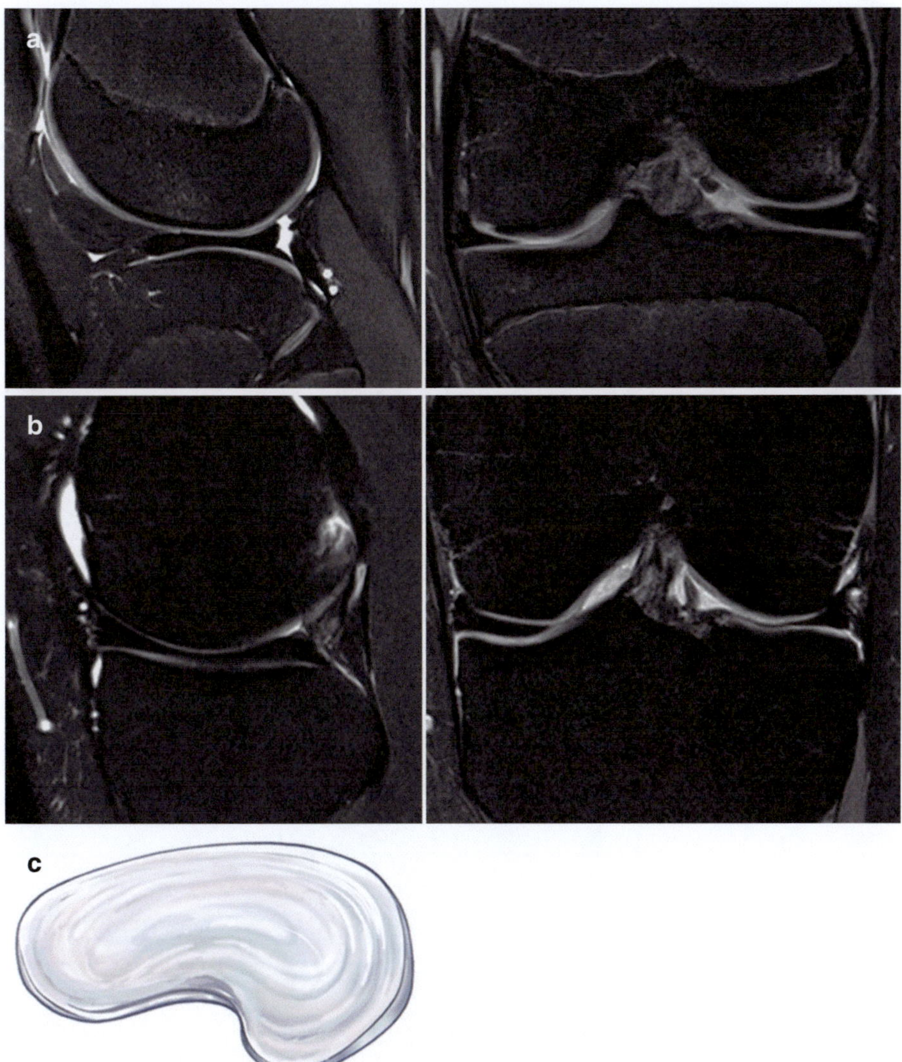

Fig. 3.10 Discoid meniscus. (**a**) Lateral discoid meniscus – T2-weighted MR images – sagittal (left) and coronal (right). (**b**) Medial discoid meniscus – T2-weighted MR images – sagittal (left) and coronal (right). (**c**) Three-dimensional diagram of a discoid meniscus

Meniscal Flounce and Meniscal Ossicle

Meniscal flounce refers to the rippled appearance of the free non-anchored inner edge of the medial meniscus, secondary to knee position and redundancy of the free edge. This does not indicate a tear, but on coronal imaging it may simulate a truncated meniscus and mimic a radial tear (Fig. 3.11).

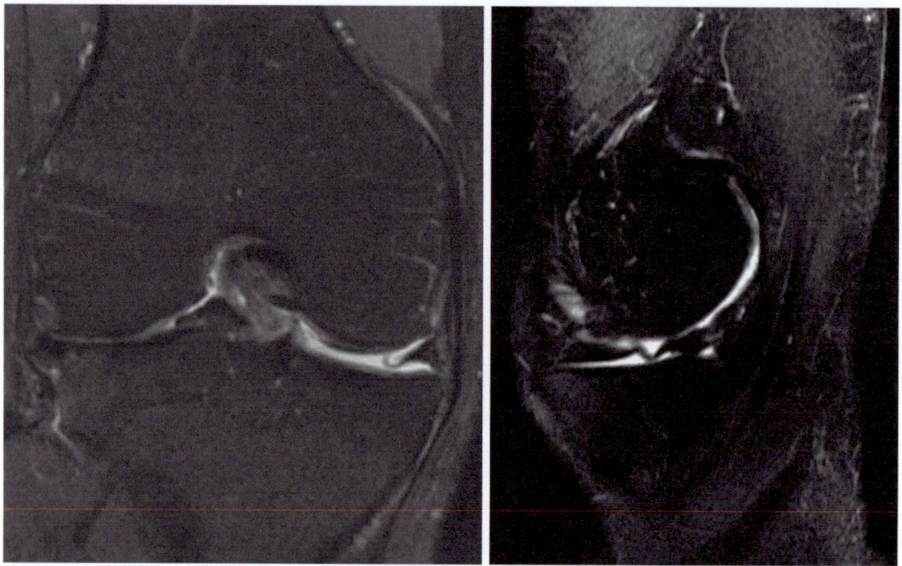

Fig. 3.11 Meniscal flounce. T2-weighted MR images – coronal (left) and sagittal (right)

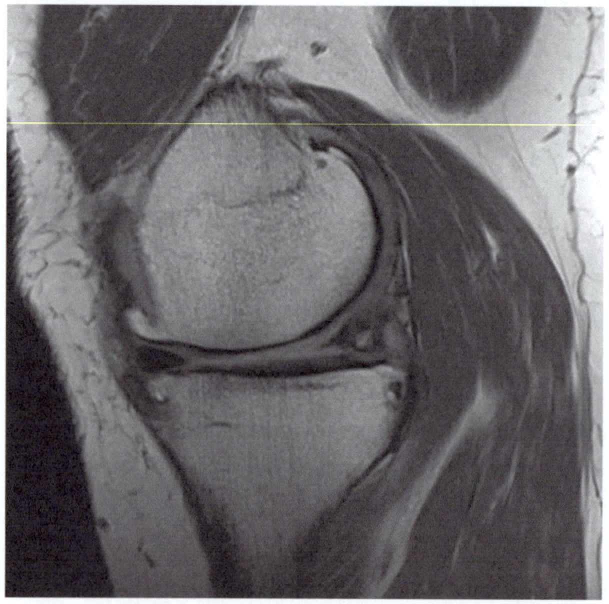

Fig. 3.12 Meniscal ossicle. Sagittal T1-weighted MR image of an ossicle in the posterior horn of the medial meniscus

A meniscal ossicle is an ossicle usually found in the posterior horn of the medial meniscus. It can be developmental, degenerative, or posttraumatic. On MRI imaging, the signal around the ossicle can be confused for a tear (Fig. 3.12).

Specific Pathology

Vertical/Longitudinal Tears

These tears are oriented perpendicular to the coronal plane and divide the meniscus into central and peripheral halves (Fig. 3.13). Unlike radial or horizontal tears, they do not involve the free edge of the meniscus. They usually occur following trauma in young patients. There is a close association of peripheral longitudinal tears and ACL tears. In one study, 90% of medial meniscus and 83% of lateral meniscus peripheral longitudinal tears had an associated ACL tear [30]. Longitudinal tears of the posterior horn may not be visible on sagittal images and can be difficult to identify due to the complex posterior attachments of the meniscus.

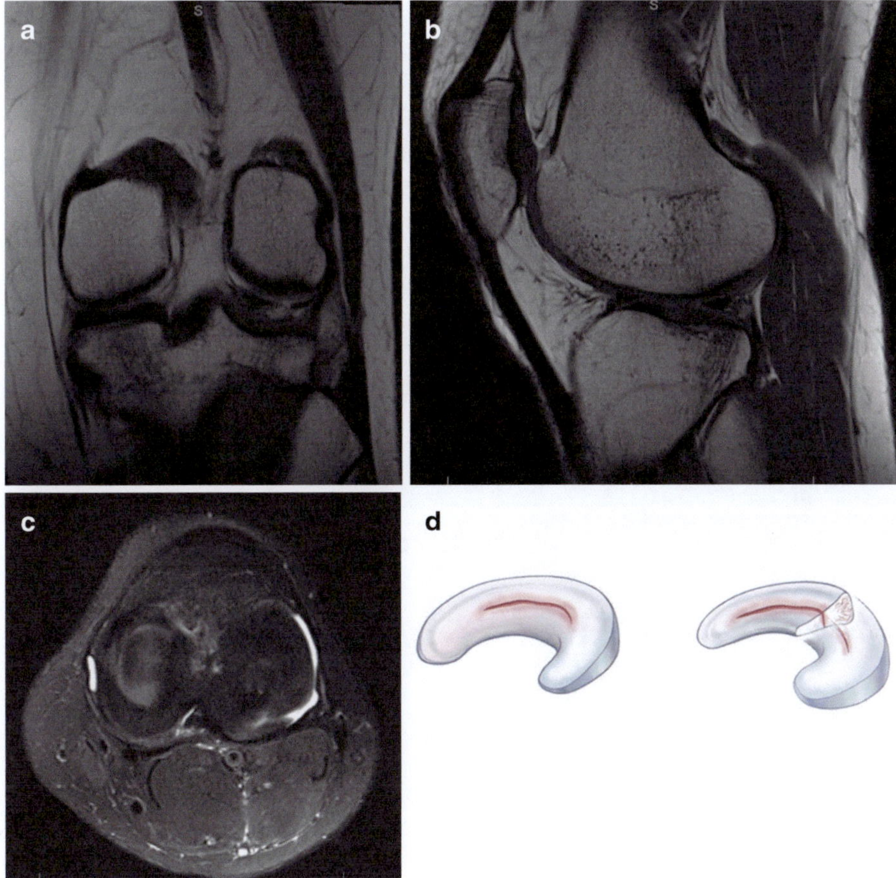

Fig. 3.13 Longitudinal tear of the posterior horn of the lateral meniscus. PD-weighted coronal (**a**) and sagittal (**b**) MR images and T2-weighted axial MR image (**c**). (**d**) Three-dimensional diagram of a longitudinal/vertical tear

Radial Tears

Radial tears, or transverse tears, run perpendicular to both the tibial plateau and the long axis of the meniscus. They start at the free edge of the meniscus and travel toward the periphery. Small tears may be difficult to see and account for many of the errors made in the interpretation of meniscal pathologies on MRI. These tears often involve the posterior horn of the medial meniscus, or the junction between the anterior horn and body of the lateral meniscus. They are best seen on sagittal images, but should also be suspected if the inner portion of the meniscal triangle is absent or blunted on one or more coronal images (Fig. 3.14). On axial imaging they appear as clefts oriented perpendicular to the free edge. Many times there are associated signs that help determine the presence of radial tears, such as a "cleft," a "ghost meniscus," and a "truncated triangle." Clefts are not specific to radial tears as they can also be seen in longitudinal/vertical tears, but the plane in which you see the cleft can

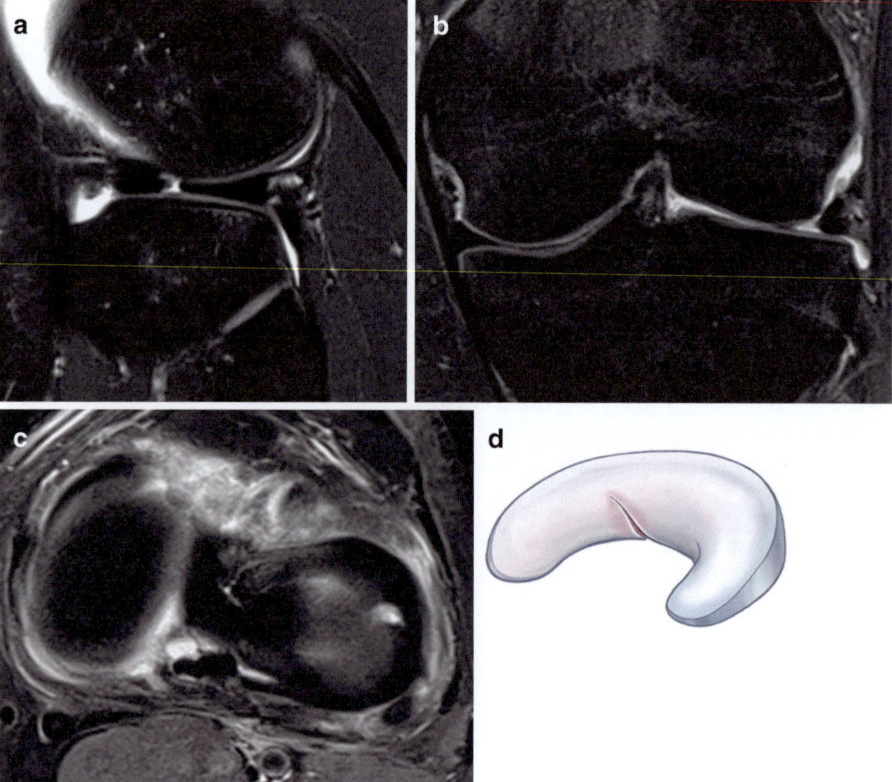

Fig. 3.14 Radial tear lateral meniscus body – T2-weighted MR images (**a**) sagittal, (**b**) coronal, and (**c**) axial. (**d**) Three-dimensional image of a radial tear

help determine the type of tear. In the coronal plane, a cleft in the body presents a longitudinal/vertical tear, while a cleft in the horn represents a radial tear. In the sagittal plane, a cleft in the body represents a radial tear, while a cleft in the horn represents a longitudinal/vertical tear.

Horizontal Tears

Horizontal tears are also called "cleavage" or "fish-mouth" tears. They run parallel to the tibial plateau and divide the meniscus into a superior half and an inferior half (Fig. 3.15). They usually begin on the undersurface of the meniscus. Horizontal tears are usually degenerative in nature and occur in older patients with osteoarthritis. On MRI, they appear as a horizontally oriented line of high signal intensity that contacts the meniscal surface or free edge. Complete horizontal tears that extend to the periphery are associated with parameniscal cyst formation.

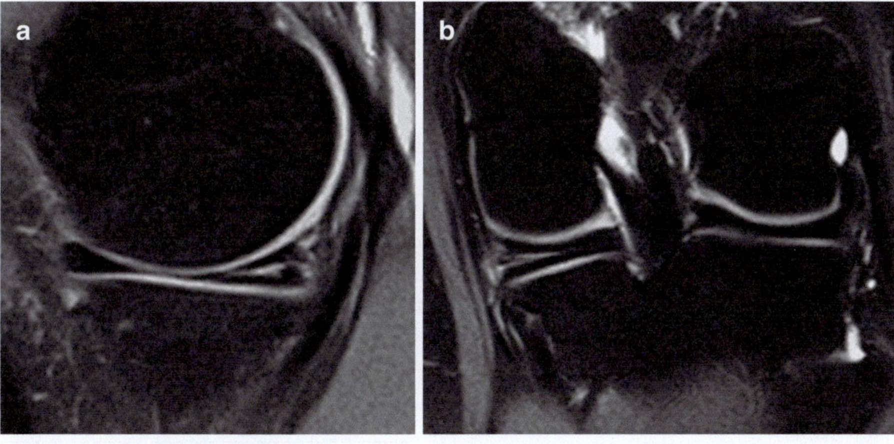

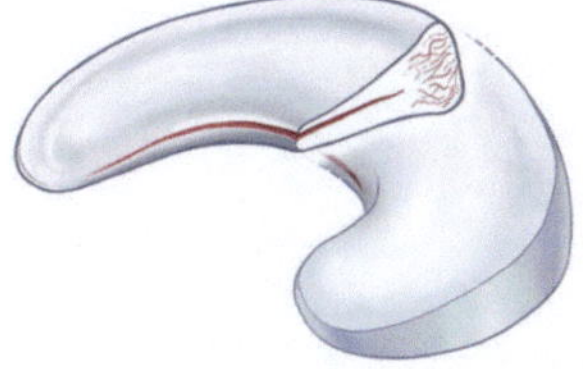

Fig. 3.15 Horizontal tear posterior horn medial meniscus – T2-weighted MR images sagittal (**a**) and coronal (**b**). Also a three-dimensional diagram of a horizontal cleavage tear (**c**)

Complex Tears

Complex tears include a combination of radial, horizontal, and longitudinal components. On MRI, the meniscus appears fragmented with tears in more than one plane (Fig. 3.16). These tears are likely degenerative in nature, commonly associated with degenerative arthritis.

Meniscal Root Tears

Tears occurring at the meniscal root usually have a radial-type morphology and have a high association with meniscal extrusion. The sensitivity and specificity for meniscal root tear detection on MRI is 86–90% and 95–96%, respectively [31]. Coronal imaging allows better visualization of the roots, and the root should course over its respective plateau on at least one image (Fig. 3.17). On sagittal imaging, if the posterior root of the medial meniscus is not detected just medial to the PCL, a root tear should be suspected. This is termed a "ghost meniscus" and is thought to represent a radial tear caught perfectly in line showing only a portion of the meniscus [6]. Lateral root tears are more commonly associated with ACL tears [32].

Displaced Meniscal Fragments/Flap Tears

Diagnosis of flap tears are usually made by MRI where one can visualize the tear with a missing part of the meniscus. Flap tears occur more frequently in the medial meniscus and fragments are usually displaced posteriorly or into the intercondylar notch (Fig. 3.18). These fragments are more commonly identified on coronal imaging.

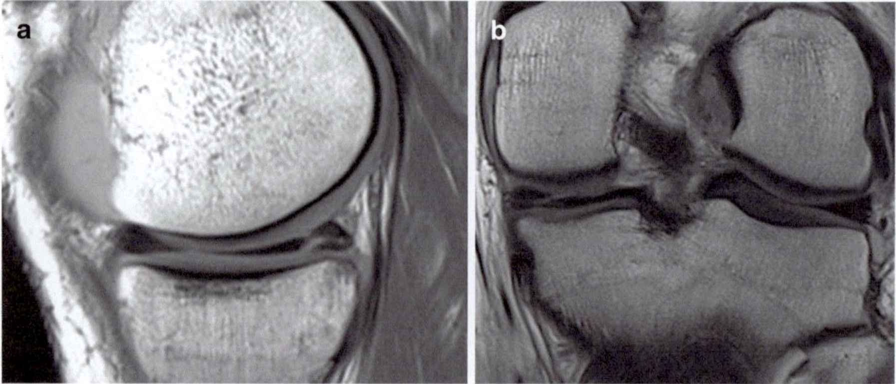

Fig. 3.16 Complex tear posterior horn medial meniscus body – PD-weighted MR images sagittal (**a**) and coronal (**b**)

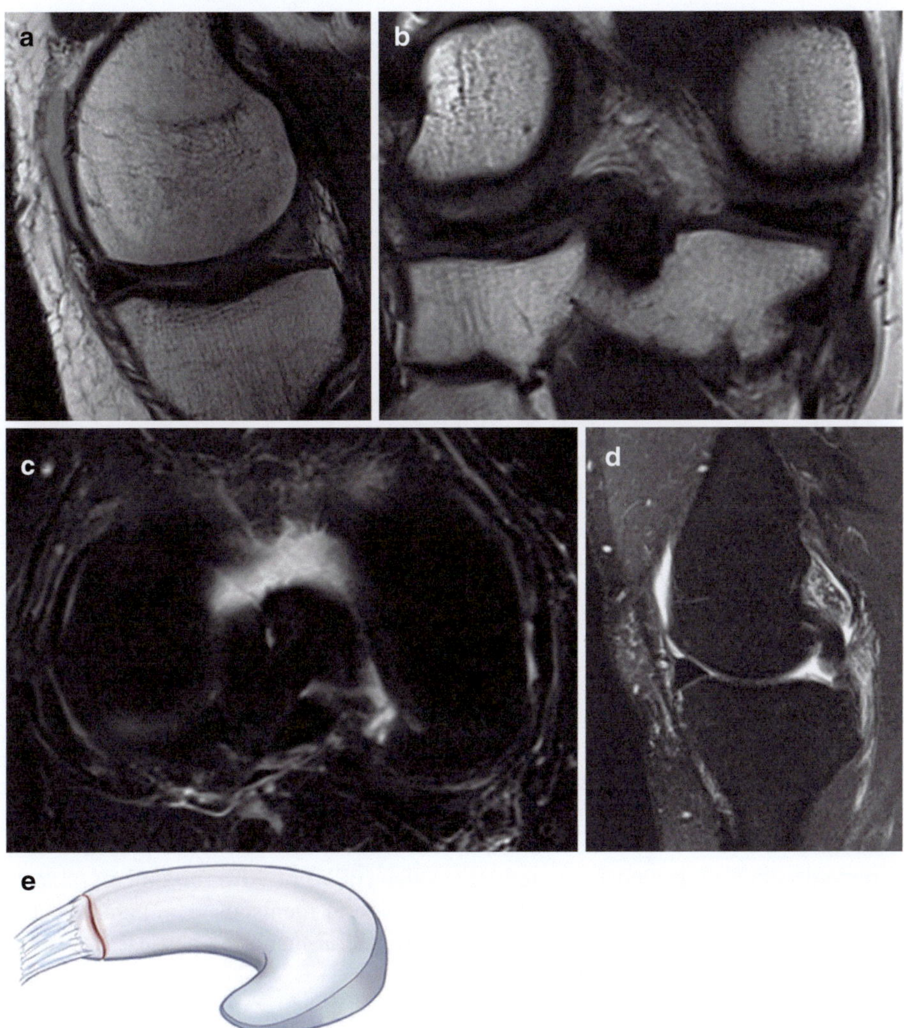

Fig. 3.17 Meniscal root tear. Complete posterior root tear – medial meniscus – PD-weighted MR images sagittal (**a**) and coronal (**b**). T2-weighted MR axial (**c**) Picture (**d**) depicts a "ghost meniscus" where the medial meniscal root is not visualized medial to the PCL. When this present a root tear should be suspected. A three-dimensional diagram of a root tear (**e**)

Bucket-Handle Tear

Bucket-handle tears are caused by full thickness vertical/longitudinal tears, where the inner fragment is usually centrally displaced (Fig. 3.19). These account for 10% of all meniscal tears and are seven times more common in the medial meniscus [33,

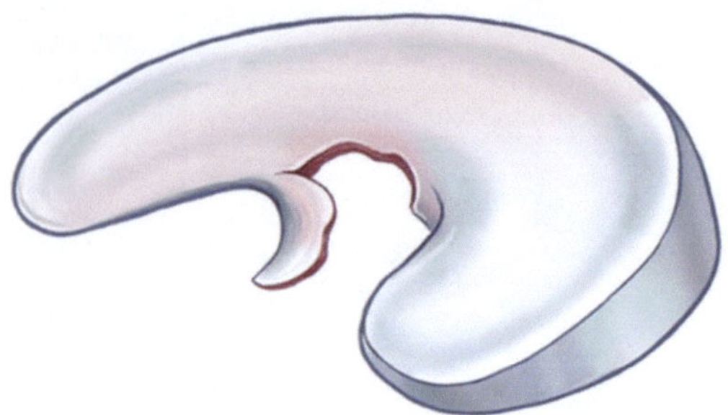

Fig. 3.18 Three-dimensional diagram of a displaced flap tear

34]. On coronal imaging, the displaced fragment can be seen in the intercondylar notch. On sagittal imaging, a "double PCL" sign can be seen. A prominent ligament of Humphreys, a meniscomeniscal ligament, and intercondylar loose bodies can sometime mimic a double PCL sign. Other signs may be seen on MRI in the setting of a bucket-handle tear including an absent bow tie, a double anterior horn or flipped meniscus, and a disproportionately small posterior horn. Rarely, a bucket-handle tear of the lateral meniscus can manifest as a "double ACL" sign as the fragment is just posterior to the ACL [35].

Parameniscal Cyst

Parameniscal cysts represent the peripheral escape of joint fluid though a meniscal tear, which usually contains a horizontal component. The cyst has direct contact with the meniscus or is connected via a fluid track (Fig. 3.20). The presence of a parameniscal cyst has a positive predictive value (PPV) of 90% for a meniscal tear, with the exception of the anterior horn of the lateral meniscus. The parameniscal cyst located adjacent to the anterior horn of the lateral meniscus has less risk of an underlying tear [36].

Meniscal Extrusion

Extrusion is when the peripheral margin of the meniscus extends 3 mm or more beyond the edge of the tibial plateau (Fig. 3.21). There is a close association between meniscal extrusion and meniscal root tears, whereas 76% of medial root tears have extrusion and 39% of extrusions have medial root tears [37]. Extrusion can also be seen in large radial tears, complex tears, and severe meniscal degeneration. In the elderly patients, some believe prior meniscal extrusion leads to increased progression of cartilage degeneration due to altered tibiofemoral contact pressures [38].

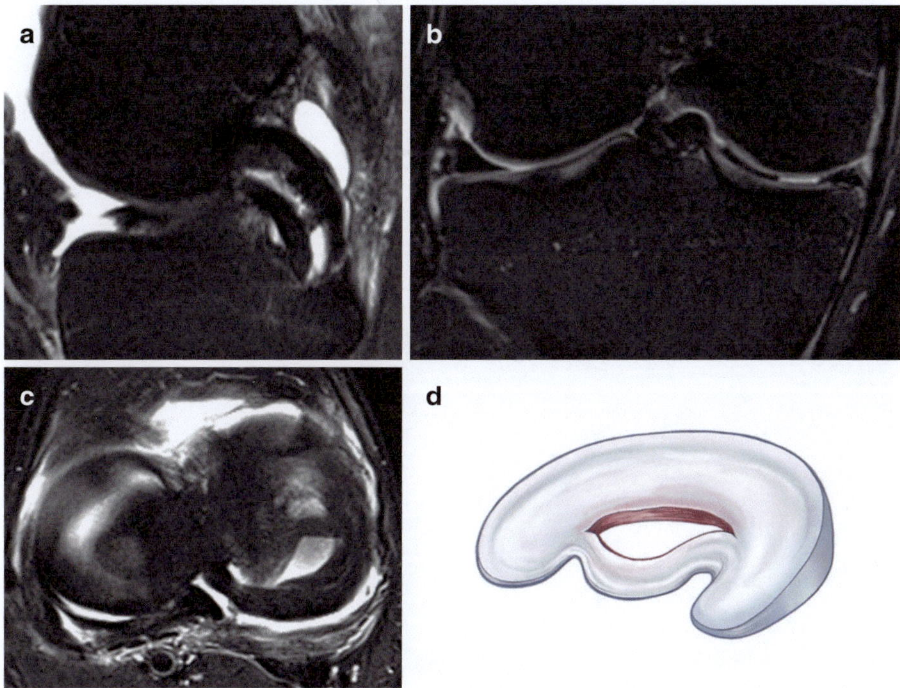

Fig. 3.19 Bucket-handle tear. Bucket-handle tear medial meniscus – T2-weighted MR images sagittal (double PCL sign) (**a**), coronal (**b**), and axial (**c**). Also a three-dimensional diagram of a bucket-handle (**d**) tear

Meniscocapsular Separation

Meniscocapsular separation is a tear of the peripheral meniscus at the meniscosynovial junction. This usually effects the posterior horn of the medial meniscus. Arthroscopy is much more reliable than MRI at detecting these injuries [39].

Key Points
- Always get standard radiographs in the acutely injured knee (AP, 45° PA, lateral, patellofemoral views). Used to rule out any other causes of knee pain such as osteoarthritis, loose bodies, or osteochondritis dissecans.
- MRI is the gold standard imaging modality used to diagnose meniscal pathology.
- MR arthrogram is useful in evaluating knees with prior meniscectomies or meniscal repair.
- High-resolution CT arthrography can be used in patients who are too large for MRI machines, suffer of claustrophobia, or have other contraindications. Claustrophobia is less of an issue nowadays due to the advent of open MRIs.

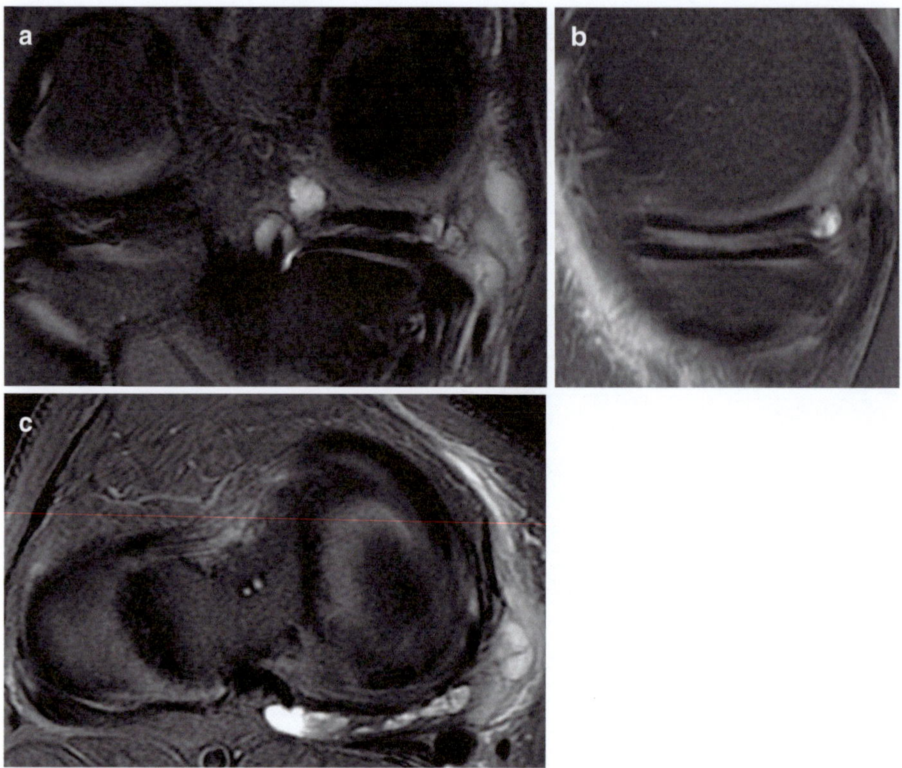

Fig. 3.20 Parameniscal cyst. Horizontal tear medial meniscus (body and posterior horn) and an associated multiloculated parameniscal cyst – T2-weighted MR images coronal (**a**), sagittal (**b**), and axial (**c**)

Fig. 3.21 Meniscal extrusion secondary to medial compartment osteoarthritis. Body extrusion medial meniscus – T2-weighted MR images coronal

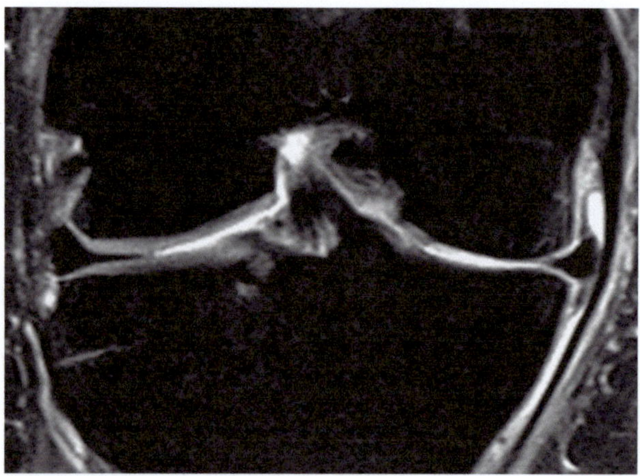

References

1. Decary S, Fallaha M, Fremont P, Martel-Pelletier J, Pelletier JP, Feldman DE, et al. Diagnostic validity of combining history elements and physical examination tests for traumatic and degenerative symptomatic meniscal tears. PM R. 2018;10(5):472–82.
2. Englund M, Guermazi A, Gale D, Hunter DJ, Aliabadi P, Clancy M, et al. Incidental meniscal findings on knee MRI in middle-aged and elderly persons. N Engl J Med. 2008;359(11):1108–15.
3. Katz JN, Smith SR, Yang HY, Martin SD, Wright J, Donnell-Fink LA, et al. Value of history, physical examination, and radiographic findings in the diagnosis of symptomatic meniscal tear among middle-aged subjects with knee pain. Arthritis Care Res (Hoboken). 2017;69(4):484–90.
4. Hagino T, Ochiai S, Senga S, Yamashita T, Wako M, Ando T, et al. Meniscal tears associated with anterior cruciate ligament injury. Arch Orthop Trauma Surg. 2015;135(12):1701–6.
5. Poehling GG, Ruch DS, Chabon SJ. The landscape of meniscal injuries. Clin Sports Med. 1990;9(3):539–49.
6. Bhatia S, LaPrade CM, Ellman MB, LaPrade RF. Meniscal root tears: significance, diagnosis, and treatment. Am J Sports Med. 2014;42(12):3016–30.
7. Stanitski CL, Harvell JC, Fu F. Observations on acute knee hemarthrosis in children and adolescents. J Pediatr Orthop. 1993;13(4):506–10.
8. Kocher MS, Klingele K, Rassman SO. Meniscal disorders: normal, discoid, and cysts. Orthop Clin North Am. 2003;34(3):329–40.
9. Kramer DE, Micheli LJ. Meniscal tears and discoid meniscus in children: diagnosis and treatment. J Am Acad Orthop Surg. 2009;17(11):698–707.
10. Ryzewicz M, Peterson B, Siparsky PN, Bartz RL. The diagnosis of meniscus tears: the role of MRI and clinical examination. Clin Orthop Relat Res. 2007;455:123–33.
11. Abdon P, Lindstrand A, Thorngren KG. Statistical evaluation of the diagnostic criteria for meniscal tears. Int Orthop. 1990;14(4):341–5.
12. Karachalios T, Hantes M, Zibis AH, Zachos V, Karantanas AH, Malizos KN. Diagnostic accuracy of a new clinical test (the Thessaly test) for early detection of meniscal tears. J Bone Joint Surg Am. 2005;87(5):955–62.
13. Ercin E, Kaya I, Sungur I, Demirbas E, Ugras AA, Cetinus EM. History, clinical findings, magnetic resonance imaging, and arthroscopic correlation in meniscal lesions. Knee Surg Sports Traumatol Arthrosc. 2012;20(5):851–6.
14. Munk B, Madsen F, Lundorf E, Staunstrup H, Schmidt SA, Bolvig L, et al. Clinical magnetic resonance imaging and arthroscopic findings in knees: a comparative prospective study of meniscus anterior cruciate ligament and cartilage lesions. Arthroscopy. 1998;14(2):171–5.
15. Boeree NR, Ackroyd CE. Assessment of the menisci and cruciate ligaments: an audit of clinical practice. Injury. 1991;22(4):291–4.
16. Akseki D, Ozcan O, Boya H, Pinar H. A new weight-bearing meniscal test and a comparison with McMurray's test and joint line tenderness. Arthroscopy. 2004;20(9):951–8.
17. Dumas JM, Edde DJ. Meniscal abnormalities: prospective correlation of double-contrast arthrography and arthroscopy. Radiology. 1986;160(2):453–6.
18. De Filippo M, Bertellini A, Pogliacomi F, Sverzellati N, Corradi D, Garlaschi G, et al. Multidetector computed tomography arthrography of the knee: diagnostic accuracy and indications. Eur J Radiol. 2009;70(2):342–51.
19. De Flaviis L, Scaglione P, Nessi R, Albisetti W. Ultrasound in degenerative cystic meniscal disease of the knee. Skelet Radiol. 1990;19(6):441–5.
20. Nguyen JC, De Smet AA, Graf BK, Rosas HG. MR imaging-based diagnosis and classification of meniscal tears. Radiographics. 2014;34(4):981–99.
21. Magee T, Williams D. 3.0-T MRI of meniscal tears. AJR Am J Roentgenol. 2006;187(2):371–5.
22. Oei EH, Nikken JJ, Verstijnen AC, Ginai AZ, Myriam Hunink MG. MR imaging of the menisci and cruciate ligaments: a systematic review. Radiology. 2003;226(3):837–48.

23. von Engelhardt LV, Schmitz A, Pennekamp PH, Schild HH, Wirtz DC, von Falkenhausen F. Diagnostics of degenerative meniscal tears at 3-Tesla MRI compared to arthroscopy as reference standard. Arch Orthop Trauma Surg. 2008;128(5):451–6.
24. Lefevre N, Naouri JF, Herman S, Gerometta A, Klouche S, Bohu Y. A current review of the meniscus imaging: proposition of a useful tool for its radiologic analysis. Radiol Res Pract. 2016;2016:8329296.
25. Ciliz D, Ciliz A, Elverici E, Sakman B, Yuksel E, Akbulut O. Evaluation of postoperative menisci with MR arthrography and routine conventional MRI. Clin Imaging. 2008;32(3):212–9.
26. Stoller DW, Martin C, Crues JV 3rd, Kaplan L, Mink JH. Meniscal tears: pathologic correlation with MR imaging. Radiology. 1987;163(3):731–5.
27. Rubin DA, Paletta GA Jr. Current concepts and controversies in meniscal imaging. Magn Reson Imaging Clin N Am. 2000;8(2):243–70.
28. Singh K, Helms CA, Jacobs MT, Higgins LD. MRI appearance of Wrisberg variant of discoid lateral meniscus. AJR Am J Roentgenol. 2006;187(2):384–7.
29. Silverman JM, Mink JH, Deutsch AL. Discoid menisci of the knee: MR imaging appearance. Radiology. 1989;173(2):351–4.
30. De Smet AA, Graf BK. Meniscal tears missed on MR imaging: relationship to meniscal tear patterns and anterior cruciate ligament tears. AJR Am J Roentgenol. 1994;162(4):905–11.
31. Lee SY, Jee WH, Kim JM. Radial tear of the medial meniscal root: reliability and accuracy of MRI for diagnosis. AJR Am J Roentgenol. 2008;191(1):81–5.
32. Brody JM, Lin HM, Hulstyn MJ, Tung GA. Lateral meniscus root tear and meniscus extrusion with anterior cruciate ligament tear. Radiology. 2006;239(3):805–10.
33. Carrino JA, Schweitzer ME. Imaging of sports-related knee injuries. Radiol Clin N Am. 2002;40(2):181–202.
34. Shakespeare DT, Rigby HS. The bucket-handle tear of the meniscus. A clinical and arthrographic study. J Bone Joint Surg Br. 1983;65(4):383–7.
35. Bui-Mansfield LT, DeWitt RM. Magnetic resonance imaging appearance of a double anterior cruciate ligament associated with a displaced tear of the lateral meniscus. J Comput Assist Tomogr. 2006;30(2):327–32.
36. De Smet AA, Graf BK, del Rio AM. Association of parameniscal cysts with underlying meniscal tears as identified on MRI and arthroscopy. AJR Am J Roentgenol. 2011;196(2):W180–6.
37. Choi CJ, Choi YJ, Lee JJ, Choi CH. Magnetic resonance imaging evidence of meniscal extrusion in medial meniscus posterior root tear. Arthroscopy. 2010;26(12):1602–6.
38. Rennie WJ, Finlay DB. Meniscal extrusion in young athletes: associated knee joint abnormalities. AJR Am J Roentgenol. 2006;186(3):791–4.
39. Rubin DA, Britton CA, Towers JD, Harner CD. Are MR imaging signs of meniscocapsular separation valid? Radiology. 1996;201(3):829–36.

Nonoperative Treatment of Meniscus Tears

4

Dennis Cardone, Lauren Borowski, and Anthony A. Essilfie

Introduction

Meniscal tears are the most common pathology found in the knee with a mean annual incidence of 66 per 100,000 [1]. In 2009, an epidemiological study found that there were over 900,000 arthroscopic knee procedures performed in the US, with over 50% involving meniscus tears [2]. However, most patients with meniscus tears do not require surgery. It is important to discern the general etiology of the meniscus tear in order to recommend the appropriate treatment for the patient. For example, the management of an acute traumatic meniscal tear that prevents full range of motion (ROM) is different than the management of a chronic degenerative meniscal tear. There have been several randomized control trials (RCTs) comparing arthroscopic partial meniscectomy (APM) to physical therapy (PT) treatment of degenerative meniscus tears that have shown no difference in functional and pain outcomes [3–9]. As a result, the first-line treatments for chronic, degenerative meniscus tears in the middle-aged adult are rest, nonsteroidal anti-inflammatory drugs (NSAIDs), and physical therapy.

Function

There are several functions of the meniscus. It plays an important role in improving stability, congruency, and lubricating the knee joint. Additionally, the menisci have an important role in dispersing the forces across the knee. The lateral and medial meniscus can encounter up to 70% and 50% of the load across the tibiofemoral joint

D. Cardone · L. Borowski (✉) · A. A. Essilfie
NYU Langone Orthopedic Center, New York, NY, USA
e-mail: Dennis.Cardone@nyulangone.org; Lauren.Borowski@nyumc.org;
Anthony.Essilfie@nyumc.org

© Springer Nature Switzerland AG 2020
E. J. Strauss, L. M. Jazrawi (eds.), *The Management of Meniscal Pathology*,
https://doi.org/10.1007/978-3-030-49488-9_4

respectively [10]. This shock-absorbing role serves to protect the cartilage of the knee joint. Roos et al. demonstrated the importance of the meniscus by showing a 14 times higher relative risk of developing osteoarthritis after a meniscectomy [11]. Unfortunately, osteoarthritis and meniscus tears are frequently seen in tandem. It is difficult to determine whether a patient's pain is a result of one or both of the ongoing pathologies. This has resulted in several studies evaluating the role of APM, particularly in the middle-aged patient population.

Mechanism of Meniscal Tears

The most common mechanism for a meniscus tear is a result of compressive and rotational forces across the tibiofemoral joint. These forces exert pressure on the meniscus and the meniscus attempts to conform to the stresses placed on it [12]. The medial meniscus has more coronary ligaments attached to the capsule making it less mobile than the lateral meniscus. Furthermore, the lateral meniscus has a hiatus to allow the popliteus to attach to its origin on the lateral femoral epicondyle. As a result, the medial meniscus is vulnerable to tears when encountering forces applied by the tibiofemoral joint [13].

Nonoperative Treatment and Outcomes

There are select circumstances warranting initial surgical intervention for meniscal tears, such as a young patient with a bucket-handle meniscus tear blocking range of motion. However, the vast majority of meniscus tears are treated with rest, NSAIDs, and PT as the first-line treatment. Weiss et al. demonstrated that stable, vertical, longitudinal tears in the red–red zone of the meniscus can be treated nonoperatively, given their good potential for healing [14]. Most would agree PT is the initial treatment for chronic degenerative meniscus tears. The evidence for this nonoperative approach is a result of multiple RCTs. The RCTs pertaining to APM versus control groups will be reviewed in this section (Table 4.1).

Osteras et al. compared APM without a structured postoperative PT program, versus PT alone, in 17 patients with degenerative meniscus tears. There were 8 patients in the APM group and 9 in the PT group. At 3-month follow-up, there was no difference between the two groups with respect to visual analogue scale (VAS) and knee injury and osteoarthritis outcome scores (KOOS).

Herrlin et al. performed two RCTs of the same cohort. The first study looked at the cohort with 6-month follow-up and the second study assessed patients at 5-year follow-up [4, 15]. The study had 96 middle-aged patients with a nontraumatic medial meniscus tears, who were randomized into APM followed by supervised PT or PT alone [4]. The PT program lasted 8 weeks, and occurred twice a week. In this study, PT included both eccentric and concentric exercises to help neuromuscular ability and muscular hypertrophy. NSAIDs in conjunction with PT were permitted to help control effusion, pain, or inflammation.

Table 4.1 A review of the randomized control trials (RCTs) where arthroscopic partial meniscectomy (APM) was compared to a control group

Study	Year	Methods	Follow Up	Conclusion
Osteras et al.	2012	APM alone vs. PT	3 months	No difference in VAS and KOOS scores
Herrlin et al.	2007, 2013	APM and PT vs. PT	5 years	No difference in KOOS, Lysholm, and VAS scores. 33% crossover to the APM group
Katz et al.	2013	APM and PT vs. PT alone	12 months	No difference in WOMAC score. 30% crossed over from the PT to the APM group
Sihvonen et al.	2013	APM vs. Sham surgery	12 months	No difference in Lysholm and WOMET scores
Yim et al.	2013	APM vs. PT	2 years	No difference in VAS, Lysholm, and Tegner scores
Vermesan et al.	2013	APM vs. corticosteroid injection	1 year	No difference in Oxford Knee Score. 22% crossover to APM
Gauffin et al.	2014, 2017	APM with PT vs. PT	3 year	No difference in KOOS pain sub score. 25% crossover to APM
Kise et al.	2016	APM vs. PT	2 years	No difference in KOOS score. Significant improvement in strength at 3 months for the PT group. 19% of patients crossed over to APM group
Van de Graaf et al.	2018	APM vs. PT	2 years	No difference in IKDC. 30% crossed over to APM group
Stensrud et al.	2015	APM vs. PT	3 months	Significant improvement in quadriceps strength favoring the PT group

At 5-year follow-up, the patients were evaluated using the Knee Injury and Osteoarthritis Score (KOOS), Lysholm Knee Score, Tegner Activity Scale, and VAS pain scale. At the conclusion of the study, Herrlin found noninferiority of the aforementioned outcome scores for the APM followed by supervised PT group, versus supervised PT alone group. By 5-year follow-up, one-third of patients in the PT group crossed over to the APM group.

Katz et al. conducted a study looking at participants 45 years and older with mild-to-moderate osteoarthritis on imaging and a meniscal tear [16]. There were 351 participants randomly assigned to APM with postoperative PT, or PT alone. The primary outcome was the Western Ontario and McMaster Universities Osteoarthritis Index (WOMAC) score. At 12-month follow-up, participants in both groups had similar baseline changes in the WOMAC and KOOS scores.

A double-blind RCT comparing APM versus sham surgery in 146 patients aged 35–65 years old with symptomatic meniscal tears and no osteoarthritis was performed by Sihvonen et al. [6]. The primary outcomes measured were the Lysholm score and the Western Ontario Meniscal Evaluation Tool (WOMET) at 12 months after procedure. Results showed no difference between APM and PT groups with respect to Lysholm and WOMET scores. A follow-up study by Sihvonen et al.

followed this cohort for an additional year. At 2-year follow-up, there was no difference in Lysholm and WOMET scores between the groups [17].

Yim et al. investigated the outcomes of APM versus PT for degenerative horizontal tears of the medial meniscus [7]. In this study, 102 patients with degenerative medial meniscus tears on MRI and knee pain were followed up as part of the study for 2 years. There were 52 participants in the PT group that participated in strengthening exercises, while 50 participants had APM. PT group participants were given NSAIDs, muscle relaxants, or analgesics for the first 2 weeks. The PT program was a supervised rehabilitation program including flexibility, endurance, and muscle strengthening exercises for 60-minute sessions, 3 times weekly for 3 weeks, followed by an unsupervised exercise program at home for the following 8 weeks. The home exercises included daily isotonic and isometric exercises. At 2-year follow-up, there was no difference in VAS pain score, satisfaction, Lysholm, and Tegner knee scores between the APM and PT groups.

A RCT comparing APM to corticosteroid injections was performed by Vermesan et al. [18]. In this study 120 consecutive patients with degenerative medial meniscus tears and early stage osteoarthritis were included. The injection consisted of 1 ml of betamethasone in 4 ml of 1% lidocaine. The Oxford Knee Score was the primary outcome assessed 1 year after intervention. At time of final follow-up, there was no difference between the APM and the corticosteroid group.

Gauffin et al. published two studies of the same cohort comparing APM with PT versus PT alone. The first study found significant difference in KOOS pain subscale favoring the APM group at a 1-year time point [19]. However, a follow-up study was performed at 3 years that showed no difference between the two cohorts [20].

Kise et al. performed a RCT to assess if PT was superior to APM in middle-aged patients with degenerative meniscus tears [8]. This study included 140 patients with an average age of 49.5 years. The patients were randomized to APM alone or a 12-week supervised PT program. The main outcome was calculated with the KOOS score at 2-year follow-up and muscle strength at 3-month follow-up. Over the course of the 2-year follow-up, 19% of patients crossed over from PT to APM group. The results showed no difference between groups with respect to KOOS. At 3 months, the muscle strength was statistically better in the PT group.

Van de Graaf et al. conducted an RCT of nonobstructive meniscal tears in patients 45–70 years old. The primary outcome was the International Knee Documentation Committee (IKDC) score at 2-year follow-up [21]. Participants were randomized and stratified by age group to either APM or PT. Participants who had APM were only referred to PT if they did not recover as predicted. Those participants who were randomized to PT completed 16 sessions over 8 weeks. If the participants in the PT group continued to have decreased ability to partake in daily activities, knee locking, or knee pain at the end of the 8 weeks, they could choose more PT sessions or APM. At 2-year follow-up, the IKDC and VAS scores improved in both the APM and PT groups. There was no difference between groups based on intention to treat

(ITT) analysis. Since one-third of PT patients crossed over to the APM group, an as-treated analysis was performed for three groups: (1) APM, (2) PT, and (3) delayed APM. The IKDC improved for all the three groups. PT was found to be noninferior to APM and delayed APM. This study is consistent with the current consensus of PT being the treatment for nonobstructive meniscal tears in middle-aged and older patients. APM should be considered in those who fail to improve their symptoms after a course of physical therapy.

In 2015, Stensrud et al. performed an RCT looking at the differences between effects of APM and a 12-week exercise program on degenerative meniscus tears in middle-aged patients [9]. These patients had greater than 2 months of unilateral knee pain without serious trauma, MRI-confirmed meniscal tear, were between ages 35 and 60 years old, and had a Kellgren–Lawrence Osteoarthritis (OA) grade 2 or less. The patients in the exercise program had at least 2 and at most 3 sessions per week for a total of 24–36 sessions. The primary outcome measured at 3 months was isokinetic knee muscle strength. There were 42 patients in the APM group and 40 patients who underwent exercise therapy. There was a 16% change in the mean difference in quadriceps strength as measured by isokinetic knee extension peak torque, favoring the PT group ($p < 0.0001$).

To summarize the available literature, Van de Graaf et al. performed a meta-analysis including five of the studies previously mentioned in this chapter [22]. After pooling the data, physical function outcomes scores and pain were significantly better in the APM group at 3 and 6 months. However, the differences resolved by 12- and 24-month follow-up. In summary, the RCTs reviewed provide support for rest, NSAIDS, and PT as the first-line treatment for degenerative meniscal tears. While there is no overall consensus on what specific regimen of PT is best, it is important all regimens include exercises that promote range of motion (ROM), flexibility, quadriceps strength, and knee proprioception.

Summary of RCT Studies

Corticosteroid Injections

A corticosteroid injection does play a role in the nonoperative management of degenerative meniscus tears with osteoarthritis. An intra-articular corticosteroid injection can relieve pain for up to 1 year after injection in the setting of osteoarthritis [23]. However, there is no consensus for the recommended amount or frequency of corticosteroid injections. These injections should be given in moderation as there is growing literature showing correlation between intra-articular corticosteroid injections and postoperative infections of total knee arthroplasty [24, 25]. A corticosteroid injection should be reserved for degenerative meniscus tears in the setting of osteoarthritis in patients that will not pursue arthroplasty in the near future.

Orthobiologics

Orthobiologics is a growing area of orthopedics increasingly used in the nonoperative management of meniscus tears. These substances are injected into the knee to help aid or enhance the body's capability to repair and regenerate musculoskeletal tissues. Intra-articular tissues, including the meniscus, have limited capacity for healing, in part due to the avascularity in some regions, which is why the use of orthobiologics continues to emerge. The topic of orthobiologics is discussed in more detail in Chap. 10.

Conclusion

The functions of the meniscus include improving stability, enhancing congruency, distributing load, and providing lubrication in the joint space to allow for articulation between the femur and tibia. Multiple RCTs have shown that there is no difference in outcomes of APM versus PT in degenerative meniscus tears at follow-up greater than 12 months. These studies provide strong evidence that nonsurgical management should be the first-line treatment for degenerative meniscal tears. Surgical intervention should be reserved for select patients who remain symptomatic despite a complete regimen of PT, young patients with bucket-handle meniscus tears that restrict ROM, and displaced flap-like tears causing mechanical symptoms, regardless of age, with minimal to no arthritis in the knee.

Acknowledgement The author would like to acknowledge Xingzi Shangguan for her contribution in this chapter.

Xingzi Shangguan
NYU Langone Orthopedic Center, New York, NY, USA
email: Xingzi.Shangguan@nyulangone.org

References

1. Hede A, Jensen DB, Blyme P, Sonne-Holm S. Epidemiology of meniscal lesions in the knee: 1,215 open operations in Copenhagen 1982–84. Acta Orthop. 1990;61(5):435–7. https://doi.org/10.3109/17453679008993557.
2. Kim S, Bosque J, Meehan JP, Jamali A, Marder R. Increase in outpatient knee arthroscopy in the United States: a comparison of national surveys of ambulatory surgery, 1996 and 2006. J Bone Joint Surg Ser A. 2011;93(11):994–1000. https://doi.org/10.2106/JBJS.I.01618.
3. Østerås H, Østerås B, Torstensen TA. Medical exercise therapy, and not arthroscopic surgery, resulted in decreased depression and anxiety in patients with degenerative meniscus injury. J Bodyw Mov Ther. 2012;16(4):456–63. https://doi.org/10.1016/j.jbmt.2012.04.003.
4. Herrlin SV, Wange PO, Lapidus G, Hållander M, Werner S, Weidenhielm L. Is arthroscopic surgery beneficial in treating non-traumatic, degenerative medial meniscal tears? A five year follow-up. Knee Surg Sports Traumatol Arthrosc. 2013;21(2):358–64. https://doi.org/10.1007/s00167-012-1960-3.
5. Katz JN, Losina E. Arthroscopic partial meniscectomy for degenerative tears: where do we stand? Osteoarthr Cartil. 2014;22(11):1749–51. https://doi.org/10.1016/j.joca.2014.07.016.

6. Sihvonen R, Paavola M, Malmivaara A, et al. Arthroscopic partial meniscectomy versus sham surgery for a degenerative meniscal tear. N Engl J Med. 2013;369(26):2515–24. https://doi.org/10.1056/NEJMoa1305189.

7. Yim JH, Seon JK, Song EK, et al. A comparative study of meniscectomy and nonoperative treatment for degenerative horizontal tears of the medial meniscus. Am J Sports Med. 2013;41(7):1565–70. https://doi.org/10.1177/0363546513488518.

8. Kise NJ, Risberg MA, Stensrud S, Ranstam J, Engebretsen L, Roos EM. Exercise therapy versus arthroscopic partial meniscectomy for degenerative meniscal tear in middle aged patients: randomised controlled trial with two year follow-up. BMJ. 2016;354:i3740. https://doi.org/10.1136/bmj.i3740.

9. Stensrud S, Risberg MA, Roos EM. Effect of exercise therapy compared with arthroscopic surgery on knee muscle strength and functional performance in middle-aged patients with degenerative meniscus tears. Am J Phys Med Rehabil. 2015;94(6):460–73. https://doi.org/10.1097/PHM.0000000000000209.

10. Seedhom BB, Dowson D, Wright V. Proceedings: functions of the menisci, a preliminary study. J Bone Joint Surg. 1974;56(B):381–2.

11. Roos H, Laurén M, Adalberth T, Roos E, Jonsson K, Lohmander LS. Knee osteoarthritis after meniscectomy. Arthritis Rheum. 1998;41(4):687–93. http://onlinelibrary.wiley.com.ezproxy.vub.ac.be:2048/store/10.1002/1529-0131(199804)41:4%3C687::AID-ART16%3E3.0.CO%5Cn2-2/asset/16_ftp.pdf?v=1&t=huiuugtz&s=a7782a91e7cf1729e0e9ed1f93fefe0658d0f5f3%5Cnpapers2://publication/uuid/3C7D6799-80D4-426D-BE50-7E1.

12. Brindle T, Nyland J, Johnson DL. The meniscus: review of basic principles with application to surgery and rehabilitation. J Athl Train. 2001;36(2):160–9.

13. Vedi V, Williams A, Tennant SJ, Spouse E, Hunt DM, Gedroyc WM. Meniscal movement: an in-vivo study using dynamic MRI. J Bone Joint Surg Br Vol. 1999;81(1):37–41.

14. Weiss CB, Lundberg M, Hamberg P, DeHaven KE, Gillquis J. Non-operative treatment of meniscal tears. J Bone Joint Surg Am Vol. 1989;71(6):811–22.

15. Herrlin S, Hållander M, Wange P, Weidenhielm L, Werner S. Arthroscopic or conservative treatment of degenerative medial meniscal tears: a prospective randomised trial. Knee Surg Sports Traumatol Arthrosc. 2007;15(4):393–401. https://doi.org/10.1007/s00167-006-0243-2.

16. Katz JN, Brophy RH, Chaisson CE, et al. Surgery versus physical therapy for a meniscal tear and osteoarthritis. N Engl J Med. 2013;368(18):1675–84. https://doi.org/10.1056/NEJMoa1301408.

17. Sihvonen R, Paavola M, Malmivaara A, et al. Arthroscopic partial meniscectomy versus placebo surgery for a degenerative meniscus tear: a 2-year follow-up of the randomised controlled trial. Ann Rheum Dis. 2018;77(2):188–95. https://doi.org/10.1136/annrheumdis-2017-211172.

18. Vermesan D, Prejbeanu R, Laitin S, et al. Arthroscopic debridement compared to intra-articular steroids in treating degenerative medial meniscal tears. Eur Rev Med Pharmacol Sci. 2013;17(23):3192–6.

19. Gauffin H, Tagesson S, Meunier A, Magnusson H, Kvist J. Knee arthroscopic surgery is beneficial to middle-aged patients with meniscal symptoms: a prospective, randomised, single-blinded study. Osteoarthr Cartil. 2014;22(11):1808–16. https://doi.org/10.1016/j.joca.2014.07.017.

20. Gauffin H, Sonesson S, Meunier A, Magnusson H, Kvist J. Knee arthroscopic surgery in middle-aged patients with meniscal symptoms: a 3-year follow-up of a prospective, randomized study. Am J Sports Med. 2017;45(9):2077–84. https://doi.org/10.1177/0363546517701431.

21. Van De Graaf VA, Noorduyn JCA, Willigenburg NW, et al. Effect of early surgery vs physical therapy on knee function among patients with nonobstructive meniscal tears: the ESCAPE randomized clinical trial. JAMA: J Am Med Assoc. 2018;320(13):1328–37. https://doi.org/10.1001/jama.2018.13308.

22. van de Graaf VA, Wolterbeek N, Mutsaerts ELAR, et al. Arthroscopic partial meniscectomy or conservative treatment for nonobstructive meniscal tears: a systematic review and meta-analysis of randomized controlled trials. Arthrosc: J Arthrosc Relat Surg. 2016;32(9):1855–1865.e4. https://doi.org/10.1016/j.arthro.2016.05.036.

23. Cheng OT, Souzdalnitski D, Vrooman B, Cheng J. Evidence-based knee injections for the management of arthritis. Pain Med (United States). 2012;13(6):740–53. https://doi.org/10.1111/j.1526-4637.2012.01394.x.
24. Papavasiliou AV, Isaac DL, Marimuthu R, Skyrme A, Armitage A. Infection in knee replacements after previous injection of intra-articular steroid. J Bone Joint Surg Ser B. 2006;88(3):321–3. https://doi.org/10.1302/0301-620X.88B3.17136.
25. Cancienne JM, Werner BC, Luetkemeyer LM, Browne JA. Does timing of previous intra-articular steroid injection affect the post-operative rate of infection in total knee arthroplasty? J Arthroplast. 2015;30(11):1879–82. https://doi.org/10.1016/j.arth.2015.05.027.

Management of Meniscal Injuries: Resection to Repair

Kevin K. Chen, Jimmy J. Chan, and James N. Gladstone

Background

Multiple studies have established a connection between the loss of meniscal tissue and the early development of osteoarthritis [1, 2]. Loss of meniscal tissue has been tied with significant long-term sequelae. These sequala are often attributed to decreases in contact area (and therefore increases in contact stresses), decreases in knee stability, and alterations in the fluid mechanics of the knee joint [3]. Altogether, these damages to the meniscal tissues are thought to have profound implications on the integrity of the cartilage and subchondral plate leading to increased risk of early osteoarthritis (OA) [4, 5]. Knee arthroscopy is the most common orthopedic procedure in the United States with its goal being the preservation of the joint, while improving subjective symptoms caused by meniscal tears, to allow for optimal return to activity [6, 7]. While the utility of this procedure has been put into question by at least one landmark study [8], the importance of meniscal preservation and management cannot be understated.

A study by Fairbanks in 1948 detailed the changes in the knee joint following total meniscectomy with up to 14-year follow-up [2]. Fairbanks concluded that loss of meniscal tissue through meniscectomy resulted in relative overloading of the articular surface on the affected side of the joint, resulting in increasing compression across the joint and ultimately damage to the underlying cartilage. The authors further remarked that these changes must be due to the loss of the weight-bearing function of the meniscus [2]. Pengas et al. noted similar findings in adolescent

K. K. Chen · J. J. Chan
Department of Orthopaedic Surgery, Icahn School of Medicine at Mount Sinai,
New York, NY, USA

J. N. Gladstone (✉)
Division of Sports Medicine, Department of Orthopaedic Surgery, Icahn School of Medicine
at Mount Sinai, New York, NY, USA
e-mail: James.Gladstone@mountsinai.org

© Springer Nature Switzerland AG 2020
E. J. Strauss, L. M. Jazrawi (eds.), *The Management of Meniscal Pathology*,
https://doi.org/10.1007/978-3-030-49488-9_5

patients' status post total meniscectomy with a mean follow-up of over 40 years [1]. Specifically, they noted a fourfold increase in the development of OA (based on Kellgren grade: >2, definite osteophytes) compared to the contralateral control knee [1]. Clearly, besides its role as a knee stabilizer, the meniscus plays a significant role in the prevention of the development of degenerative arthritis of the knee. In fact, it has been reported that loss of the inner third of the medial meniscus may result in decreased contact areas of 10% and increased stresses of 65% [5]. The amount of stress increase has also been shown to directly correlate to the degree of meniscal tissue loss. In a series of progressively increased meniscectomies, Lee et al. found the stress increased proportionally to the degree of meniscus tissue removed [4]. In addition, they noted contact area and mean contact stress increased more significantly as the resection extended more peripherally, suggesting the peripheral portion of the meniscus plays a greater role in increasing contact area and decreasing mean contact stresses. Finally, segmental resections resulted in outcomes similar to that of patients where the entire meniscus was removed (total meniscectomy) [4].

Besides the impact on knee contact area and stress, loss of meniscus tissue may alter the natural fluid mechanics within the knee, specifically articular cartilage [3]. This may result in an increase in the maximum fluid pressure within the knee and a reduction in the rate of pressure dissipation; both factors are thought to lead to decreased knee mobility and increased stiffness of the joint. As with contact stresses, these changes were noted to be correlated with the amount of meniscal resection [3].

Overall, it is apparent that the meniscus plays a vital role in the function and protection of the knee joint. Loss or damage to the meniscal tissue can have profound implications in the development of early OA. Accordingly, the role of meniscal preservation surgeries must be thoroughly examined. Here we review the anatomy, treatment, techniques, indications, and outcomes of meniscal injuries.

Anatomy, Function, and Diagnosis

Baseline knowledge of the meniscus' anatomy and function is important in order to fully understand the role of this structure and of the effect of meniscectomy. Each knee has one lateral and one medial meniscus. The menisci are crescent-shaped with triangular cross-sections. The menisci are composed of fibers that run circumferentially with radial fibers "presenting longitudinal splits" [9]. Typically, the medial meniscus is "C-shaped," while the lateral meniscus is described as being circular. Both menisci have attachments (root attachments) anteriorly and posteriorly to the tibia which prevent meniscal subluxation during movement or load-bearing. In addition, they are attached via the transverse inter-meniscal ligament anteriorly. The lateral meniscus has two femoral attachments: the posterior meniscofemoral ligament (ligament of Wrisberg) posteriorly and the anterior meniscofemoral ligament (ligament of Humphrey) anteriorly. The medial meniscus is tethered by the deep medial collateral ligament (MCL), allowing for less motion as compared to the lateral meniscus. In general, the lateral meniscus covers a greater percentage of the condylar surface (84% vs. 64%) than the medial meniscus.

The function of the meniscus is to act to cushion forces across the knee joint by increasing contact area, reducing contract stress and articular wear. The menisci also function to increase the stability of the knee.

Proper diagnosis of meniscal injury requires a thorough history and physical examination, which in turn can then be supplemented with advanced imaging. History of pain localized to a single knee compartment should be noted. Mechanical symptoms, including locking or catching sensations, with associated swelling, may point to meniscal pathology. Joint line tenderness, along with positive special tests, can be used to increase likelihood of meniscal tear diagnosis. Of these tests, the McMurray Test, Thessaly Test, and the deep squat test have been shown to have variable results in terms of sensitivity and specificity but tend to be helpful in the diagnosis. Finally, MRI has long been considered the gold standard for diagnosis. A meta-analysis looking at the overall accuracy of MRI in the diagnosis of meniscal tears of the knee estimated it can be as sensitive and specific as 89% (95% CI: 83–94%) and 88% (95% CI: 82–93%) respectively for medial meniscal tears; and 78% (95% CI: 66–87%) and 95% (95% CI: 91–97%) respectively for lateral meniscal tears [10]. Alternatively, studies suggest ultrasound may also have some diagnostic utility in the correct hands. Reliance on advanced imaging should be tempered as it has recently been suggested a high rate of asymptomatic tears are found on MRI, which may prematurely direct patients and surgeons to more invasive interventions than required [11]. As mentioned before, it is imperative a good history and physical exam be clinically correlated with what is seen on imaging.

Treatment

Conservative Management

When evaluating patients with meniscal tears, it is important to distinguish which patients may benefit from nonoperative management. Conservative management of meniscal tears can include physical therapy, bracing, weight loss, ice, and use of nonsteroidal anti-inflammatory drugs (NSAIDs). Katz et al. performed a study drawing data from the Meniscal Tear in Osteoarthritis Research (MeTeOR) trial, looking at subjects ≥45 years old who either had arthroscopic partial meniscectomy (APM) with physical therapy (PT), or PT alone. Patients who crossed over from the PT alone group to the APM group had shorter symptom duration and greater baseline pain than those who did not cross over from PT [12]. The authors also conclude patients who undergo conservative therapy prior to APM did not end up with worse outcomes [12]. A trial of conservative therapy may not ultimately decrease the efficacy of APM to improve symptoms should conservative therapy fail. This study suggests patients with stable tears should receive a trial of conservative therapy prior to opting for APM.

The determination of proper management of a meniscal injury is contingent upon appropriate characterization of the type and severity of the tear, while considering patient-specific factors. Additionally, an important consideration is the integrity and stability of the anterior cruciate ligament (ACL) [13]. In the US, many ACL injuries are treated operatively to provide stability and avoid further meniscal and cartilaginous injuries to the knee joint [13]. Patients with ACL stable knees tend to have better outcomes with regard to radiographic and clinical symptoms following meniscal injury.

Not all tears are symptomatic, and not all symptomatic tears require operative intervention. In general, the location of the tear and type of tear have been shown to be good prognostic factors for its ability to heal. Specifically, tears that are more stable are thought to have a better likelihood to heal and are less likely to result in rapid degeneration of the osteochondral surface. Multiple studies have documented a noninferior outcome in patients with meniscal tears who undergo nonoperative management compared to APM [14]. In a classic paper by Weiss and DeHaven, only 80 out of 1316 tears were defined as stable [15]. Of these stable tears, 70 were vertical longitudinal tears near the periphery, which have healing potential and may be successfully treated by leaving the tear in situ [15].

In knees where ACL reconstruction is undertaken, peripheral, lateral-sided, stable tears may be left in situ [16, 17]. Fitzgibbons and Shelbourne suggest that lateral meniscal tears with posterior horn avulsion, vertical tears posterior to the popliteus tendon, vertical longitudinal tears, radial tears, or anterior vertical tears tend to be asymptomatic if left in situ [17]. In their study, 189 posterior horn avulsions of the lateral meniscus all remained asymptomatic. In contrast, tears which tend to occur in the avascular inner third of the meniscus (including most radial tears) portend a poorer likelihood for healing. It is these tears that likely require more aggressive intervention [15].

Arthroscopic Partial Meniscectomy (APM)

Despite the success of conservative therapy, many patients still remain symptomatic and may be candidates for APM. First introduced in the 1960–1970s by Ikeuchi [18], APM was developed to remove free fragments, preserve the outer rim, and clear loose tissue with the hopes of preventing further irritation and worsening of symptoms. Restoration of meniscal anatomy is crucial for proper knee biomechanics and facilitates rapid rehabilitation of the knee [19]. Large, unstable tears left in situ may introduce a greater inflammatory response secondary to the free fragments, further damaging the overlying or underlying articular cartilage. Symptomatic tears which are not responsive to conservative treatment and not amenable to repair require partial resection.

Technique

Originally an open procedure, arthroscopic partial meniscectomy has become one of the most prevalent orthopedic procedures in the United States [6]. Anteromedial and anterolateral portals are the standard primary workhorse portals for APM. All free fragments identified that can be displaced with a probe should be removed. If necessary, an ancillary medial or lateral portal can be used to allow for an additional grasper to pull the fragment forward, thus allowing resection at the base of the tear. The technique of using an auxiliary portal and a grasper can be particularly helpful for free meniscal fragments that are attached posteriorly. This allows the fragment to be removed at its base and avoids leaving a tag of meniscus that may be harder to access.

Tighter knees may require narrower instruments or additional techniques to allow for better access to the medial joint in particular. If necessary, persistent valgus stress (applied carefully) can lead to incremental opening of the compartment over time. If this does not help, a targeted pie-crusting of the MCL can be performed. With a valgus stress applied to the knee, a spinal needle can be used at the joint line. Two techniques have been described. In the first, the spinal needle is placed from the contralateral portal just beneath the meniscus, beginning mid-joint and moving posteriorly. Small punctures to the deep MCL are repeated until the joint space opens adequately. The other described technique uses the spinal needle from outside-in and peppers the superficial MCL at the level of the tibia until the joint opens adequately. Studies have shown no detrimental effect of this technique [20, 21].

At this point, it is useful to appreciate the normal texture of the meniscus and resect damaged or degenerative portions where the meniscal tissue is notably different (i.e., mushy, soft, or fibrotic). It is typically recommended to leave a smooth, contoured border to avoid catching or re-tearing; however, a perfectly smooth rim is not necessary as remodeling typically occurs regardless [19] (Fig. 5.1a–c). In order to preserve the longitudinal circumferential fibers, which protect against hoop stresses, it is important to attempt to preserve as much of the peripheral tissue as possible. At the conclusion of the procedure, copious lavage and suctioning of the joint should be performed to remove any loose debris. Following the procedure, proper postoperative follow-up and education is critical for optimal recovery and return to activity in a timely and successful manner.

Rehabilitation Following APM

Appropriate expectations are important in order to achieve optimum and expedient recoveries following APM. Patients should be encouraged to rest during the first 3–4 days after surgery, elevating and icing often. In addition, they should perform quad sets, straight leg raises, and ankle range of motion four to five times a day. This helps reduce or minimize swelling, reduce quadriceps atrophy, and reduce the chance of deep vein thrombosis (DVT). Rates of DVT following APM are thought to be negligible (less than 1% in older populations) [22]; however if there is any concern, aspirin or another form of DVT prophylaxis should be used until normal activity is resumed. While formal physical therapy is not essential, it is often helpful, for most patients in the first 4 weeks.

At our institution, we prospectively evaluated patients who underwent APM for their functional improvement and monitored overall recovery patterns. In a total of 67 patients we found it took an average of 15 days (median 10.5 days, range 2–84) for patients to return to work following APM, with half discontinuing use of assistive devices by 8 days. In this cohort, patients stopped use of narcotic medications

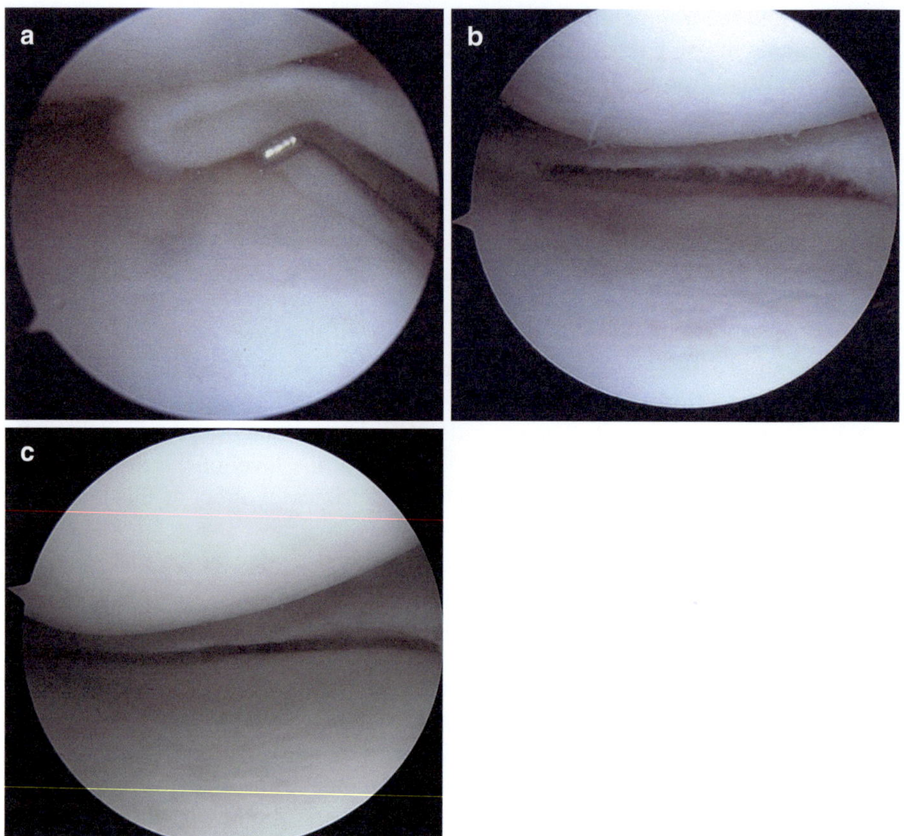

Fig. 5.1 (**a**) Meniscus tear noted in arthroscopic view of knee. (**b**) Post-meniscus resection view of meniscus: resection is clean but not entirely smooth. (**c**) 3-year follow-up of knee demonstrating smooth contours despite not having left smooth edge 3 years prior

and over-the-counter pain medications at a mean of 7.37 days (range 2–56) and 12.01 days (range 2–84), respectively.

Return to Activity

Return to activity following APM differs depending on the patient characteristics and the type of tear. Clinical data can help guide physicians to educate their patients on their expected recovery. In general, patients are able to return to full activity relatively quickly with minimal restrictions. Specifically, recreational athletes, who undergo two and three portal knee arthroscopies have been shown to be able to return to work and normal activities in an average of 9 and 19 days, respectively [23]. In addition, Lubowitz et al. reported that 82% of patients who underwent knee arthroscopy were able to return to light activity at the 1-week post-op time point, and 94% at 2 weeks. By 4 weeks, all patients were transitioned to full activity [24].

In addition, while 88% of patients indicated knee-related activity restriction preoperatively, only 74%, 38%, and 4% of patients described knee-related activity restriction at 2, 4, and 20 weeks postoperatively [24].

Indications and Outcomes of APM

Multiple studies have examined outcomes following APM to determine if there is a subset of patients where APM is more effective. In general, clinical outcomes tend to be favorable (at short- to mid-term follow-up) [25–28], whereas radiographic findings have been more concerning [29, 30]. A cross-sectional study performed by Aaron et al. noted an improvement in the mean pain score from 11.9 to 30.8 points (using the Knee Society Severity Score), and 72 (65%) of the 110 patients were considered to have substantial improvement [27].

Age/Preoperative OA

Of note, they also found that 52 (90%) knees with radiographically mild arthritis were associated with clinical improvement, while only 5 (25%) knees with severe arthritis were noted to have clinical improvement [27]. In addition, patients of older age (generally above 40 years old) tend to have worse clinical outcomes than younger patients who undergo APM [28, 31]. These results may be confounded by the fact that older patients tend to have more significant preoperative OA than their younger counterparts.

Total Versus Partial Meniscectomy

As mentioned previously, the amount of meniscal tissue preserved is directly correlated with radiographic outcomes. Unsurprisingly, APM has been shown to have better radiographic and clinical outcomes when compared to total or subtotal meniscectomy [31, 32]. Englund et al. found that patients who underwent partial meniscectomy had significantly higher Lysholm scores ($p = 0.03$) and were found to be more stable with less mediolateral laxity as compared to patients who underwent total meniscectomy [31]. These studies go hand in hand with the concept that greater preservation of meniscal tissue is critical to the prevention of development of OA. When directly comparing a contralateral knee without meniscectomy to the knee with meniscectomy, it appears patients who undergo APM have a greater progression of radiographic signs of OA [12, 14, 33–38]. Likewise, greater degrees of meniscectomy are associated with earlier and more severe progression of OA [33–35]. In a systematic review of patients who underwent ACL repair, there was a fivefold increase in radiographic findings associated with OA in the patients who underwent APM compared to those with an intact meniscus [38].

Laterality

There is some literature suggesting that medial meniscus tears are thought to perform worse after meniscectomy when compared to a lateral meniscectomy [35]. This is thought to be due to the dynamic loading pattern of the knee, where the center of pressure for a normal knee is in the medial compartment during maximum loading transmission [35, 39, 40]. This has been put into question by at least one other study which found while subjective and clinical results are similar, radiologic results were significantly worse in patients who underwent lateral meniscectomy [37]. To further complicate this matter, studies have simultaneously suggested more rapid progression of OA [37] and higher reoperation rates [41], following loss of or damage to the lateral meniscus. Others, however, suggested no difference in outcomes between medial and lateral meniscectomy with regard to radiographic outcomes [30, 34].

Body Mass Index

As with the preexisting degenerative changes, patients with preoperative obesity tend to have worse radiographic outcomes than those not classified as obese [26, 42, 43]. Englund et al. found patients with obesity (BMI $\geq$30) and APM had a greater likelihood of tibiofemoral radiographic OA than those who had undergone partial meniscal resection with a BMI <25 [42]. More recently, Klucyznski et al. measured various patient-reported outcomes in a randomized controlled trial of 256 patients who underwent APM and found obese patients had significantly worse pain, physical functioning, and quality of life scores when compared with their nonobese cohorts [43]. These results are altogether not surprising as this patient population at baseline tend to be at higher risk for the development of OA, given the increased demand placed on their joints.

Degenerative Versus Nondegenerative Tears

It is important to distinguish acute traumatic tears from degenerative tears which are typically considered in a different category. Degenerative tear patterns are usually characterized as complex, horizontal cleavage, or shredded, as opposed to the more well-defined tears of acute meniscal injuries. Degenerative tears are often associated with older age and tend to have additional features including chondral damage and radiographic findings of OA [44]. It is important to consider the benefit potential in these situations as alternative options such as arthroplasty might be more benefitial [45]. Menetrey et al. evaluated the mid-term outcomes in patients over 50 years of age after APM of the medial meniscus and determined that patients with nondegenerative tears had significantly better outcomes when compared to degenerative tears (90% rated excellent or good results versus only 20%, respectively) [25].

Radiographic Progression of OA

In contrast, there is some concern that a correlation between APM and progression of OA may exist. Partial meniscectomy has been shown to increase stresses by an average of 67%, while total meniscectomy increased stresses by 236% [5]. Similarly, cadaveric studies have demonstrated significantly decreased contact areas and therefore increased contact stresses after partial posterior medial meniscectomy [4]. Rockborn et al. found post-meniscectomy knees had substantially more Fairbanks changes when compared to the contralateral knee (20 versus 5 out of 33 total knees). Hulet et al. found that in 74 stable knees with 12-year follow-up, 21% of operative knees had radiographic signs of narrowing as compared to 11% in the contralateral knee [36]. Accordingly, there is movement toward extending the indications and tear patterns for meniscal repair with the goal of preserving more meniscal tissue and thus protecting the biomechanical function of the meniscus. A systematic review comparing meniscal repair and partial meniscectomy found that meniscal repairs were associated with less radiologic degeneration than partial meniscectomy [41]. Despite this, it is important to remember that radiographic outcomes need to be correlated with the patient's clinical picture as many of these changes may not be clinically symptomatic or significant. Longer-term follow-up of the results of APM will help define these findings of radiographic changes.

Discussion

Despite evidence to suggest poor long-term radiographic findings, it is important to understand while many of these studies suggest meniscal resection portends arthritis, this is not altogether an accurate statement. Rather, it is the occurrence of the tear itself which creates changes to the biomechanical capabilities of the meniscus leading to early arthritis. In meniscus-deficient or -injured patients, damage to the articular surface is more frequent and tends to be more aggressive, but this appears to occur even without additional meniscectomy [46]. The goal of APM is to decrease morbidity related to the tear and allow for early return to function. Overall, despite the controversy surrounding the efficacy and indications for APM, there appears to be a subset of patients where APM is preferable. Proper patient selection and education are essential in creating optimal outcomes [47].

Meniscal tears which are not amenable to repair (those with damage to poorly vascularized areas of the meniscus unlikely to remain viable following repair), and those which cause mechanical symptoms, or restrictions in range of motion of the patient's knee, may be candidates for APM [48, 49]. In addition, APM may be an option in patients with acute, simple, yet symptomatic tears where there is less concern for meniscal healing potential. In older patients, it may be better to perform the least morbid procedure (APM) with the goal of mitigating symptoms without the concern for development of OA, as these patients tend to develop OA and have similar outcomes regardless of treatment modality [50]. This must be weighed carefully with data suggesting preexisting degenerative changes impact the postoperative outcomes. While it is unclear if age is an independent risk factor for worse outcomes, it does seem apparent patients who have worse preoperative radiographic signs of OA may have less satisfactory results compared to patients with radiographically healthier knees [27, 51]. Patients with greater body mass index (BMI) seem to have worse outcomes after meniscectomy, and therefore the physician must be careful when discussing this elective procedure with their patients. Data regarding laterality of meniscus injury is unclear and requires further research.

Overall, the role for APM in the treatment of meniscal tears is an area of some controversy. Considering the concerns related to meniscectomy outlined above, a preservation of the maximum amount of meniscal tissue should be the ultimate goal in the treatment of meniscal tear. Accordingly, meniscal repair is often preferred whenever possible. This includes tears at the meniscocapsular junction, red–red zone, and red–white zone, especially in the acute setting where the meniscus appears healthy and has an appropriate tear pattern (typically longitudinal tear without shearing). Additionally, radial tears extending to the periphery (complete radial tears) should be considered for repair, especially in younger individuals, as loss of the circumferential fiber hoop stresses simulates total meniscectomy. Clearly, meniscal repair is not always possible and there are certainly circumstances where APM can offer both symptomatic and clinical benefit to the patient [52]. APM appears to provide more favorable outcomes in patients who are not obese (BMI <30), in the setting of an acute tear, and for patients who have better preoperative cartilage integrity [45].

Summary

Meniscus tear is one of the most common injuries in the knee and accordingly, APM is among the most common procedures performed in the United States (approximately 700,000 procedures a year in the USA) [7, 53]. Removal of meniscal tissue inherently leads to decreases in contact area, and therefore increases contact stresses. In addition, this loss of tissue confers biomechanical and structural changes to the articular cartilage and subchondral plate. The degeneration of articular cartilage is a logical extension of these processes. Meniscal repair should be undertaken whenever possible and longer-term outcomes appear to be better than with partial meniscectomy. Despite this, mid-term functional results of partial meniscectomy are generally very good. It is possible that the rapid availability of advanced imaging and improvements in their techniques has led to an increased "overreading" of damage without clinical significance.

In terms of the structure of the meniscus itself, the peripheral rim of the meniscus plays a significantly greater role in force distribution and should be preserved whenever possible. ACL stability is critical to long-term preservation of joint space, and meniscal integrity, and a smooth and well-balanced meniscus should be the goal of a partial meniscectomy.

It is important to remember that APM, when performed properly, does not cause arthritis. Rather a torn meniscus creates the biomechanical abnormalities that, with or without surgery, can lead to the development of arthritis. APM, in the appropriately indicated knee, can lead to the rapid amelioration of symptoms and improvement in function.

References

1. Pengas IP, Assiotis A, Nash W, Hatcher J, Banks J, McNicholas MJ. Total meniscectomy in adolescents: a 40-year follow-up. J Bone Joint Surg Br. 2012;94:1649–54. Available at: http://www.ncbi.nlm.nih.gov/pubmed/23188906.
2. Fairbank TJ. Knee joint changes after meniscectomy. J Bone Joint Surg Br. 1948;30B:664–70. Available at: http://www.ncbi.nlm.nih.gov/pubmed/18894618.

3. Kazemi M, Li LP, Buschmann MD, Savard P. Partial meniscectomy changes fluid pressurization in articular cartilage in human knees. J Biomech Eng. 2012;134:021001. Available at: http://www.ncbi.nlm.nih.gov/pubmed/22482668.

4. Lee SJ, Aadalen KJ, Malaviya P, Lorenz EP, Hayden JK, Farr J, Kang RW, Cole BJ. Tibiofemoral contact mechanics after serial medial meniscectomies in the human cadaveric knee. Am J Sports Med. 2006;34:1334–44. Available at: http://www.ncbi.nlm.nih.gov/pubmed/16636354.

5. Baratz ME, Fu FH, Mengato R. Meniscal tears: the effect of meniscectomy and of repair on intraarticular contact areas and stress in the human knee. A preliminary report. Am J Sports Med. 1986;14:270–5. Available at: http://www.ncbi.nlm.nih.gov/pubmed/3755296.

6. Abrams GD, Frank RM, Gupta AK, Harris JD, McCormick FM, Cole BJ. Trends in meniscus repair and meniscectomy in the United States, 2005–2011. Am J Sports Med. 2013;41:2333–9.

7. Cullen KA, Hall MJ, Golosinskiy A. Ambulatory surgery in the United States, 2006. Natl Health Stat Rep. 2009:1–25. Available at: http://www.ncbi.nlm.nih.gov/pubmed/19294964.

8. Sihvonen R, Paavola M, Malmivaara A, Itälä A, Joukainen A, Nurmi H, Kalske J, Järvinen TLN, and Finnish Degenerative Meniscal Lesion Study (FIDELITY) Group. Arthroscopic partial meniscectomy versus sham surgery for a degenerative meniscal tear. N Engl J Med. 2013;369:2515–24. Available at: http://www.ncbi.nlm.nih.gov/pubmed/24369076.

9. Canale ST, Beaty JH. Campell's operative orthopaedics. 12th ed. Philadelphia: Mosby; 2012.

10. Phelan N, Rowland P, Galvin R, O'Byrne JM. A systematic review and meta-analysis of the diagnostic accuracy of MRI for suspected ACL and meniscal tears of the knee. Knee Surg Sports Traumatol Arthrosc. 2016;24(5):1525–39.

11. Boden SD, Davis DO, Dina TS, Stoller DW, Brown SD, Vailas JC, Labropoulos PA. A prospective and blinded investigation of magnetic resonance imaging of the knee. Abnormal findings in asymptomatic subjects. Clin Orthop Relat Res. 1992:177–85. Available at: http://www.ncbi.nlm.nih.gov/pubmed/1516310.

12. Katz JN, Wright J, Spindler KP, Mandl LA, Safran-Norton CE, Reinke EK, Levy BA, Wright RW, Jones MH, Martin SD, et al. Predictors and outcomes of crossover to surgery from physical therapy for meniscal tear and osteoarthritis: a randomized trial comparing physical therapy and surgery. J Bone Joint Surg Am. 2016;98:1890–6. Available at: http://www.ncbi.nlm.nih.gov/pubmed/27852905.

13. Ekås GR, Ardern C, Grindem H, Engebretsen L. New meniscal tears after ACL injury: what is the risk? A systematic review protocol. Br J Sports Med. 2018;52:386. Available at: http://www.ncbi.nlm.nih.gov/pubmed/28647718.

14. van de Graaf VA, Noorduyn JCA, Willigenburg NW, Butter IK, de Gast A, Mol BW, Saris DBF, Twisk JWR, Poolman RW, and ESCAPE Research Group. Effect of early surgery vs physical therapy on knee function among patients with nonobstructive meniscal tears: the ESCAPE randomized clinical trial. JAMA. 2018;320:1328–37. Available at: http://www.ncbi.nlm.nih.gov/pubmed/30285177.

15. Weiss CB, Lundberg M, Hamburg P, DeHaven KE, Gillquist J. Non-operative treatment of meniscal tears. J Bone Joint Surg Ser A. 1989;71:811–22.

16. Shelbourne KD, Gray T. Anterior cruciate ligament reconstruction with autogenous patellar tendon graft followed by accelerated rehabilitation. A two- to nine-year followup. Am J Sports Med. 1997;25:786–95. Available at: http://www.ncbi.nlm.nih.gov/pubmed/9397266.

17. Fitzgibbons RE, Shelbourne KD. "Aggressive" nontreatment of lateral meniscal tears seen during anterior cruciate ligament reconstruction. Am J Sports Med. 1995;23:156–9. Available at: http://www.ncbi.nlm.nih.gov/pubmed/7778698.

18. Ikeuchi H. Meniscus surgery using the Watanabe arthroscope. Orthop Clin North Am. 1979;10:629–42. Available at: http://www.ncbi.nlm.nih.gov/pubmed/460837.

19. Jeong H-J, Lee S-H, Ko C-S. Meniscectomy. Knee Surg Relat Res. 2012;24:129–36. Available at: http://www.ncbi.nlm.nih.gov/pubmed/22977789.

20. Bert JM. First, do no harm: protect the articular cartilage when performing arthroscopic knee surgery! Arthroscopy. 2016;32:2169–74. Available at: http://www.ncbi.nlm.nih.gov/pubmed/27593535. Accessed 10 July 2019.

21. Claret G, Montañana J, Rios J, Ruiz-Ibán MÁ, Popescu D, Núñez M, Lozano L, Combalia A, Sastre S. The effect of percutaneous release of the medial collateral ligament in arthroscopic medial meniscectomy on functional outcome. Knee. 2016;23(2):251–5.
22. Hame SL, Nguyen V, Ellerman J, Ngo SS, Wang JC, Gamradt SC. Complications of arthroscopic meniscectomy in the older population. Am J Sports Med. 2012;40(6):1402–5.
23. Stetson WB, Templin K. Two-versus three-portal technique for routine knee arthroscopy. Am J Sports Med. 2002;30:108–11. Available at: http://www.ncbi.nlm.nih.gov/pubmed/11799005.
24. Lubowitz JH, Ayala M, Appleby D. Return to activity after knee arthroscopy. Arthroscopy. 2008;24:58–61.e4. Available at: http://www.ncbi.nlm.nih.gov/pubmed/18182203.
25. Ménétrey J, Siegrist O, Fritschy D. Medial meniscectomy in patients over the age of fifty: a six year follow-up study. Swiss Surg. 2002;8:113–9. Available at: http://www.ncbi.nlm.nih.gov/pubmed/12125334.
26. Lee B-S, Bin S-I, Kim J-M, Park M-H, Lee S-M, Bae K-H. Partial meniscectomy for degenerative medial meniscal root tears shows favorable outcomes in well-aligned, nonarthritic knees. Am J Sports Med. 2019:363546518819225. Available at: http://www.ncbi.nlm.nih.gov/pubmed/30673297.
27. Aaron RK, Skolnick AH, Reinert SE, Ciombor DM. Arthroscopic débridement for osteoarthritis of the knee. J Bone Joint Surg Am. 2006;88:936–43. Available at: http://www.ncbi.nlm.nih.gov/pubmed/16651566.
28. Bolano LE, Grana WA. Isolated arthroscopic partial meniscectomy. Functional radiographic evaluation at five years. Am J Sports Med. 1993;21:432–7. Available at: http://www.ncbi.nlm.nih.gov/pubmed/8346759.
29. Petty CA, Lubowitz JH. Does arthroscopic partial meniscectomy result in knee osteoarthritis? A systematic review with a minimum of 8 years' follow-up. Arthroscopy. 2011;27:419–24. Available at: http://www.ncbi.nlm.nih.gov/pubmed/21126847.
30. Englund M, Roos EM, Lohmander LS. Impact of type of meniscal tear on radiographic and symptomatic knee osteoarthritis: a sixteen-year followup of meniscectomy with matched controls. Arthritis Rheum. 2003;48:2178–87. Available at: http://www.ncbi.nlm.nih.gov/pubmed/12905471.
31. Englund M, Roos EM, Roos HP, Lohmander LS. Patient-relevant outcomes fourteen years after meniscectomy: influence of type of meniscal tear and size of resection. Rheumatology (Oxford). 2001;40:631–9. Available at: http://www.ncbi.nlm.nih.gov/pubmed/11426019.
32. Andersson-Molina H, Karlsson H, Rockborn P. Arthroscopic partial and total meniscectomy: a long-term follow-up study with matched controls. Arthroscopy. 2002;18:183–9. Available at: http://www.ncbi.nlm.nih.gov/pubmed/11830813.
33. Rockborn P, Hamberg P, Gillquist J. Arthroscopic meniscectomy: treatment costs and postoperative function in a historical perspective. Acta Orthop Scand. 2000;71:455–60. Available at: http://www.ncbi.nlm.nih.gov/pubmed/11186400.
34. Burks RT, Metcalf MH, Metcalf RW. Fifteen-year follow-up of arthroscopic partial meniscectomy. Arthroscopy. 1997;13:673–9. Available at: http://www.ncbi.nlm.nih.gov/pubmed/9442319.
35. Higuchi H, Kimura M, Shirakura K, Terauchi M, Takagishi K. Factors affecting long-term results after arthroscopic partial meniscectomy. Clin Orthop Relat Res. 2000;377:161–8.
36. Hulet CH, Locker BG, Schiltz D, Texier A, Tallier E, Vielpeau CH. Arthroscopic medial meniscectomy on stable knees. J Bone Joint Surg Br. 2001;83:29–32. Available at: http://www.ncbi.nlm.nih.gov/pubmed/11245533.
37. Chatain F, Adeleine P, Chambat P, Neyret P, and Société Française d'Arthroscopie. A comparative study of medial versus lateral arthroscopic partial meniscectomy on stable knees: 10-year minimum follow-up. Arthroscopy. 2003;19:842–9. Available at: http://www.ncbi.nlm.nih.gov/pubmed/14551546.
38. Magnussen RA, Mansour AA, Carey JL, Spindler KP. Meniscus status at anterior cruciate ligament reconstruction associated with radiographic signs of osteoarthritis at 5- to 10-year follow-up: a systematic review. J Knee Surg. 2009;22:347–57. Available at: http://www.ncbi.nlm.nih.gov/pubmed/19902731.

39. Johnson F, Leitl S, Waugh W. The distribution of load across the knee. A comparison of static and dynamic measurements. J Bone Joint Surg Br. 1980;62:346–9. Available at: http://www.ncbi.nlm.nih.gov/pubmed/7410467.
40. Harrington IJ. Static and dynamic loading patterns in knee joints with deformities. J Bone Joint Surg Am. 1983;65:247–59. Available at: http://www.ncbi.nlm.nih.gov/pubmed/6822587.
41. Paxton ES, Stock MV, Brophy RH. Meniscal repair versus partial meniscectomy: a systematic review comparing reoperation rates and clinical outcomes. Arthroscopy. 2011;27:1275–88. Available at: http://www.ncbi.nlm.nih.gov/pubmed/21820843.
42. Englund M, Lohmander LS. Risk factors for symptomatic knee osteoarthritis fifteen to twenty-two years after meniscectomy. Arthritis Rheum. 2004;50:2811–9. Available at: http://www.ncbi.nlm.nih.gov/pubmed/15457449.
43. Kluczynski MA, Marzo JM, Wind WM, Fineberg MS, Bernas GA, Rauh MA, Zhou Z, Zhao J, Bisson LJ. The effect of body mass index on clinical outcomes in patients without radiographic evidence of degenerative joint disease after arthroscopic partial meniscectomy. Arthroscopy. 2017;33:2054–2063.e10. Available at: http://www.ncbi.nlm.nih.gov/pubmed/28969948.
44. Christoforakis J, Pradhan R, Sanchez-Ballester J, Hunt N, Strachan RK. Is there an association between articular cartilage changes and degenerative meniscus tears? Arthroscopy. 2005;21:1366–9. Available at: http://www.ncbi.nlm.nih.gov/pubmed/16325089.
45. Salata MJ, Gibbs AE, Sekiya JK. A systematic review of clinical outcomes in patients undergoing meniscectomy. Am J Sports Med. 2010;38:1907–16. Available at: http://www.ncbi.nlm.nih.gov/pubmed/20587698.
46. Englund M, Guermazi A, Roemer FW, Aliabadi P, Yang M, Lewis CE, Torner J, Nevitt MC, Sack B, Felson DT. Meniscal tear in knees without surgery and the development of radiographic osteoarthritis among middle-aged and elderly persons: the Multicenter Osteoarthritis Study. Arthritis Rheum. 2009;60:831–9. Available at: http://www.ncbi.nlm.nih.gov/pubmed/19248082.
47. Thompson SR. Diagnostic knee arthroscopy and partial meniscectomy. JBJS Essent Surg Tech. 2016;6:e7. Available at: http://www.ncbi.nlm.nih.gov/pubmed/30237917.
48. Vautrin M, Schwartz C. Future of 34 meniscectomies after bucket-handle meniscus tear: a retrospective study with a follow-up over 22 years. Eur J Orthop Surg Traumatol. 2016;26:435–40. Available at: http://www.ncbi.nlm.nih.gov/pubmed/26940211.
49. Shelbourne KD, Dersam MD. Comparison of partial meniscectomy versus meniscus repair for bucket-handle lateral meniscus tears in anterior cruciate ligament reconstructed knees. Arthroscopy. 2004;20:581–5. Available at: http://www.ncbi.nlm.nih.gov/pubmed/15241307.
50. Stein T, Mehling AP, Welsch F, von Eisenhart-Rothe R, Jäger A. Long-term outcome after arthroscopic meniscal repair versus arthroscopic partial meniscectomy for traumatic meniscal tears. Am J Sports Med. 2010;38:1542–8. Available at: http://www.ncbi.nlm.nih.gov/pubmed/20551284.
51. Crevoisier X, Munzinger U, Drobny T. Arthroscopic partial meniscectomy in patients over 70 years of age. Arthroscopy. 2001;17:732–6. Available at: http://www.ncbi.nlm.nih.gov/pubmed/11536092.
52. Stuart MJ, Lubowitz JH. What, if any, are the indications for arthroscopic debridement of the osteoarthritic knee? Arthroscopy. 2006;22:238–9. Available at: http://www.ncbi.nlm.nih.gov/pubmed/16523583.
53. Carr A. Arthroscopic surgery for degenerative knee. BMJ. 2015;350:h2983. PMID: 26080046. Available at: https://pubmed.ncbi.nlm.nih.gov/26080046/.

Meniscus Repair

6

Robert Meislin and Darryl Whitney

Meniscal repair is becoming a commonly performed procedure [1] due to the increasing recognition of the functional importance of the meniscus and evidence of long-term complications associated with meniscectomy. In their classic biomechanical study, Baratz et al. showed a decrease in contact area by 10% and increased peak local contact pressures by 65% in cadaveric knees following partial medial meniscectomy [2]. More recently, others have found significantly increased contact pressures following the creation of horizontal cleavage tears [3, 4], with a further increase following subtotal meniscectomy and reduction to near normal pressures after meniscus repair [4].

Despite favorable short-term clinical outcomes in 90% of patients undergoing partial meniscectomy, long-term follow-up studies have raised concern for the development or progression of osteoarthritis. One study found that 35% of patients had progression of radiographic osteoarthritis 5-years following partial medial meniscectomy [5]. Similarly, another showed that 53% of patients developed osteoarthritis after partial meniscectomy at a mean of 8.5-year follow-up [6]. A study of 147 athletes who underwent partial meniscectomy demonstrated an increase in radiographic arthritic changes from 40% at 4.5 years to 89% at 14.5 years after surgery, with 46% of patients no longer participating in their previous sport [7]. These concerning findings have led surgeons to perform an increasing number of meniscal repairs when indicated.

R. Meislin (✉) · D. Whitney
NYU Langone Orthopedic Center, New York, NY, USA
e-mail: Robert.Meislin@nyulangone.org; Darryl.Whitney@nyulangone.org

© Springer Nature Switzerland AG 2020
E. J. Strauss, L. M. Jazrawi (eds.), *The Management of Meniscal Pathology*,
https://doi.org/10.1007/978-3-030-49488-9_6

Indications for Meniscal Repair

Historically, meniscal repair was reserved for peripheral tears in young patients, but repair indications are expanding with improvements in technique and understanding of meniscal healing. Tear characteristics (pattern, size, location, stability) as well patient factors (age, activity level, symptoms) and knee stability need to be considered when attempting repair. Ideal conditions for the healing of a meniscal repair include reducible vertical tears in the red–red or red–white zones, with good tissue integrity and in the setting of concomitant anterior cruciate ligament (ACL) reconstruction [1].

The blood supply [8] and neural innervation [9] of the human meniscus reaches only the outer third and, therefore, peripheral tears have significantly higher healing rates. Retrospective studies using second-look arthroscopy have shown significant differences in healing rates based on tear location, with partial or no healing occurring more often with central tears than peripheral tears [10, 11]. Although they heal less reliably, many authors still advocate attempting repair of red–white zone tears in younger patients given the aforementioned concerns about meniscectomy. One series showed a 62% success rate with the repair of longitudinal red–white tears in patients under 20 years of age at 10-year follow-up [12]. Attempts to encourage bleeding in avascular zones may be of benefit, as evidenced by a study [13] showing that the addition of trephination of vascular channels led to significantly lower re-tear rates. There is also some literature to support that bone marrow stimulation from the drilling of bone tunnels at the time of ACL reconstruction improves healing rates [14]. In terms of size, length greater than 4 cm is a negative prognostic factor since these tears are unstable and often don't heal, especially in the chronic setting [15]. Furthermore, medial meniscal repairs have a higher rate of failure than lateral tears [16, 17].

The tear pattern is also an important factor to consider, with vertically oriented tears that do not disrupt the circumferential fibers of the meniscus being more amenable to repair. Conversely, radial and oblique tears involve mostly the avascular portions of the meniscus, are often unstable, and have traditionally been treated with meniscectomy. However, newer techniques have shown promise for repair of radial tears, both biomechanically [18–20] and clinically [21, 22]. A matched cohort study by Wu et al. [21] demonstrated no difference in reoperation rate or clinical outcome scores between patients undergoing repair of radial and bucket-handle tears. Therefore, repair of radial tears should be considered in younger patients, especially in tears extending to the periphery. Horizontal cleavage meniscal tears are often degenerative and usually treated with meniscectomy due to their poor healing potential. However, in younger patients with acute horizontal cleavage tears, meniscal repair has shown promising results in several recent studies [23–25].

Knee stability can also have a significant impact on repair success. Meniscal repairs performed in the setting of ACL-deficiency have been shown to have significantly lower healing rates, with only 67% of repairs healed on second-look arthroscopy in knees with a torn ACL compared to 92% when the ACL was concurrently reconstructed [26–28]. Despite these concerns, some authors have had success with isolated meniscal repair in ACL-deficient knees, with satisfactory clinical outcomes in 87% of 23 patients in one case series [29]. Nevertheless, strong consideration should be given to restoring knee stability when indicating a patient for repair of a torn meniscus.

Timing of surgery may also affect healing. Tears that are repaired within 6 weeks of the injury were found to have higher rates of successful outcomes and reparability than those repaired after 6 weeks [30, 31]. With regards to staging the ACL reconstruction in the setting of meniscal repair, it is generally recommended to perform both procedures concurrently, as an unstable knee often precludes healing of the meniscus. This concept is supported by a study by Gallacher et al. [32], who found higher failure rates of the meniscal repair when ACL reconstruction was delayed. Our preferred sequence is to perform both procedures in the same sitting and to repair the meniscus prior to ACL reconstruction.

Several patient factors can influence meniscus repair outcomes. Older patients have been shown in some studies to have lower rates of healing [33, 34], while other studies have found either no difference based on age [10, 35], or improved outcomes in older patients [17]. Steadman et al. [36] performed a large, single-surgeon cohort study comparing their 10-year outcomes of meniscus repair with patients stratified based on age (>40 vs. <40 years) and found no difference between groups in repair failure rate or clinical outcome scores. Obesity may be a factor, as patients with a higher BMI have been shown to have worse outcomes after posterior root repairs [37] and higher rates of advanced chondral lesions seen at the time of arthroscopy [38]. Lastly, smoking has also been shown to significantly reduce the healing rates of meniscal repair [33].

Meniscus Repair Techniques

Repair of a torn meniscus can be performed open or arthroscopically. Open meniscal repair is now reserved for tears occurring in conjunction with tibial plateau fractures or horizontal tears extending to the periphery in young athletes [23, 25, 39]. Arthroscopic techniques include inside-out, outside-in, and all-inside approaches. Regardless of the technique, several general principles should be followed, including removal of loose fragments or unstable segments, abrasive perforation/rasping of the tear edges, and perimeniscal vascular stimulation/trephination to promote a healing response [40]. These steps should be performed before suture or device placement.

Inside-out meniscal repair has long been considered the gold standard for tears in the posterior and middle third of the meniscus [41]. The technique involves the use of long, flexible needles and open incisions either medially or laterally to retrieve the needles and tie sutures to the capsule while avoiding neurovascular injury. Success rates have been reported to be up to 80% for isolated repairs and 90% when performed with concurrent ACL reconstruction [1]. Concerns have been raised regarding increased surgical time, more invasive incisions, and risk of neurovascular injury with this approach compared to all-inside techniques [42]. A systematic review found a significantly higher incidence (9% vs. 2%) of nerve injury/irritation following inside-out repair than all-inside repair [43].

Outside-in repair techniques are particularly useful for anterior to mid-body meniscal tears that are difficult to reach with inside-out or all-inside approaches [44]. A spinal needle is passed through the skin and across the meniscus tear under visualization with the arthroscope [45]. A looped wire or suture shuttle can then be used to pass sutures in a mattress fashion with the use of a second spinal needle also placed from outside-in. A small incision is then made between the suture limbs and the sutures are tied over the capsule to reduce the tear. Various modifications of this technique have been described in efforts to make anterior horn repairs time- and cost-efficient and technically reproducible [46, 47]. Unrepaired anterior horn tears have been found to increase peak contact pressures by 78%, while repaired ones result in a near-complete restoration of pressures [48].

All-inside meniscal repair techniques were developed to decrease surgical time, risk to neurovascular structures, and technical skill required (Fig. 6.1). These

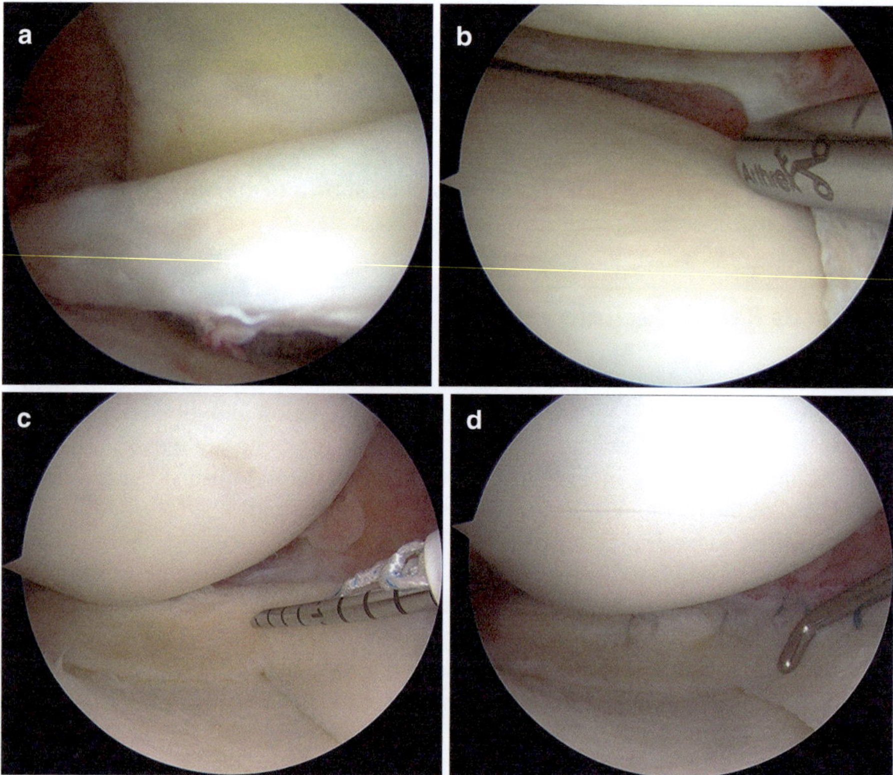

Fig. 6.1 Example of a repair of a bucket-handle medial meniscus tear. (**a**) A large bucket-handle-type tear is noted in the red–white zone. (**b**) The torn flipped fragment is reduced with a blunt instrument and the capsule and tear edges are abraded with shaver and meniscal rasp. (**c**) A suture passing/retrieving device is used to place sutures circumferentially in a vertical mattress configuration. (**d**) The meniscus is probed to assess the stability of the repair

techniques have evolved in recent years with improvements in device technology and surgeon comfort with knee arthroscopy. Earlier generation devices such as arrows, screws, harpoons, and staples have been replaced with newer generations of "hybrid" devices that feature sutures that can slide and tension through small retrocapsular implants that are introduced through the meniscus tear arthroscopically with needles of varying caliber, curvature, and orientation [39]. These newer devices have been shown to have similar failure loads and restoration of contact pressures as traditional meniscus suturing techniques [49–51], while obviating the concern of implant loosening/chondral damage [52–54] and high failure rates [55–57] seen with earlier generation devices. At 5-year follow-up, successful repair was seen in 84% of the 81 patients treated with an all-inside hybrid suture device [58]. A meta-analysis comparing all-inside techniques to inside-out and outside-in repairs showed lower operative times with the all-inside technique and comparable clinical outcome scores and overall complication rates [59].

Various suture repair configurations have been described including vertical, horizontal, and oblique mattress techniques. Vertical mattress configurations have historically been considered the gold standard, as numerous biomechanical studies have demonstrated better fixation than the horizontal mattress technique [60–63]. Conversely, other studies have found no difference between the two with regards to load to failure, pullout strength, or knot resistance [49, 63, 64]. In a recent meta-analysis of 41 studies, the authors found that vertical mattress repairs had higher load-to-failure rates and were stiffer than horizontal repairs [65]. Since most of these biomechanical studies were performed on vertically orientated tear patterns, it is important to consider tear pattern as well and to individualize each repair technique based on tear configuration.

Repair of radial meniscus repair requires different technical considerations, with all-inside, inside-out, and transtibial tunnel techniques all described for this tear pattern [18, 19, 21]. Both inside-out and all-inside techniques were found to have comparable success rates for radial tears as for bucket-handle tears in one study [21]. Another study found high success rates (91%) for posterior horn radial tears extending to the periphery repaired with an inside-out horizontal mattress suture technique [22]. A cadaveric study showed improved biomechanical properties with an all-inside, vertical mattress fixation device compared to an inside-out, horizontal mattress technique [19]. A crossed suture configuration was found to have higher load-to-failure and greater stiffness than a double horizontal mattress for radial tears in cadaveric menisci [20]. In another biomechanical study, complete mid-body tears of the medial meniscus showed less gap formation and a significantly higher load-to-failure when repaired with two transtibial tunnels compared to a double horizontal mattress technique [18].

Horizontal cleavage tears were historically treated with open techniques due to difficulty passing sutures perpendicular to the tear with traditional techniques and devices. Several studies demonstrated excellent short- and long-term results of combined arthroscopic partial meniscectomy and open repair of horizontal cleavage tears in young athletes [23–25]. A newer technique allows for all-inside repair of these lesions with the use of a self-retrieving suture-passing device to place a circumferential compression stitch in what is known as a "hay bale" technique [66,

67]. This technique allows for all the advantages of all-inside repair, with a theoretically even lower risk of neurovascular injury, as the device does not pass sutures beyond the capsule. However, no outcome study has yet compared this technique with open repair.

Medial meniscus meniscocapsular (Ramp) lesions are associated with 15–30% of ACL tears and require specific techniques for successful repair [39]. These lesions often do not show up on anterior arthroscopy and require visualization of the posteromedial compartment through the modified Gillquist maneuver, with some lesions requiring an additional posteromedial portal for diagnosis and treatment [68, 69]. Ramp lesions cannot be repaired through traditional inside-out or all-inside techniques as they require a posteromedial instrument portal for instrument and suture passage given the retrocondylar location of the tear (Fig. 6.2). Various techniques have been described, including the use of a suture-passer hook inserted through a posteromedial cannula, with re-approximation of the torn posterior capsule to the posterior horn of the medial meniscus through a knotted repair [70].

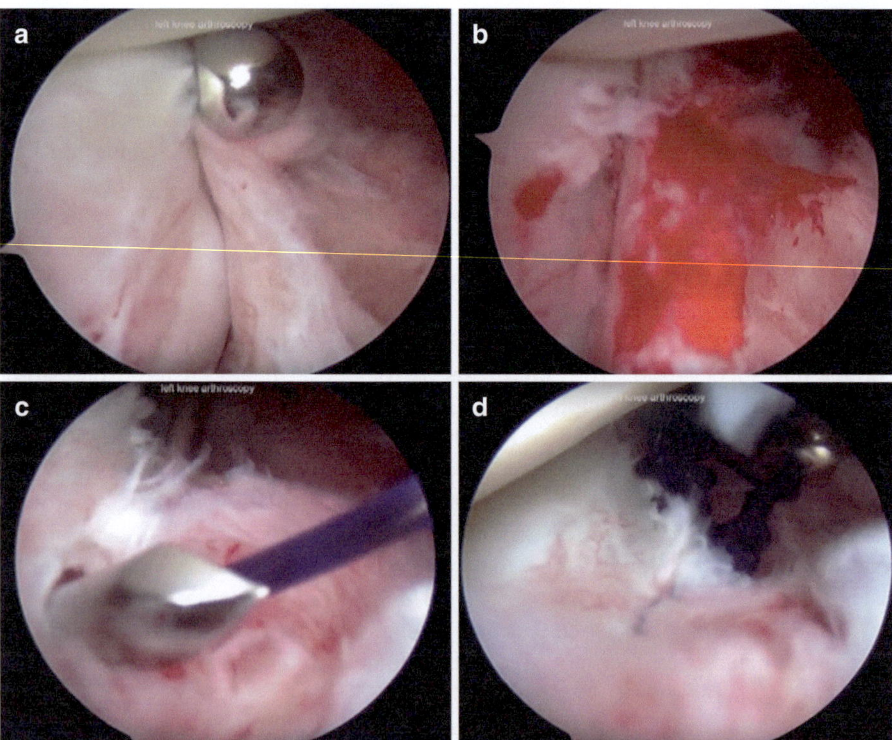

Fig. 6.2 Example of medial meniscal ramp lesion repair. (**a**) Tear is identified and posteromedial portal is created for instrument passage. (**b**) The meniscal and capsular attachments are debrided to create bleeding for biologic healing response. (**c**) Curved lasso suture passers are used to pass sutures through the peripheral meniscus and capsule. (**d**) Arthroscopic knot-tying techniques are utilized to complete the repair

Another recently described technique uses an arthroscopic grasper to hold the meniscotibial ligament in place for subsequent fixation to the meniscus using an all-inside suture device [71].

Outcomes of Meniscal Repair

Studies comparing meniscal repair to meniscectomy are limited as they are difficult to perform. Different tear patterns and tear severity may be more amenable to repair versus meniscectomy, and randomization may not be practical or ethical [1]. Stein et al. [72] performed a cohort study of 81 patients with isolated traumatic medial meniscus tears who underwent either partial meniscectomy or repair. At long-term follow-up (mean 8.5 years), a significantly higher percentage of patients had no evidence of osteoarthritic progression in the repair group (80%) than in the meniscectomy group (40%). Meniscal repair also significantly improved the rate of return-to-sport compared with meniscectomy.

In a systematic review of 95 studies comparing meniscectomy to meniscal repair, Paxon et al. [73] found that although meniscectomy had a lower reoperation rate than repair (3% vs. 20%), long-term clinical outcome scores and evidence of radiographic deterioration were significantly improved in patients who were treated with meniscal repair. Repairs performed at the time of ACL reconstruction had a significantly lower failure rate than isolated repairs (14% vs. 24%). A recent meta-analysis by Xu et al. [74] showed a lower failure rate and improved clinical outcomes scores in patients undergoing meniscal repair compared to partial meniscectomy. The importance of long-term follow-up of these patients is highlighted in a recent meta-analysis by Nepple et al. [75], who found a pooled failure rate of 24% 5 years after meniscal repair, compared to only 30% at 2 years.

Using the latest techniques with all-inside newer generation devices, an overall success rate of 84% was demonstrated at a minimum of 5-years follow-up in a recent study [58]. The authors found no difference in failure rates in isolated repairs compared to those performed in conjunction with ACL reconstruction. Another recent study found successful outcomes following meniscal repair using the same all-inside device in 73% of 63 patients at a minimum of 12-years follow-up, with half of the failures attributable to subsequent traumatic episode [76].

Tear location and type can also affect outcomes after meniscus repair. In small case series, several authors have noted a high rate of return to previous level-of-sport after repair of anterior horn meniscus tears in soccer players [77, 78]. Osti et al. [79] reported good-to-excellent results in a series of patients undergoing anterior horn repairs with a suture anchor technique at 1-year follow-up. Radial tears were historically felt to be less repairable and more amenable to meniscectomy; however, recent studies have found success rates up to 90% following repair of radial tears [22, 80], with results comparable to a matched cohort of bucket-handle repairs [21]. Furthermore, follow-up MRIs demonstrated at least partial healing in 93% of menisci after repair of mid-body radial tears [81]. Horizontal cleavage tears treated with partial meniscectomy of unstable flaps as well as open repairs were found to have high clinical outcomes scores, a 91% return to same level of sport, and an 85% success rate at long-term follow-up [24]. These results have been corroborated by other authors [23, 25], with better outcomes observed in patients under the age of 30.

Tibial plateau fractures are often associated with meniscus tears. Repairs performed at the time of open reduction internal fixation of fracture were shown to have excellent results in a recent study [82]. In the same study, patients reported no meniscal symptoms at 4-year follow-up, and 92% of menisci demonstrated complete healing at second-look arthroscopy. In another study, meniscus tears were seen in 52% of tibial plateau fractures, with follow-up MRIs showing healing of all menisci after repair [83]. The degree of plateau depression has also been shown to be predictive of meniscal injury, with an average 12.3 mm of depression seen in the 55% of patients with associated meniscal tears compared to 5.4 mm in the 45% without meniscal pathology [84]. In the same study, meniscal repair at the time of tibial plateau fixation produced outcomes similar to patients with intact menisci. These findings suggest the menisci should be inspected and repaired at the time of tibial plateau surgery whenever possible.

Failure of meniscus repair can be treated with either partial meniscectomy or revision repair, depending on the residual condition of the meniscus. Krych et al. [85] performed revision meniscus repair in 34 patients at an average of 2-years after the index procedure. They demonstrated successful revision repair in 79% of patients at 6-year follow-up, with the remaining patients undergoing subsequent partial meniscectomy. Patient age was the only independent risk factor for failure of revision repair. In another case series, Imade et al. [86] showed meniscal re-tear in 5/15 patients undergoing revision repair, with all 5 failures showing degenerative changes in the meniscus at the time of attempted repair. They concluded that revision repair should be attempted only in the absence of degenerative changes of the meniscus.

Postoperative evaluation of meniscal repair can include unenhanced MRI, MR arthrography, or CT arthrography. A recent review concluded that MR arthrography is superior to conventional MRI and CT arthrography to evaluate meniscal integrity after repair [87]. However, it is important for radiologists to be able to recognize the normal MR appearance of a repaired meniscus versus recurrent or residual tear [88], and the differential signal provided by intra-articular contrast is beneficial [89]. With repeat arthroscopy being the gold standard for evaluation of a prior meniscus repair, there may be a role for in-office needle arthroscopy in patients with recurrent pain, as this technique has been found to be safe and cost-effective when compared to MRI in evaluation of the meniscus [90, 91].

Biologic Augmentation of Repair

Given our knowledge of the mechanism of healing in the vascular portion of the meniscus, attempts should be made to enhance the healing response by trephination of the peripheral meniscus and rasping of the tear edges. There has also been a growing interest in the direct application of pluripotent stem cells to augment the repair and enhance the rate of healing following repair [92]. This section will discuss the scientific evidence behind various augmentation techniques, including trephination/abrasion, fibrin clot, platelet-rich plasma, and cerclage with collagen membranes.

After successful experiments in animal models, Zhang and Arnold [13] compared suture alone with suture and trephination in patients undergoing meniscal repair and found a significantly lower re-tear rate in the trephination group (6%) compared to the suture only group (25%). Numerous other studies [93–96] have demonstrated good-to-excellent clinical results following trephination alone without suture repair of meniscus, especially if performed at the time of ACL reconstruction. These studies, however, have often lacked control groups and did not evaluate healing with MRI or second-look arthroscopy. Several other studies found excellent clinical results [97, 98] and high healing rates at second-look arthroscopy [99] after rasping and synovial abrasion without suture repair.

Fibrin and blood clots have been used clinically in an attempt to clinically augment the repair. In a randomized control trial, Biedert et al. [100] showed only 43% healing on MRI following augmentation of suture repair with fibrin clot, which compared poorly to suture repair alone, partial meniscectomy, and conservative treatment. Ishimura et al. [101–103] used fibrin glue with or without sutures to treat longitudinal and bucket-handle tears, and found successful repair in 85–94% of patients clinically and at second-look arthroscopy. Similarly, success rates over 90% were reported for repair of radial tears augmented by exogenous fibrin clot in several studies [104–106]. Kamimura and Kimura [107, 108] augmented all-inside suture repairs of horizontal cleavage tears and found excellent clinical results, with 70% of tears completely healed at second-look arthroscopy.

Platelet-rich plasma (PRP) has received considerable attention for various applications in orthopedics. Animal studies, however, showed equivocal results for PRP augmentation of meniscus repairs [92]. In a clinical trial, Griffin et al. [109] performed meniscus repairs with and without PRP and found similar clinical outcomes and failure rates between groups. Pujol et al. [110] demonstrated similar failure rates, but improved clinical outcome scores and MRI findings of complete healing in meniscal repairs augmented with PRP. Kemmochi et al. [111] utilized a novel device for injection of PRP and platelet-rich fibrin for augmentation of meniscal repairs and found no significant differences in clinical outcome scores or MRI findings. These studies suffer from issues such as low sample sizes and inconsistent PRP preparation, and more research is indicated before PRP can be recommended for routine use in meniscal repair surgery.

Meniscal cerclage with fascial or collagen scaffolds has also been described in augmenting meniscal repairs. Henning et al. [112] reported lower failure rates in repairs augmented with a fascial sheath and fibrin clot compared to isolated repairs (8% vs. 24%). Piontek et al. [113] treated complex meniscus tears with a collagen matrix wrap combined with bone marrow blood injection and an all-inside repair device. They demonstrated a low failure rate (4%) in 53 patients treated with this technique and an 87% rate of clinical improvement. Their MRI findings demonstrated non-homogeneous signal and tear absence in 76% of menisci. Concerns for this technique include that it is technically challenging, costly, and can increase operative times.

Rehab After Meniscal Repair

Unlike meniscectomies, most surgeons performing meniscal repair instruct their patients to be non- or partial-weight-bearing on crutches postoperatively for 4–6 weeks, with a return to normal activity after 3–6 months. However, rehabilitation protocols vary considerably, with some surgeons advocating for an accelerated protocol and early weight-bearing. Tear pattern also plays a role in determining the rehab protocol since radial tears are subject to distraction forces under axial loading, compared to vertical tears which experience compressive forces at the repair site [114]. A systematic review [115] of various rehabilitation protocols including accelerated, weight restriction, and motion restriction protocols demonstrated no difference in clinical outcomes between the groups. They concluded that early range of motion and immediate weight-bearing have no detrimental effect on the success of isolated meniscus repair. In a randomized controlled trial, Lind et al. [116] compared accelerated and restricted protocols after isolated meniscal repairs and showed no differences in failure rates, clinical outcome scores, or appearance on repeat arthroscopy. Our preferred rehabilitation protocol includes partial weight-bearing in full extension for 6 weeks, flexion limited to 100° for the first 6 weeks after isolated meniscal repair, and consideration of the use of a continuous passive motion machine following combined meniscal repair and ACL reconstruction. Further research is needed to define optimal protocols based on tear type and biologic factors.

Conclusions

Meniscal repair is a reliable and reproducible procedure, with overall success rates of 80–90% when properly indicated. Biomechanically, the preservation of meniscal tissue is preferable to meniscectomy whenever possible. Advancement in surgical techniques, including all-inside devices and biological augmentation, may allow for expanded indications, decreased difficulty, and improved success rates of meniscus repair.

References

1. Mordecai SC, Al-Hadithy N, Ware HE, Gupte CM. Treatment of meniscal tears: an evidence based approach. World J Orthop. 2014;5(3):233–41.
2. Baratz ME, Fu FH, Mengato R. Meniscal tears: the effect of meniscectomy and of repair on intraarticular contact areas and stress in the human knee. A preliminary report. Am J Sports Med. 1986;14(4):270–5.

3. Arno S, Bell CP, Uquillas C, Borukhov I, Walker PS. Tibiofemoral contact mechanics following a horizontal cleavage lesion in the posterior horn of the medial meniscus. J Orthop Res. 2015;33(4):584–90.
4. Beamer BS, Walley KC, Okajima S, Manoukian OS, Perez-Viloria M, DeAngelis JP, et al. Changes in contact area in meniscus horizontal cleavage tears subjected to repair and resection. Arthroscopy. 2017;33(3):617–24.
5. Han SB, Shetty GM, Lee DH, Chae DJ, Seo SS, Wang KH, et al. Unfavorable results of partial meniscectomy for complete posterior medial meniscus root tear with early osteoarthritis: a 5- to 8-year follow-up study. Arthroscopy. 2010;26(10):1326–32.
6. Faunø P, Nielsen AB. Arthroscopic partial meniscectomy: a long-term follow-up. Arthroscopy. 1992;8(3):345–9.
7. Jørgensen U, Sonne-Holm S, Lauridsen F, Rosenklint A. Long-term follow-up of meniscectomy in athletes. A prospective longitudinal study. J Bone Joint Surg Br. 1987;69(1):80–3.
8. Arnoczky SP, Warren RF. Microvasculature of the human meniscus. Am J Sports Med. 1982;10(2):90–5.
9. Day B, Mackenzie WG, Shim SS, Leung G. The vascular and nerve supply of the human meniscus. Arthroscopy. 1985;1(1):58–62.
10. Scott GA, Jolly BL, Henning CE. Combined posterior incision and arthroscopic intra-articular repair of the meniscus. An examination of factors affecting healing. J Bone Joint Surg Am. 1986;68(6):847–61.
11. Tenuta JJ, Arciero RA. Arthroscopic evaluation of meniscal repairs. Factors that effect healing. Am J Sports Med. 1994;22(6):797–802.
12. Noyes FR, Chen RC, Barber-Westin SD, Potter HG. Greater than 10-year results of red-white longitudinal meniscal repairs in patients 20 years of age or younger. Am J Sports Med. 2011;39(5):1008–17.
13. Zhang Z, Arnold JA. Trephination and suturing of avascular meniscal tears: a clinical study of the trephination procedure. Arthroscopy. 1996;12(6):726–31.
14. Cannon WD, Vittori JM. The incidence of healing in arthroscopic meniscal repairs in anterior cruciate ligament-reconstructed knees versus stable knees. Am J Sports Med. 1992;20(2):176–81.
15. Laible C, Stein DA, Kiridly DN. Meniscal repair. J Am Acad Orthop Surg. 2013;21(4):204–13.
16. Logan M, Watts M, Owen J, Myers P. Meniscal repair in the elite athlete: results of 45 repairs with a minimum 5-year follow-up. Am J Sports Med. 2009;37(6):1131–4.
17. Lyman S, Hidaka C, Valdez AS, Hetsroni I, Pan TJ, Do H, et al. Risk factors for meniscectomy after meniscal repair. Am J Sports Med. 2013;41(12):2772–8.
18. Bhatia S, Civitarese DM, Turnbull TL, LaPrade CM, Nitri M, Wijdicks CA, et al. A novel repair method for radial tears of the medial meniscus: biomechanical comparison of transtibial 2-tunnel and double horizontal mattress suture techniques under cyclic loading. Am J Sports Med. 2016;44(3):639–45.
19. Beamer BS, Masoudi A, Walley KC, Harlow ER, Manoukian OS, Hertz B, et al. Analysis of a new all-inside versus inside-out technique for repairing radial meniscal tears. Arthroscopy. 2015;31(2):293–8.
20. Matsubara H, Okazaki K, Izawa T, Tashiro Y, Matsuda S, Nishimura T, et al. New suture method for radial tears of the meniscus: biomechanical analysis of cross-suture and double horizontal suture techniques using cyclic load testing. Am J Sports Med. 2012;40(2):414–8.
21. Wu IT, Hevesi M, Desai VS, Camp CL, Dahm DL, Levy BA, et al. Comparative outcomes of radial and bucket-handle meniscal tear repair: a propensity-matched analysis. Am J Sports Med. 2018;46(11):2653–60.
22. Anderson L, Watts M, Shapter O, Logan M, Risebury M, Duffy D, et al. Repair of radial tears and posterior horn detachments of the lateral meniscus: minimum 2-year follow-up. Arthroscopy. 2010;26(12):1625–32.
23. Pujol N, Bohu Y, Boisrenoult P, Macdes A, Beaufils P. Clinical outcomes of open meniscal repair of horizontal meniscal tears in young patients. Knee Surg Sports Traumatol Arthrosc. 2013;21(7):1530–3.

24. Billières J, Pujol N, and the U45 Committee of ESSKA. Meniscal repair associated with a partial meniscectomy for treating complex horizontal cleavage tears in young patients may lead to excellent long-term outcomes. Knee Surg Sports Traumatol Arthrosc. 2019;27(2):343–8.
25. Sallé de Chou E, Pujol N, Rochcongar G, Cucurulo T, Potel JF, Dalmay F, et al. Analysis of short and long-term results of horizontal meniscal tears in young adults. Orthop Traumatol Surg Res. 2015;101(8 Suppl):S317–22.
26. Barber FA, Click SD. Meniscus repair rehabilitation with concurrent anterior cruciate reconstruction. Arthroscopy. 1997;13(4):433–7.
27. Morgan CD, Wojtys EM, Casscells CD, Casscells SW. Arthroscopic meniscal repair evaluated by second-look arthroscopy. Am J Sports Med. 1991;19(6):632–7; discussion 7–8.
28. Steenbrugge F, Van Nieuwenhuyse W, Verdonk R, Verstraete K. Arthroscopic meniscus repair in the ACL-deficient knee. Int Orthop. 2005;29(2):109–12.
29. Hanks GA, Gause TM, Handal JA, Kalenak A. Meniscus repair in the anterior cruciate deficient knee. Am J Sports Med. 1990;18(6):606–11; discussion 12–3.
30. Tengrootenhuysen M, Meermans G, Pittoors K, van Riet R, Victor J. Long-term outcome after meniscal repair. Knee Surg Sports Traumatol Arthrosc. 2011;19(2):236–41.
31. Sood A, Gonzalez-Lomas G, Gehrmann R. Influence of health insurance status on the timing of surgery and treatment of bucket-handle meniscus tears. Orthop J Sports Med. 2015;3(5):2325967115584883.
32. Gallacher PD, Gilbert RE, Kanes G, Roberts SN, Rees D. Outcome of meniscal repair prior compared with concurrent ACL reconstruction. Knee. 2012;19(4):461–3.
33. Haklar U, Donmez F, Basaran SH, Canbora MK. Results of arthroscopic repair of partial- or full-thickness longitudinal medial meniscal tears by single or double vertical sutures using the inside-out technique. Am J Sports Med. 2013;41(3):596–602.
34. Eggli S, Wegmüller H, Kosina J, Huckell C, Jakob RP. Long-term results of arthroscopic meniscal repair. An analysis of isolated tears. Am J Sports Med. 1995;23(6):715–20.
35. Everhart JS, Higgins JD, Poland SG, Abouljoud MM, Flanigan DC. Meniscal repair in patients age 40 years and older: a systematic review of 11 studies and 148 patients. Knee. 2018;25(6):1142–50.
36. Steadman JR, Matheny LM, Singleton SB, Johnson NS, Rodkey WG, Crespo B, et al. Meniscus suture repair: minimum 10-year outcomes in patients younger than 40 years compared with patients 40 and older. Am J Sports Med. 2015;43(9):2222–7.
37. Brophy RH, Wojahn RD, Lillegraven O, Lamplot JD. Outcomes of arthroscopic posterior medial meniscus root repair: association with body mass index. J Am Acad Orthop Surg. 2019;27(3):104–11.
38. Haviv B, Bronak S, Thein R. Correlation between body mass index and chondral lesions in isolated medial meniscus tears. Indian J Orthop. 2015;49(2):176–80.
39. Beaufils P, Pujol N. Meniscal repair: technique. Orthop Traumatol Surg Res. 2018;104(1S):S137–S45.
40. Barber FA, McGarry JE. Meniscal repair techniques. Sports Med Arthrosc Rev. 2007;15(4):199–207.
41. Cannon WD. Arthroscopic meniscal repair. Inside-out technique and results. Am J Knee Surg. 1996;9(3):137–43.
42. Nelson CG, Bonner KF. Inside-out meniscus repair. Arthrosc Tech. 2013;2(4):e453–60.
43. Grant JA, Wilde J, Miller BS, Bedi A. Comparison of inside-out and all-inside techniques for the repair of isolated meniscal tears: a systematic review. Am J Sports Med. 2012;40(2):459–68.
44. Menge TJ, Dean CS, Chahla J, Mitchell JJ, LaPrade RF. Anterior horn meniscal repair using an outside-in suture technique. Arthrosc Tech. 2016;5(5):e1111–e6.
45. Warren RF. Arthroscopic meniscus repair. Arthroscopy. 1985;1(3):170–2.
46. Silberberg Muiño JM, Nilo Fulvi A, Gimenez M, Muina Rullan JR. Outside-in single-lasso loop technique for meniscal repair: fast, economic, and reproducible. Arthrosc Tech. 2018;7(11):e1191–e6.

47. Serrano PM, Amorim-Barbosa T, Santos Silva M, Sousa R. Alternative method of outside-in meniscal repair for anterior horn tears. Open Access J Sports Med. 2018;9:167–70.
48. Prince MR, Esquivel AO, Andre AM, Goitz HT. Anterior horn lateral meniscus tear, repair, and meniscectomy. J Knee Surg. 2014;27(3):229–34.
49. Aros BC, Pedroza A, Vasileff WK, Litsky AS, Flanigan DC. Mechanical comparison of meniscal repair devices with mattress suture devices in vitro. Knee Surg Sports Traumatol Arthrosc. 2010;18(11):1594–8.
50. Barber FA, Herbert MA, Bava ED, Drew OR. Biomechanical testing of suture-based meniscal repair devices containing ultrahigh-molecular-weight polyethylene suture: update 2011. Arthroscopy. 2012;28(6):827–34.
51. Marchetti DC, Phelps BM, Dahl KD, Slette EL, Mikula JD, Dornan GJ, et al. A contact pressure analysis comparing an all-inside and inside-out surgical repair technique for bucket-handle medial meniscus tears. Arthroscopy. 2017;33(10):1840–8.
52. Calder SJ, Myers PT. Broken arrow: a complication of meniscal repair. Arthroscopy. 1999;15(6):651–2.
53. Kumar A, Malhan K, Roberts SN. Chondral injury from bioabsorbable screws after meniscal repair. Arthroscopy. 2001;17(8):34.
54. Gunes T, Bostan B, Erdem M, Asci M, Sen C, Kelestemur MH. Biomechanical evaluation of arthroscopic all-inside meniscus repairs. Knee Surg Sports Traumatol Arthrosc. 2009;17(11):1347–53.
55. Gifstad T, Grøntvedt T, Drogset JO. Meniscal repair with biofix arrows: results after 4.7 years' follow-up. Am J Sports Med. 2007;35(1):71–4.
56. Kurzweil PR, Tifford CD, Ignacio EM. Unsatisfactory clinical results of meniscal repair using the meniscus arrow. Arthroscopy. 2005;21(8):905.
57. Järvelä S, Sihvonen R, Sirkeoja H, Järvelä T. All-inside meniscal repair with bioabsorbable meniscal screws or with bioabsorbable meniscus arrows: a prospective, randomized clinical study with 2-year results. Am J Sports Med. 2010;38(11):2211–7.
58. Bogunovic L, Kruse LM, Haas AK, Huston LJ, Wright RW. Outcome of all-inside second-generation meniscal repair: minimum five-year follow-up. J Bone Joint Surg Am. 2014;96(15):1303–7.
59. Elmallah R, Jones LC, Malloch L, Barrett GR. A meta-analysis of arthroscopic meniscal repair: inside-out versus outside-in versus all-inside techniques. J Knee Surg. 2019;32(8):750–7.
60. Rimmer MG, Nawana NS, Keene GC, Pearcy MJ. Failure strengths of different meniscal suturing techniques. Arthroscopy. 1995;11(2):146–50.
61. Kocabey Y, Chang HC, Brand JC, Nawab A, Nyland J, Caborn DN. A biomechanical comparison of the FasT-Fix meniscal repair suture system and the RapidLoc device in cadaver meniscus. Arthroscopy. 2006;22(4):406–13.
62. Kocabey Y, Taser O, Nyland J, Doral MN, Demirhan M, Caborn DN, et al. Pullout strength of meniscal repair after cyclic loading: comparison of vertical, horizontal, and oblique suture techniques. Knee Surg Sports Traumatol Arthrosc. 2006;14(10):998–1003.
63. Tabrizi A, Shariyate MJ. Biomechanical study of meniscal repair using horizontal sutures and vertical loop techniques. Adv Biomed Res. 2018;7:144.
64. Borden P, Nyland J, Caborn DN, Pienkowski D. Biomechanical comparison of the FasT-Fix meniscal repair suture system with vertical mattress sutures and meniscus arrows. Am J Sports Med. 2003;31(3):374–8.
65. Buckland DM, Sadoghi P, Wimmer MD, Vavken P, Pagenstert GI, Valderrabano V, et al. Meta-analysis on biomechanical properties of meniscus repairs: are devices better than sutures? Knee Surg Sports Traumatol Arthrosc. 2015;23(1):83–9.
66. Saliman JD. The circumferential compression stitch for meniscus repair. Arthrosc Tech. 2013;2(3):e257–64.
67. Woodmass JM, Johnson JD, Wu IT, Saris DBF, Stuart MJ, Krych AJ. Horizontal cleavage meniscus tear treated with all-inside circumferential compression stitches. Arthrosc Tech. 2017;6(4):e1329–e33.

68. Sonnery-Cottet B, Conteduca J, Thaunat M, Gunepin FX, Seil R. Hidden lesions of the posterior horn of the medial meniscus: a systematic arthroscopic exploration of the concealed portion of the knee. Am J Sports Med. 2014;42(4):921–6.

69. Peltier A, Lording TD, Lustig S, Servien E, Maubisson L, Neyret P. Posteromedial meniscal tears may be missed during anterior cruciate ligament reconstruction. Arthroscopy. 2015;31(4):691–8.

70. Ahn JH, Yoo JC, Lee SH. Posterior horn tears: all-inside suture repair. Clin Sports Med. 2012;31(1):113–34.

71. Negrín R, Reyes NO, Iñiguez M, Pellegrini JJ, Wainer M, Duboy J. Meniscal ramp lesion repair using an all-inside technique. Arthrosc Tech. 2018;26(7(3)):e265–e70.

72. Stein T, Mehling AP, Welsch F, von Eisenhart-Rothe R, Jäger A. Long-term outcome after arthroscopic meniscal repair versus arthroscopic partial meniscectomy for traumatic meniscal tears. Am J Sports Med. 2010;38(8):1542–8.

73. Paxton ES, Stock MV, Brophy RH. Meniscal repair versus partial meniscectomy: a systematic review comparing reoperation rates and clinical outcomes. Arthroscopy. 2011;27(9):1275–88.

74. Xu C, Zhao J. A meta-analysis comparing meniscal repair with meniscectomy in the treatment of meniscal tears: the more meniscus, the better outcome? Knee Surg Sports Traumatol Arthrosc. 2015;23(1):164–70.

75. Nepple JJ, Dunn WR, Wright RW. Meniscal repair outcomes at greater than five years: a systematic literature review and meta-analysis. J Bone Joint Surg Am. 2012;94(24):2222–7.

76. Zimmerer A, Sobau C, Nietschke R, Schneider M, Ellermann A. Long-term outcome after all inside meniscal repair using the FasT-Fix system. J Orthop. 2018;15(2):602–5.

77. Choi NH, Victoroff BN. Anterior horn tears of the lateral meniscus in soccer players. Arthroscopy. 2006;22(5):484–8.

78. Hagino T, Ochiai S, Sato E, Watanabe Y, Senga S. Footballer's lateral meniscus: anterior horn tears of the lateral meniscus with a stable knee. ISRN Surg. 2011;2011:170402.

79. Osti L, Del Buono A, Maffulli N. Anterior medial meniscal root tears: a novel arthroscopic all inside repair. Transl Med UniSa. 2015;12:41–6.

80. Moulton SG, Bhatia S, Civitarese DM, Frank RM, Dean CS, LaPrade RF. Surgical techniques and outcomes of repairing meniscal radial tears: a systematic review. Arthroscopy. 2016;32(9):1919–25.

81. Choi NH, Kim TH, Son KM, Victoroff BN. Meniscal repair for radial tears of the midbody of the lateral meniscus. Am J Sports Med. 2010;38(12):2472–6.

82. Ruiz-Ibán M, Diaz-Heredia J, Elías-Martín E, Moros-Marco S, Cebreiro Martinez Del Val I. Repair of meniscal tears associated with tibial plateau fractures: a review of 15 cases. Am J Sports Med. 2012;40(10):2289–95.

83. Tekin A, Çakar M, Esenyel CZ, Adaş M, Bayraktar MK, Özcan Y, et al. An evaluation of meniscus tears in lateral tibial plateau fractures and repair results. J Back Musculoskelet Rehabil. 2016;29(4):845–51.

84. Forman JM, Karia RJ, Davidovitch RI, Egol KA. Tibial plateau fractures with and without meniscus tear--results of a standardized treatment protocol. Bull Hosp Joint Dis. 2013;71(2):144–51.

85. Krych AJ, Reardon P, Sousa P, Levy BA, Dahm DL, Stuart MJ. Clinical outcomes after revision meniscus repair. Arthroscopy. 2016;32(9):1831–7.

86. Imade S, Kumahashi N, Kuwata S, Kadowaki M, Ito S, Uchio Y. Clinical outcomes of revision meniscal repair: a case series. Am J Sports Med. 2014;42(2):350–7.

87. Baker JC, Friedman MV, Rubin DA. Imaging the postoperative knee meniscus: an evidence-based review. AJR Am J Roentgenol. 2018;211(3):519–27.

88. Russo A, Capasso R, Varelli C, Laporta A, Carbone M, D'Agosto G, et al. MR imaging evaluation of the postoperative meniscus. Musculoskelet Surg. 2017;101(Suppl 1):37–42.

89. Chapin R. Imaging of the postoperative meniscus. Radiol Clin N Am. 2018;56(6):953–64.

90. Gill TJ, Safran M, Mandelbaum B, Huber B, Gambardella R, Xerogeanes J. A prospective, blinded, multicenter clinical trial to compare the efficacy, accuracy, and safety of in-office

diagnostic arthroscopy with magnetic resonance imaging and surgical diagnostic arthroscopy. Arthroscopy. 2018;34(8):2429–35.

91. Amin N, McIntyre L, Carter T, Xerogeanes J, Voigt J. Cost-effectiveness analysis of needle arthroscopy versus magnetic resonance imaging in the diagnosis and treatment of meniscal tears of the knee. Arthroscopy. 2019;35(2):554–62.e13.

92. Ghazi Zadeh L, Chevrier A, Farr J, Rodeo SA, Buschmann MD. Augmentation techniques for meniscus repair. J Knee Surg. 2018;31(1):99–116.

93. Fox JM, Rintz KG, Ferkel RD. Trephination of incomplete meniscal tears. Arthroscopy. 1993;9(4):451–5.

94. Shelbourne KD, Rask BP. The sequelae of salvaged nondegenerative peripheral vertical medial meniscus tears with anterior cruciate ligament reconstruction. Arthroscopy. 2001;17(3):270–4.

95. Shelbourne KD, Heinrich J. The long-term evaluation of lateral meniscus tears left in situ at the time of anterior cruciate ligament reconstruction. Arthroscopy. 2004;20(4):346–51.

96. Shelbourne KD, Benner RW, Nixon RA, Gray T. Evaluation of peripheral vertical nondegenerative medial meniscus tears treated with trephination alone at the time of anterior cruciate ligament reconstruction. Arthroscopy. 2015;31(12):2411–6.

97. Talley MC, Grana WA. Treatment of partial meniscal tears identified during anterior cruciate ligament reconstruction with limited synovial abrasion. Arthroscopy. 2000;16(1):6–10.

98. Tetik O, Kocabey Y, Johnson DL. Synovial abrasion for isolated, partial thickness, undersurface, medial meniscus tears. Orthopedics. 2002;25(6):675–8.

99. Uchio Y, Ochi M, Adachi N, Kawasaki K, Iwasa J. Results of rasping of meniscal tears with and without anterior cruciate ligament injury as evaluated by second-look arthroscopy. Arthroscopy. 2003;19(5):463–9.

100. Biedert RM. Treatment of intrasubstance meniscal lesions: a randomized prospective study of four different methods. Knee Surg Sports Traumatol Arthrosc. 2000;8(2):104–8.

101. Ishimura M, Tamai S, Fujisawa Y. Arthroscopic meniscal repair with fibrin glue. Arthroscopy. 1991;7(2):177–81.

102. Ishimura M, Ohgushi H, Habata T, Tamai S, Fujisawa Y. Arthroscopic meniscal repair using fibrin glue. Part I: experimental study. Arthroscopy. 1997;13(5):551–7.

103. Ishimura M, Ohgushi H, Habata T, Tamai S, Fujisawa Y. Arthroscopic meniscal repair using fibrin glue. Part II: clinical applications. Arthroscopy. 1997;13(5):558–63.

104. Jang SH, Ha JK, Lee DW, Kim JG. Fibrin clot delivery system for meniscal repair. Knee Surg Relat Res. 2011;23:180–3.

105. Ra HJ, Ha JK, Jang SH, Lee DW, Kim JG. Arthroscopic inside-out repair of complete radial tears of the meniscus with a fibrin clot. Knee Surg Sports Traumatol Arthrosc. 2013;21(9):2126–30.

106. van Trommel MF, Simonian PT, Potter HG, Wickiewicz TL. Arthroscopic meniscal repair with fibrin clot of complete radial tears of the lateral meniscus in the avascular zone. Arthroscopy. 1998;14(4):360–5.

107. Kamimura T, Kimura M. Repair of horizontal meniscal cleavage tears with exogenous fibrin clots. Knee Surg Sports Traumatol Arthrosc. 2011;19(7):1154–7.

108. Kamimura T, Kimura M. Meniscal repair of degenerative horizontal cleavage tears using fibrin clots: clinical and arthroscopic outcomes in 10 cases. Orthop J Sports Med. 2014;2(11):2325967114555678.

109. Griffin JW, Hadeed MM, Werner BC, Diduch DR, Carson EW, Miller MD. Platelet-rich plasma in meniscal repair: does augmentation improve surgical outcomes? Clin Orthop Relat Res. 2015;473(5):1665–72.

110. Pujol N, Salle De Chou E, Boisrenoult P, Beaufils P. Platelet-rich plasma for open meniscal repair in young patients: any benefit? Knee Surg Sports Traumatol Arthrosc. 2015;23(1):51–8.

111. Kemmochi M, Sasaki S, Takahashi M, Nishimura T, Aizawa C, Kikuchi J. The use of platelet-rich fibrin with platelet-rich plasma support meniscal repair surgery. J Orthop. 2018;15(2):711–20.

112. Henning CE, Yearout KM, Vequist SW, Stallbaumer RJ, Decker KA. Use of the fascia sheath coverage and exogenous fibrin clot in the treatment of complex meniscal tears. Am J Sports Med. 1991;19(6):626–31.
113. Piontek T, Ciemniewska-Gorzela K, Naczk J, Jakob R, Szulc A, Grygorowicz M, et al. Complex meniscus tears treated with collagen matrix wrapping and bone marrow blood injection: a 2-year clinical follow-up. Cartilage. 2016;7(2):123–39.
114. Jones RS, Keene GC, Learmonth DJ, Bickerstaff D, Nawana NS, Costi JJ, et al. Direct measurement of hoop strains in the intact and torn human medial meniscus. Clin Biomech (Bristol, Avon). 1996;11(5):295–300.
115. O'Donnell K, Freedman KB, Tjoumakaris FP. Rehabilitation protocols after isolated meniscal repair: a systematic review. Am J Sports Med. 2017;45(7):1687–97.
116. Lind M, Nielsen T, Faunø P, Lund B, Christiansen SE. Free rehabilitation is safe after isolated meniscus repair: a prospective randomized trial comparing free with restricted rehabilitation regimens. Am J Sports Med. 2013;41(12):2753–8.

Meniscal Root Repair

Michael Alaia and David Klein

Introduction

Disruption of the meniscal root describes an injury to the posterior horn of the meniscus within 1 cm of the root attachment. This can be in the form of a bony or soft tissue avulsion, or a radial tear just adjacent to the root attachment onto the tibia [1, 2].

Detachment of the meniscal root results in a break in the ring or "hoop" of the circumferential fibers of the meniscus. If the meniscus is thought of as a ring of tissue that nestles the respective femoral condyle within it, a complete break in the ring causes a total breakdown of the ability of the meniscus to dissipate tibiofemoral contact stresses [2]. Repair of the meniscal root restores its ability to reduce contact pressure of the tibiofemoral joint and normalizes contact mechanics. [3]

The most common injury pattern is a medial meniscal posterior root disruption (Figs. 7.1 and 7.2), accounting for up to 10% of all meniscal tears requiring surgery [4]. Lateral root tears are less common and are more likely seen in conjunction with ACL injuries. [5] A lateral root tear is 10 times more likely to coexist with an ACL tear than is a medial root tear [6], and repairing the lateral meniscal root tear improves knee stability after ACL reconstruction [7]. Medial meniscal posterior root tears (MMPRTs) are almost six times more likely to have a concomitant chondral injury [8]. Laprade et al. studied coexisting knee pathology in patients with meniscal root tears and found that MMPRTs can also have a significant degenerative component. They found that up to 55% of their MMPRT patients also had at least Outerbridge grade II chondral changes [8]. Although uncommon, iatrogenic

M. Alaia (✉) · D. Klein
Department of Orthopedic Surgery, Sports Medicine Division, NYU Langone Orthopedic Hospital, New York, NY, USA
e-mail: Michael.Alaia@NYULangone.org; David.Klein3@NYULangone.org

© Springer Nature Switzerland AG 2020
E. J. Strauss, L. M. Jazrawi (eds.), *The Management of Meniscal Pathology*,
https://doi.org/10.1007/978-3-030-49488-9_7

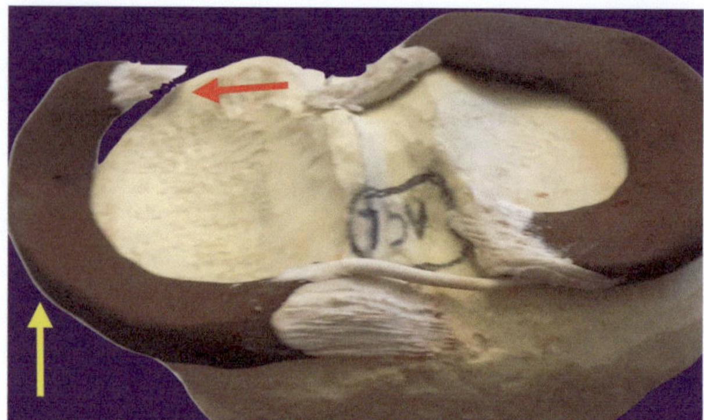

Fig. 7.1 Disruption of the posterior root of the medial meniscus (red arrow) and associated meniscal extrusion (yellow arrow)

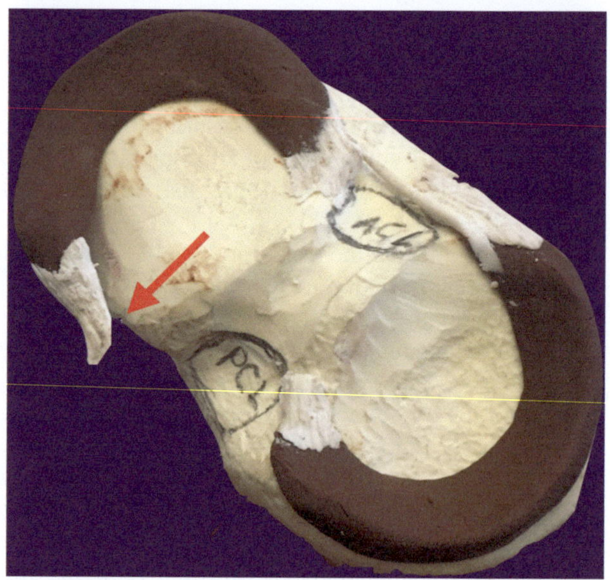

Fig. 7.2 Superior view of disruption of the medial meniscal posterior root

injury to the meniscal roots can happen, and has been reported with aberrant PCL tunnel drilling [9]. Another less appreciated form of iatrogenic injury to the meniscal roots involves the anterior roots which are often injured during ACL tunnel reaming and placement of tibial intramedullary nails [9–11].

While the mainstay of treatment of meniscal injury in the past was meniscectomy, a new understanding of the biomechanical protective role of the menisci has led to the development and improvement of repair techniques. Meniscectomy results were generally poor [12], with a high degree of progression to arthrosis. Meniscal repair outcomes have been more promising, in some series cutting the rate of progression to osteoarthritis (OA) in half [13]. Long-term outcomes of meniscal root repair, however, have not been studied extensively, and most research consists of series limited to short- to mid-term follow-up [14, 15].

Anatomy

The menisci are a pair of C-shaped fibrocartilage rings that deepen and protect the articulation by reducing joint contact pressures and increasing the peak contact area. The menisci have also been shown to have proprioceptive function [16]. They do not, however, have nociceptive capability since they lack neural elements [17]. The circumferential fibers of the meniscus provide tensile strength and resistance to elongation of the menisci. These fibers terminate at the anterior and posterior root attachments as Sharpey's fibers that insert directly into bone of the tibial plateau (Fig. 7.3). Detailed anatomy of the menisci and their attachments are described by Johannsen et al. [18] In their anatomic study, the posterior meniscal roots were shown to be intimately related to the cruciate ligaments. The distances from intra-articular structures are outlined in Table 7.1.

The figures by Johansen et al. show the intimate relationships the meniscal roots have with the surrounding structures (Fig. 7.4). The anatomic dissections by Johansen show the pertinent arthroscopic anatomy (Fig. 7.5).

Medial Meniscus

The medial meniscus is a C-shaped cartilage ring that acts to deepen the congruity of the medial tibiofemoral joint. It has attachments to the capsule surrounding it, as well as its two root attachments (Fig. 7.3). The medial meniscus has a larger radius than the lateral meniscus, but it tends to be somewhat thinner in cross-section. The posterior root is quite close to the PCL insertion. There have been anatomical studies showing the importance of the "shiny white fibers" of the root attachment. These

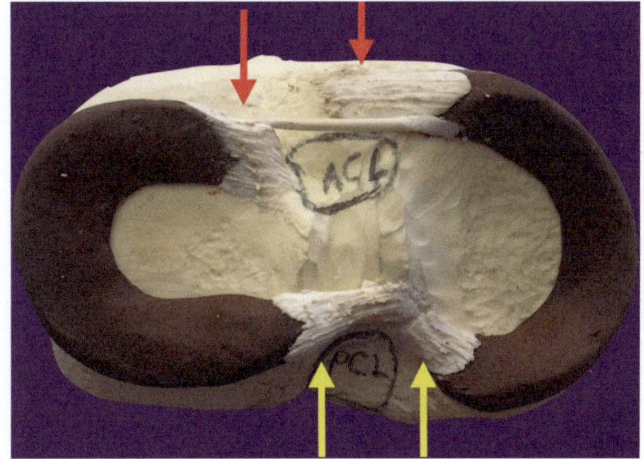

Fig. 7.3 Superior view of anterior meniscal root attachments (red arrows), posterior root attachments (yellow arrows). (Left knee)

Table 7.1 Measurements of medial and lateral meniscal root proximity to pertinent arthroscopic landmarks

	Average distance ± SEM, mm	Direction
To medial meniscus posterior root attachment center from:		
Medial tibial eminence apex	11.5 ± 0.9	Posterior/inferior/lateral
Medial tibial eminence apex (medial–lateral distance)	0.7 ± 0.4	Lateral
Medial tibial eminence apex (anterior–posterior distance)	9.6 ± 0.8	Posterior
Medial tibial eminence apex (inferior–superior distance)	6.0 ± 0.6	Inferior
Medial articular edge inflection point (medial–lateral distance)	3.5 ± 0.4	Lateral
Nearest PCL edge	8.2 ± 0.7	Superior/anterior/medial
To lateral posterior root attachment center from:		
Lateral tibial eminence apex	5.3 ± 0.3	Medial/posterior/inferior
Lateral tibial eminence apex (medial–lateral distance)	4.2 ± 0.4	Medial
Lateral tibial eminence apex (anterior–posterior distance)	1.5 ± 0.7	Posterior
Lateral tibial eminence apex (inferior–superior distance)	1.4 ± 0.2	Inferior
Nearest lateral articular cartilage edge (medial–lateral distance)	4.3 ± 0.5	Medial
Nearest posterior cruciate ligament edge	12.7 ± 1.1	Anterior/superior/medial
Posterior edge of the anterior root attachment of lateral meniscus	10.1 ± 0.8	Posterior/superior/medial

[a]*SEM* standard error of the mean

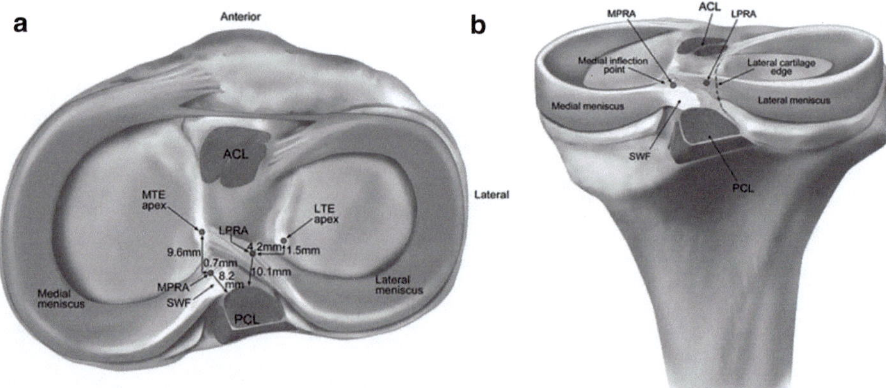

Fig. 7.4 Illustration demonstrating the medial and lateral posterior root attachments and relevant arthroscopic anatomy (right knee). (**a**) Superior view and (**b**) posterior view. ACL anterior cruciate ligament bundle attachments, LPRA lateral meniscus posterior root attachment, LTE lateral tibial eminence, MPRA medial meniscus posterior root attachment, MTE medial tibial eminence, PCL posterior cruciate ligament, SWF shiny white fibers of posterior horn of medial meniscus

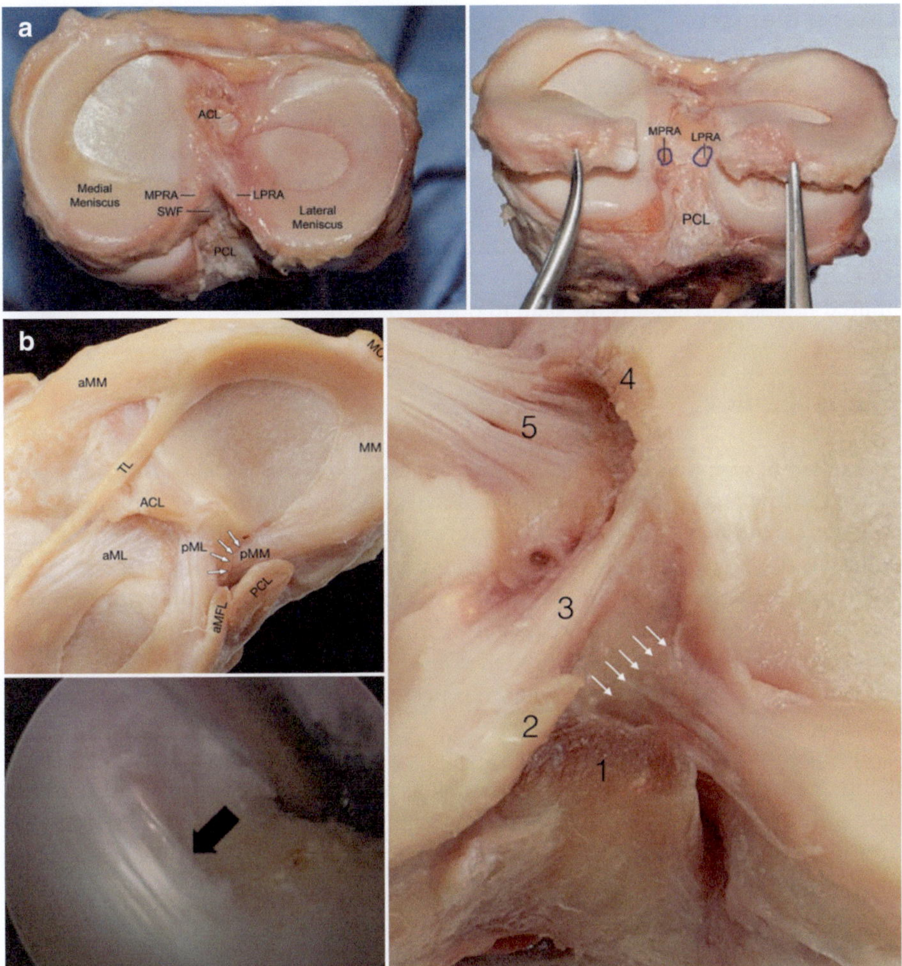

Fig. 7.5 Photographs of the medial and lateral meniscus posterior root attachments and relevant arthroscopic anatomy. (**a**) Superior view and (**b**) posterior view. ACL anterior cruciate ligament bundle attachments, LPRA lateral meniscus posterior root attachment, LTE lateral tibial eminence, MPRA medial meniscus posterior root attachment, MTE medial tibial eminence, PCL posterior cruciate ligament, SWF shiny white fibers of posterior horn of medial meniscus **b**: The white arrows depict a cadaveric dissection of the "shiny white fibers" of the posterior medial meniscal root. Note the fibrous nature of these fibers which are also visible arthroscopically (black arrow). (Photo credits of cadaveric dissection: Smigielski et al. [19])

fibers are important for the overall integrity of the repair, and, if possible, effort should be made to have sutures go through these fibers in the repair [20]. Notice the fibrous nature of the shiny white fibers on the cadaveric dissection by Smigielski et al. [19] shown in Fig. 7.5b, as well as the arthroscopic representation of this anatomic landmark shown in the figure.

Lateral Meniscus

The lateral meniscus is less constrained than the medial meniscus. It has capsular attachments, but a significant amount of the meniscus is free from the capsule at the popliteal hiatus. The lateral meniscus also covers relatively more of the tibial plateau than the medial meniscus. Both roots of the lateral meniscus are located between the tibial spines. The anterior root attachment is found intimately related to the ACL tibial footprint and is used as an anatomic landmark when placing the tibial ACL tunnel. Both the anterior and posterior roots of the lateral meniscus can be injured if close attention is not paid to operative technique.

Biomechanics

A detailed description of meniscal biomechanics is found in Chap. 1 of this book. When the meniscal root is incompetent, the entire meniscus is nonfunctional.

Root function was apparent as early as the1940s, when Fairbank stated that meniscus roots prevent extrusion "like an orange pip squeezed through the fingers." Extrusion is demonstrated by the model in Fig. 7.1. This same phenomenon was described arthroscopically by Pagnani et al. in 1991 [21], and demonstrated in cadaveric study by Hein and Marzo in 2009 [22], showing biomechanical equivalence of a total meniscectomy when the posterior root of the medial meniscus is compromised.

In situations where the root is intact, but it is otherwise disrupted from the rest of the meniscus by a radial tear, it can function as a root disruption. This clinical entity deserves mention in this chapter since it has the same biomechanical activity; however, the reader is referred to Chap. 6 of this book for details on management and repair of radial meniscal tear treatment.

Mechanism of Injury

Although acute meniscal root tears can occur from axial loading and noncontact injuries, by far the most common type of meniscal root tear is degenerative [23], accounting for some 70% of these. Meniscal root injury only occurs in approximately 3% of multi-ligament injured knees [23, 24]. The incidence of lateral meniscal root tear in association with ACL injury was estimated at 6.6% in a large series by Praz et al. [25] Since the medial meniscal root attachment is more constrained, it is more likely to be injured. As many as 80% of patients with spontaneous osteonecrosis of the knee (SONK) also have a coexisting medial meniscal root tear [26].

History and Physical Exam

Since meniscal root injury can happen in many clinical settings, the clinician must maintain a high index of suspicion for this injury, both in and out of the operating room. Mechanical symptoms such as clicking, popping, and catching can occur, but are not necessary to make the diagnosis. Often times, patients present after feeling a pop in the knee from something as benign as getting up from a squatted or seated position, and, in our experience, this happens more frequently in overweight women in their 40–60s. When there is suspicion of a root tear, patients should be screened for overall coronal malalignment. Pain can be medial, lateral, or, very often, posterior. The most common physical exam findings are joint line tenderness, significant pain with deep flexion, and a positive McMurray test. [27] At times, an extruded meniscus can be palpated at the anteromedial joint line with varus stress in full extension [28]. A complete ligament exam should be done as well since injury of these structures can coexist with meniscal root tears.

Imaging

Standard four-view radiographs, consisting of AP, PA flexion, lateral, and sunrise views are obtained. Additionally, a full leg–length alignment film is helpful in determining alignment and can also be used to help with prognosis, as significant coronal malalignment may subject the compartment to more load than usual. The presence (or lack thereof) of osteoarthritis is important to assess, since meniscal root repair may not provide durable pain relief or joint preservation in this setting. Instead, the discussion may focus on other joint preserving or replacing options. Varus alignment of greater than 5°, and presence of Outerbridge grade 3 chondromalacia have been shown to lead to poorer outcomes [29].

MRI is the mainstay of meniscal imaging [23, 30]. The entire substance of the meniscus should be evaluated, especially when a root tear is suspected. Identifying root tears can be challenging but can be simplified with certain assessments. The "ghost sign" of a meniscal root tear can be appreciated on T2 and T1 sagittal imaging (Fig. 7.6a and b). Instead of a solid black insertion, the meniscal root "disappears" as the MRI sections reach the expected insertion point, rendering that area of expected meniscal tissue white. Additionally, this can be seen on coronal and axial images (Figs. 7.7 and 7.8). Often, radial tears juxtaposed to the roots can also be visualized on axial images. Three T MRI has been shown to have improved diagnostic accuracy over conventional 1.5 T MRI and provides a 77% specificity, 73% sensitivity, positive predictive value of 22%, and negative predictive value of 97% [6]. Additionally, any extrusion on midcoronal sequence of greater than 3 mm is associated with more severe meniscal pathology and, frequently, chondral damage [31, 32].

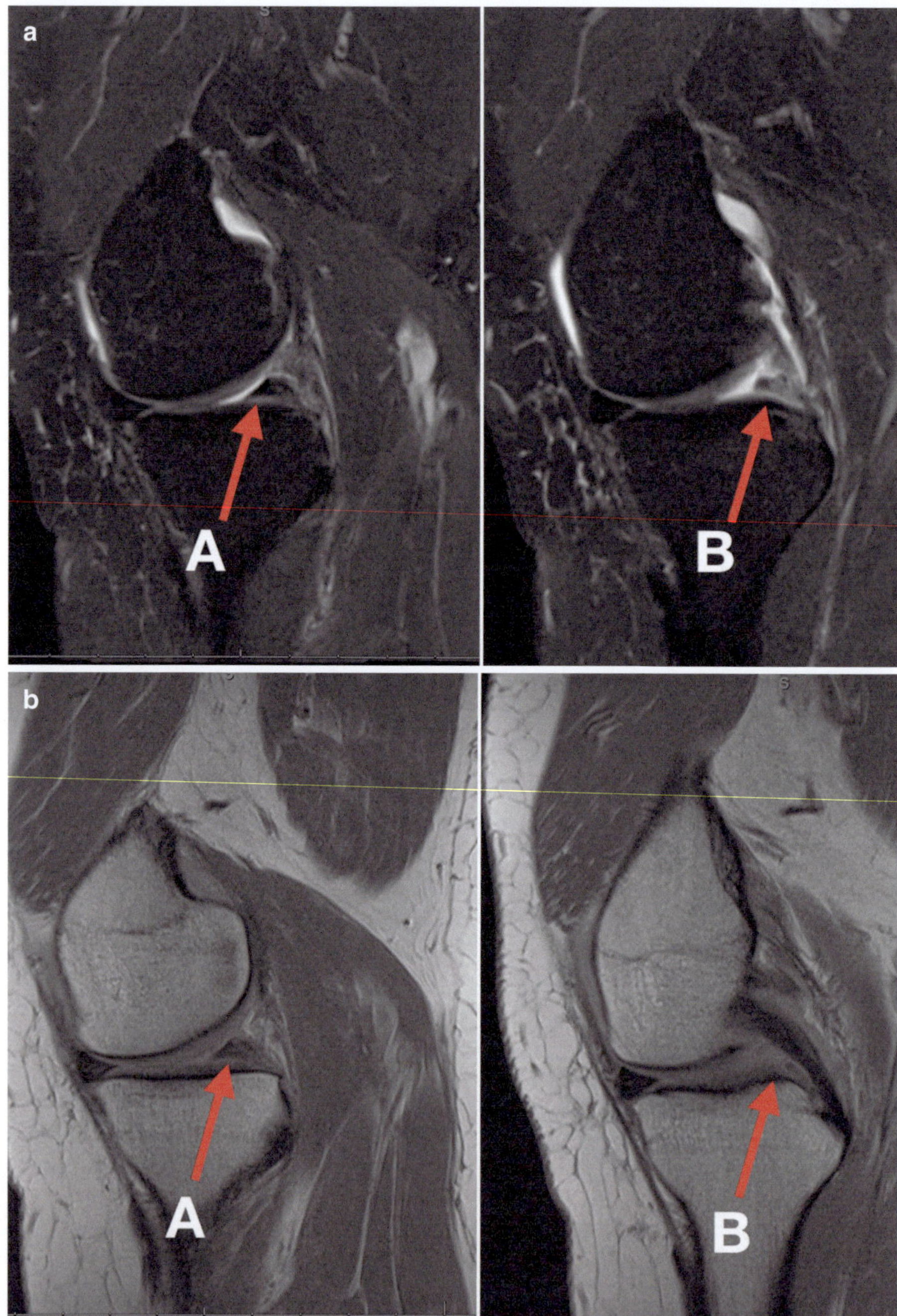

Fig. 7.6 (**a**) Sagittal T2-weighted MRI showing (A) visible posterior horn medial meniscal tissue in a cut through the middle of the medial plateau and (B) "ghost sign" of meniscal tissue disappearing more medially as it inserts at the root. (**b**) Sagittal T1-weighted MRI showing (A) visible posterior horn medial meniscal tissue in a cut through the middle of the medial plateau and (B) "ghost sign" of meniscal tissue disappearing more medially as it inserts at the root

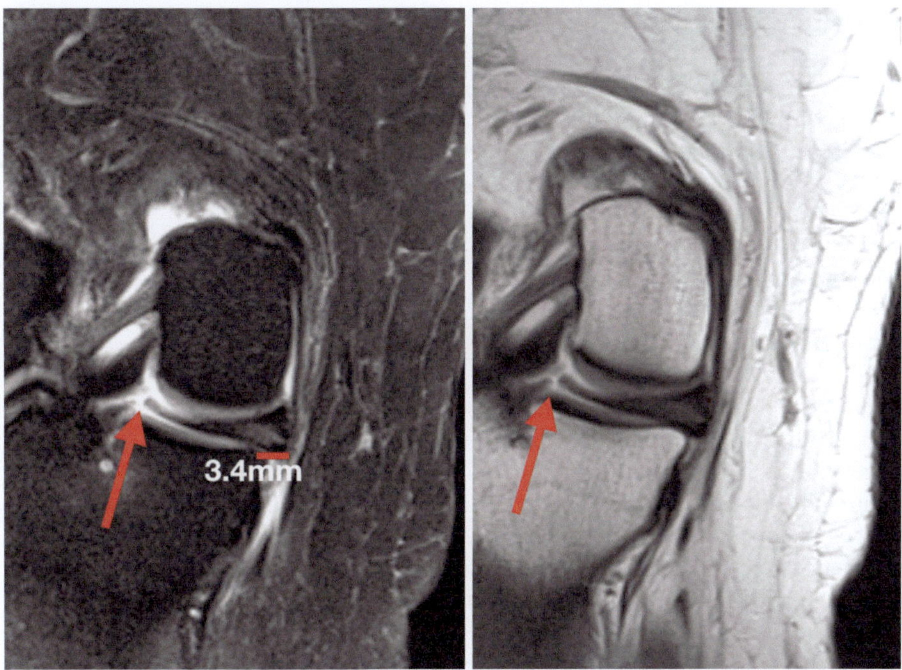

Fig. 7.7 Red arrow: T2- and T1-weighted coronal MRI showing disruption of meniscal tissue at the root, a sign of meniscal root tear. Also noted is meniscal extrusion of 3.4 mm

Fig. 7.8 Red arrow: Axial T2-weighted MRI showing disruption of meniscal tissue at the root, a sign of meniscal root tear

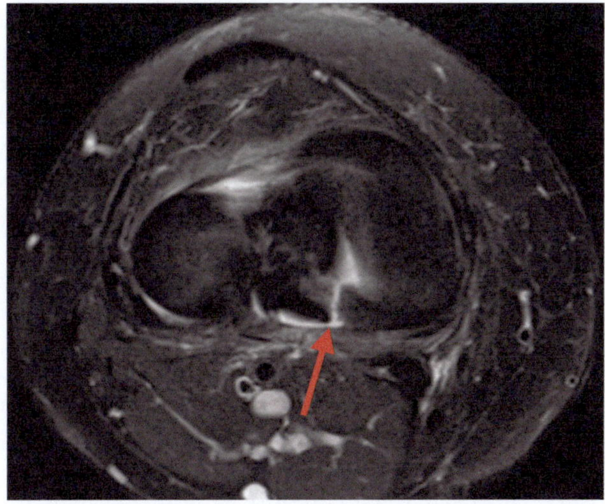

Classification

Laprade et al. classified meniscus posterior root tear (MPRT) by location and morphology [33]. Tears within 9 mm from the posterior attachment are considered root tears based on biomechanical data, and outcomes have not been reported based on tear type. Data on this classification scheme and overall outcomes are lacking.

Management Options

Nonoperative Management

We often recommend repair for patients without contraindications to surgery since nonoperative management of MPRT is associated with significant increases in degeneration [34]. However, nonoperative management is offered to patients with contraindications to surgery and to patients with significant osteoarthritis, significant extrusion, or moderate-to-severe varus deformity. Additionally, if the quality of the meniscus appears poor, a repair may not be possible. Young patients with irreparable root tears may be candidates for meniscal transplantation if symptoms persist despite meniscal debridement.

Patients who are treated nonoperatively should undergo physical therapy and be offered nonnarcotic oral and topical medication for pain control. Assistive devices such as a cane can provide pain relief. The cane should be held in the contralateral hand, and the patient should be instructed to lean on the cane while weight-bearing on the affected leg. This helps offload the knee and has been shown to provide significant pain relief in patients with degenerative knees [35, 36].

While data is lacking to support the use of unloader bracing in patients with meniscal root injury, enough data exists in the context of unicompartmental osteoarthritis to consider this noninvasive management option to offload an essentially meniscus-deficient knee [37–39]. Patients can be offered a brace to help reduce pain if they are not surgical candidates, or offered a brace while awaiting surgery, but should be counseled that this is not an equivalent treatment to meniscal root repair, when indicated.

Operative Management

While it is known that meniscectomy can result in symptomatic improvement, it does not halt the progression of osteoarthritis. Kim et al. [30] found that meniscal root repair resulted in better clinical and radiographic outcomes compared with partial meniscectomy at an average of 56- and 48.5-month follow-up, respectively. However, when carefully scrutinizing their results, they had a heterogeneous data set, and their patient-reported outcome measures likely failed to reach clinical significance despite showing a statistically significant improvement. A study by Krych et al. [40] redemonstrated that while partial meniscectomy can relieve pain in the short term, this does not portend a decreased rate of osteoarthritis and showed significant radiographic degeneration of the knee at 5-year follow-up.

Subjective outcomes have been shown to improve following meniscal root repair. In a meta-analysis performed by Chung et al., meniscal root repair resulted in significantly improved patient-reported outcomes [41, 42]. Chung et al. also found that repair had significantly improved clinical and radiographic outcomes at 5 years when compared with meniscectomy, and that radiographic OA did not progress at the 30-month follow-up. Feucht et al. did a systematic review of meniscal root repair and found that 84% of patients had no progression of OA when assessed with the Kellgren–Lawrence grading system. In terms of repair technique, one study showed no clinical difference between suture anchor repair and pullout suture repair of medial meniscal root tears at 2 years [27].

A retrospective study by Laprade et al. with level III evidence found that there were significant improvements in patient satisfaction, pain, and clinical outcomes following meniscal root repairs [15]. This study also found that age and side did not affect failure rate of repair, suggesting that failures may be more common in patients with higher degrees of degenerative changes, higher BMI, or inability to participate in appropriate postoperative rehab [15]. Patients with a higher BMI have also been found to have poorer outcomes [43].

One of the worst prognosticators of meniscal pathology is the presence of meniscal extrusion. An extruded meniscus is essentially nonfunctional [31, 32]. While the relationship between an extruded meniscus at follow-up after meniscal root repair and outcome has not been fully delineated, it can be assumed that reduction of the meniscus and avoidance of extrusion is an important goal of repair.

Kaplan et al., however, demonstrated worsening International Cartilage Repair Society (ICRS) scores on MRI at 2-year follow-up after medial meniscus posterior root repair. Additionally, although the majority of repairs demonstrated at least partial healing, meniscal extrusion was unable to be anatomically restored. Despite these findings, clinical scores were improved significantly [14]. Kwak et al. [44] also demonstrated that extrusion is associated with poor prognosis, and concluded that early meniscal root repair in knees that exhibit a high degree of meniscal extrusion should be performed whenever possible.

The rate of failure of meniscal root repair has not been well documented in the literature. In a series by Cho et al., where 13/20 knees underwent second-look arthroscopies after meniscal root repair, the authors showed that clinical improvement correlated with stout healing of the meniscal tissue. To optimize the success of repair, some suture repair configurations have been shown to be biomechanically superior than others. For example, a simple cinch stitch has been shown to be stronger than a Mason–Allen-type repair in a study by Krych et al. [45] Additionally, the meniscus can be fixed with either suture anchors or a transtibial repair with cortical fixation. Suture anchor repair is technically demanding, and transtibial repair has the advantage of being performed through two familiar anterior arthroscopic portals. However, no clinical differences have been shown when comparing the two techniques [27].

The most common complication of meniscal root repair, malposition of the tibial tunnel, is related to surgical error. Small deviations in tunnel placement can lead to drastic changes in tibiofemoral contact stresses [46]. Additionally, in situations where access to the medial compartment is restricted, iatrogenic chondral damage can occur if care is not taken when inserting the guide and reamer. In such instances, we routinely perform pie-crusting of the deep medial collateral ligament (MCL), as this will improve the working space by several millimeters and improve access to the meniscal root. Conversely, it is not possible to perform a similar pie-crusting release of the lateral compartment given the rope-like structure of the lateral collateral ligament (LCL), nor would it be advisable due to the proximity of the common peroneal nerve. Healing rates following surgical repair in the literature have been variable and reported to range from 0 to 100% on MRI or second-look arthroscopy [14, 47]. A study by Lee et al. used a homogeneous arthroscopic measurement method and MRI evaluation to determine meniscal root-healing rates in a series of 56 patients. Thirty-three patients underwent second-look arthroscopies, and in this subset the rate of meniscal root healing was 70%.

Medial Meniscus Root Repair Surgical Technique

Our preferred technique is suture repair of the meniscal root with transtibial fixation over a cortical button using a single tunnel [14]. The operative extremity is positioned in a leg holder and a tourniquet placed high on the thigh. The distal aspect of the leg holder should be about two to three fingerbreadths proximal to the proximal pole of the patella in order to best visualize the medial compartment when applying valgus stress, while also minimizing hip internal rotation. Standard anteromedial and anterolateral portals are made, and a diagnostic arthroscopy is performed. The anteromedial portal is established using spinal needle localization, ensuring a direct trajectory to the posterior horn of the medial meniscus can be achieved. This portal tends to be more lateral and inferior than a standard anteromedial arthroscopic portal. Once the portals are established, the root is examined and the nature of the tear is assessed.

Maximal valgus stress and external rotation of the tibia can provide a better view of the meniscal root. As previously mentioned, we often piecrust and release the deep MCL fibers to allow for medial joint space opening. This is done percutaneously using an 18-gauge spinal needle. The needle pierces the skin approximately 1 cm below the joint line just anterior to the posteromedial border of the tibia. The needle is used to make several passes through the deep MCL fibers while providing consistent valgus stress to the knee. As the MCL fibers are pierced, the tissue will gradually release. Occasionally, there will be a palpable and audible pop as the MCL releases completely. Releasing the deep MCL fibers facilitates suture passage and helps minimize iatrogenic damage to the femoral and tibial cartilage, and is associated with minimal morbidity in our experience.

Figures 7.9 and 7.10 show a step-by-step repair of an unstable medial meniscal posterior root tear. The root tear is first debrided with a shaver. If an unstable root is identified (Fig. 7.10a), debride the edges, and then pass two #0 nonabsorbable sutures using a self-retrieving suture passer (Fig. 7.10b and c) (Meniscal Scorpion, Arthrex,

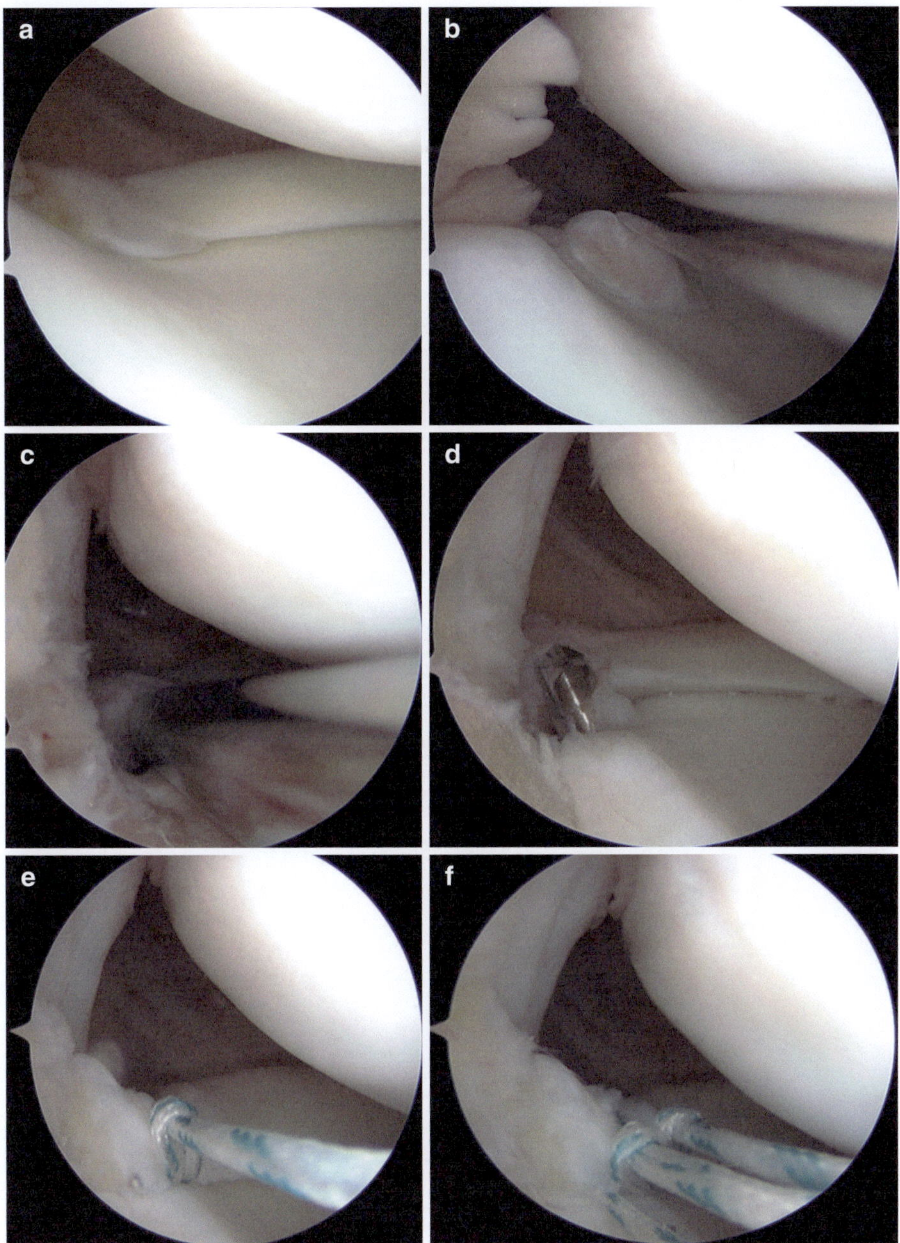

Fig. 7.9 Step-by-step arthroscopic repair of a MMPRT. (**a**) View of the meniscus prior to probing; (**b**) the meniscus is probed revealing the tear; (**c**) view of the meniscal root aiming guide in the correct position prior to reaming; (**d**) the tip of the flip cutter is seen after drilling through the tibia; (**e**) the first cinch stitch is placed; (**f**) the second cinch stitch is placed; (**g**, **h**) the meniscus root and body is probed for stability after tying the sutures over the cortical button

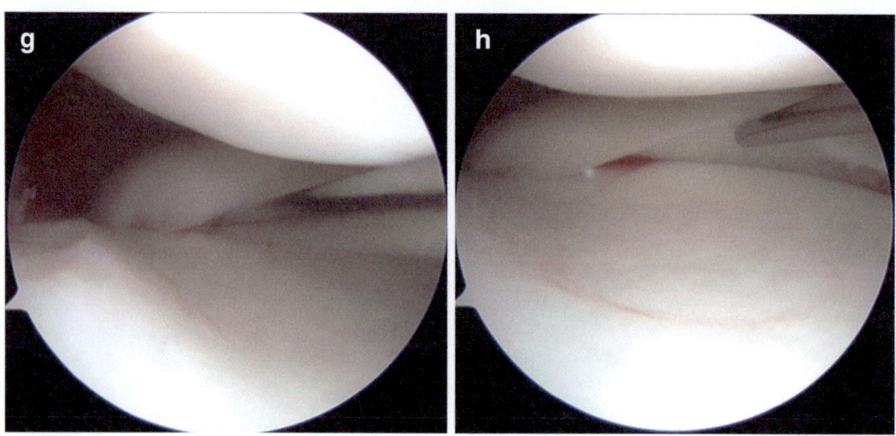

Fig. 7.9 (continued)

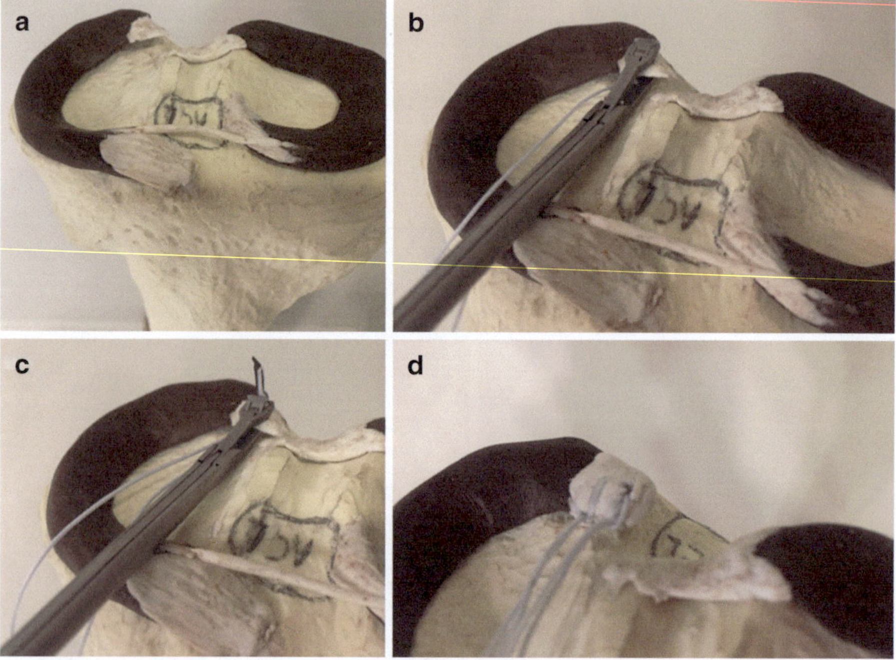

Fig. 7.10 An unstable meniscal root tear is identified (**a**), the knee scorpion is used to pass two #0 nonabsorbable sutures in the root in a cinch fashion (**b, c**). The sutures are cinched against the root (**d**)

Naples, FL) approximately 5 mm apart in a cinch configuration (Fig. 7.10d). Often times, the more medially based suture is passed first and can be used as a traction suture to draw the meniscus anteriorly and allow better tissue purchase for the second suture, which is subsequently placed 2–3 mm from the root edge. Although a more complex suture configuration increases the pullout strength of the repair [48], we

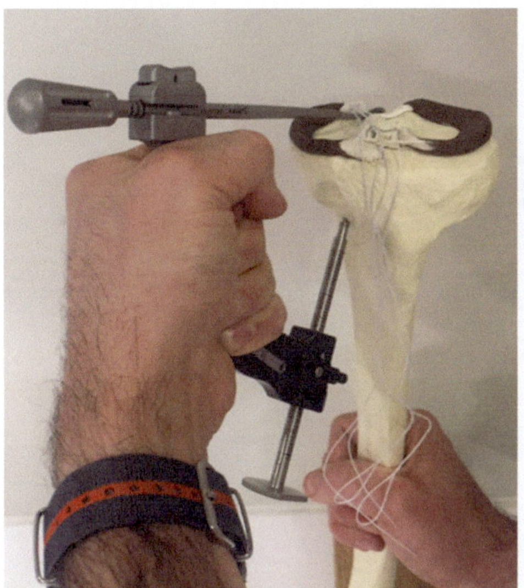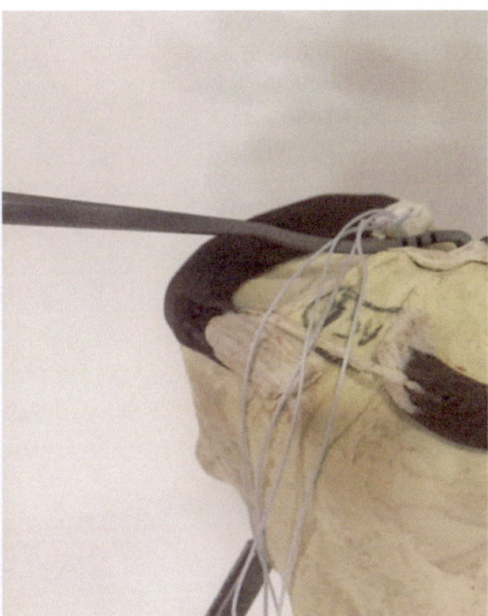

Fig. 7.11 Meniscal retrograde drill guide in position prior to retrograde drilling of the tibial tunnel. The sutures are held out of the way using the guide, so they do not get wrapped up in the drill as it comes through the subchondral bone

Fig. 7.12 Retrograde drill used for drilling the tibial tunnel. (Flipcutter, Arthrex, Naples FL)

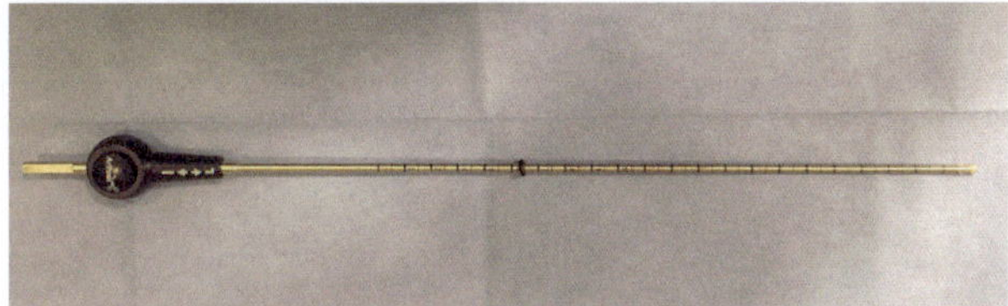

have found it not to be necessary in our practice as the strength of the construct outweighs the loads borne on the repair with a standard rehabilitation protocol [49].

A meniscus root retrograde drill guide (Fig. 7.11) (Arthrex, Naples, FL) is placed at the anatomic insertion site of the meniscus root. Care is taken not to err too anterior or medial, given the previously raised concerns about the effects of a nonanatomic repair. A 6 mm retrograde reamer (Fig. 7.12) (Flipcutter, Arthrex, Naples, FL) is then used to create a blind-ended socket in the anatomic footprint of the meniscal root. Upon entry into the joint, the reamer is deployed (Fig. 7.13a and b) and the guide is used to lift the meniscus to improve visualization and protect the previously placed sutures. The socket is reverse-reamed to a depth of 10 mm, and a passing suture is then passed through the tunnel (Fig. 7.14), into the joint, and retrieved out the anteromedial portal.

Next, a looped arthroscopic grasper is used to retrieve all sutures through the anteromedial portal. This step is critical to prevent the formation of a soft tissue bridge between the cinch suture and the passing suture. The sutures are then shuttled through the tunnel and out of the anterior tibia (Fig. 7.15a, b, and c) and tied over a cortical button (Fig. 7.16a and b) on the anterior tibial cortex with the knee in full extension. The meniscus is then probed to check the stability of the repair.

Fig. 7.13 (**a**) Retrograde drill tip within the joint at the footprint of the medial meniscal posterior root. After drilling into the joint, the drill tip is deployed, and the tunnel is reamed approximately 10 mm deep. (**b**) Posterior view of the retrograde drill tip within the joint at the footprint of the medial meniscal posterior root

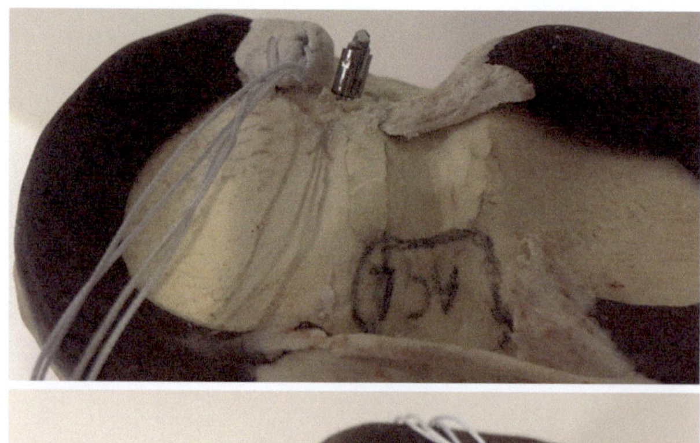

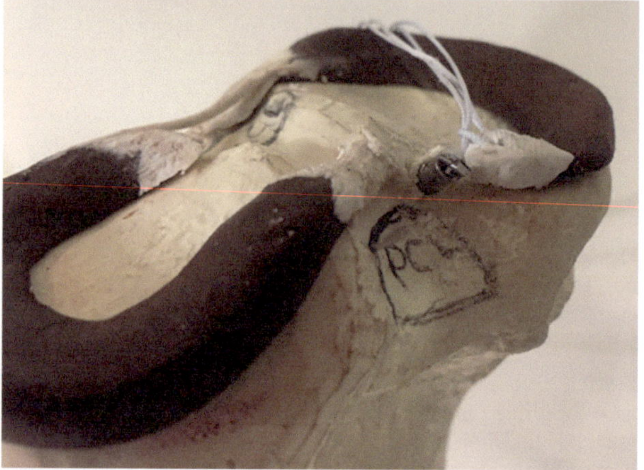

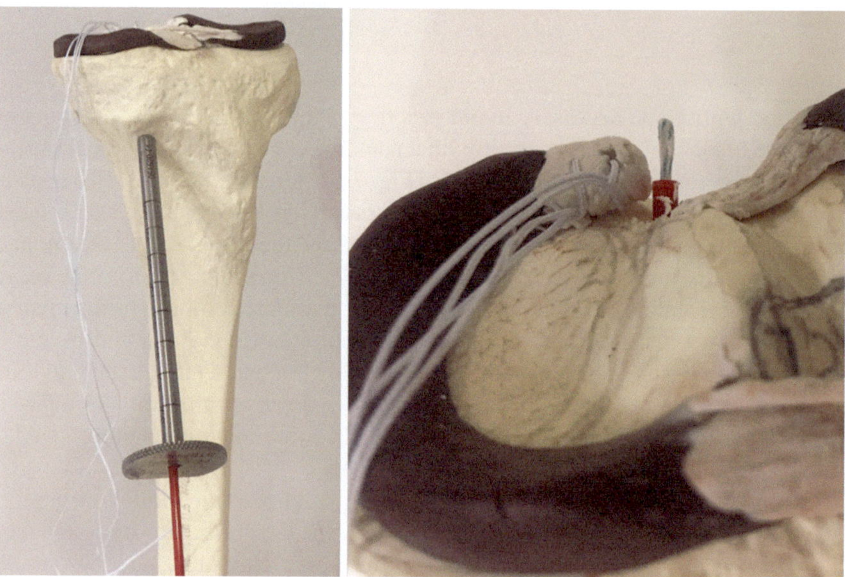

Fig. 7.14 A loop-ended suture is passed into the joint and is used to shuttle the meniscal sutures into the tunnel

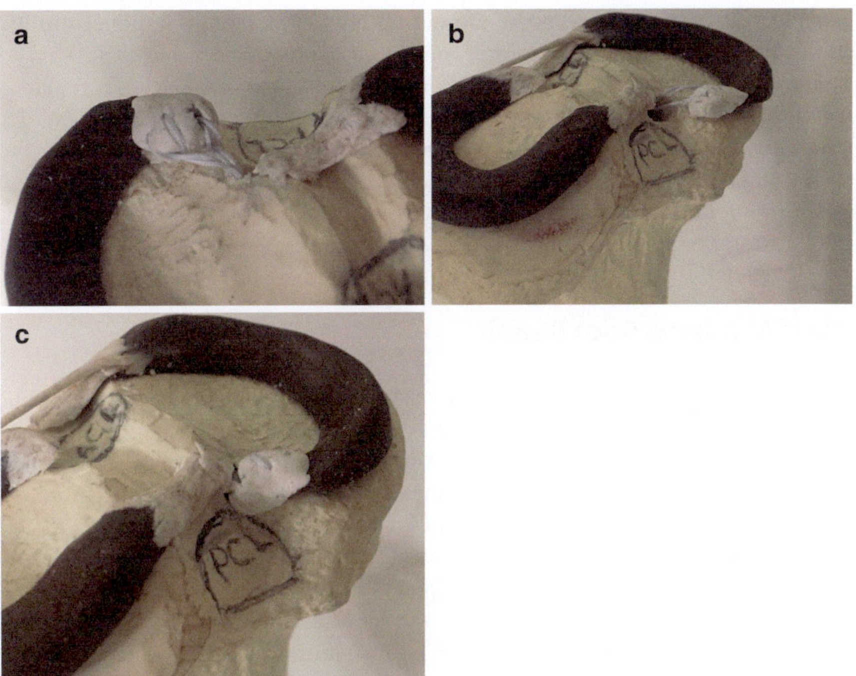

Fig. 7.15 (**a**) The meniscal sutures shuttled into the tunnel. (**b**) posterior view of meniscal sutures shuttled into the tunnel, compressing it against cancellous bone. (**c**) Pulling on the sutures brings the root partially into the tunnel

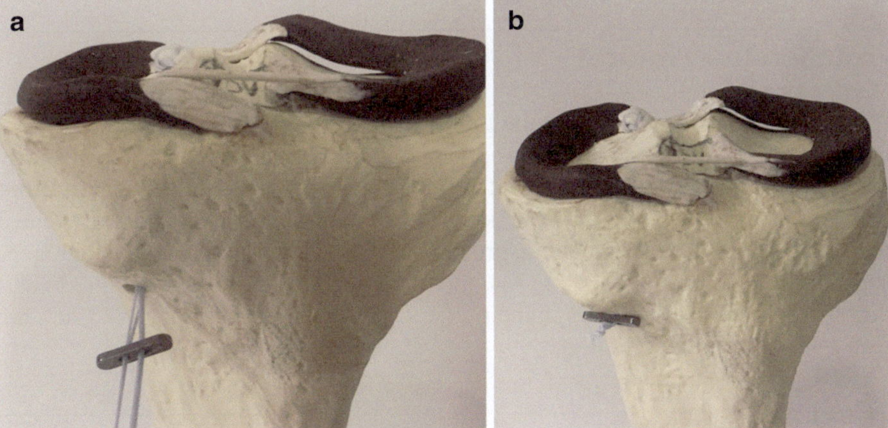

Fig. 7.16 (**a**) The sutures are individually passed through the cortical button. (**b**) The completed meniscal root repair construct. The sutures are independently tied over the cortical button so that if one fails, the other one remains intact maintaining integrity of the repair

As previously mentioned, nonanatomic placement of the tibial tunnel results in significant increases in tibiofemoral contact pressures. In an anatomic study by Laprade et al., nonanatomic placement of the tibial tunnel resulted in a repair that essentially functioned like a subtotal meniscectomy. In this cadaveric study, a meniscal root tear was simulated and repaired nonanatomically. The knees were then tested in varying degrees of knee flexion and compared to anatomic repairs. The authors found that anatomic placement of the tibial tunnel resulted in a near-normal restoration of tibiofemoral contact mechanics [50].

Lateral Meniscus Root Repair

The lateral meniscus root can be repaired in similar fashion to the medial root, understanding that LCL pie-crusting should be avoided in all cases. The surgical assistant can provide additional varus stress by positioning the knee in a figure-of-4 position to improve visualization of the lateral compartment. The remainder of the procedure is performed in a similar fashion as medial meniscus posterior root repair. Our preference, however, is to exit the tunnel on the anterolateral aspect of the tibia given the improved vector of pull of the sutures. When performing lateral meniscal root repair in conjunction with ACL reconstruction, the meniscal repair sutures can be passed through the ACL tunnel along with the ACL graft, if desired. This avoids the creation of a separate tibial tunnel, which poses the risk of tunnel convergence given the intimate relationship of the lateral meniscus root to the ACL tibial footprint. If this technique is chosen, it is important to debride the tibial ACL insertion of remnant fibers to ensure easy passage of the repair sutures and ACL graft. After the ACL reconstruction is completed, the limbs of the meniscus repair are tensioned, loaded into a knotless anchor, and placed about 2–3 cm distal to the ACL tunnel.

Postoperative Protocol

A hinged knee brace is used for the first 4 weeks postoperatively, and patients are instructed to remain partial weight-bearing with crutches with the knee locked in extension. Range of motion restricted to 0–90° may be started immediately postoperatively and progressed at 4–6 weeks. After 6 weeks, patients begin a graduated weight-bearing and strengthening protocol as tolerated, focusing on quadriceps activation and core strengthening. At 6 months, patients are allowed to return to cutting sports if their strength is symmetric (at least 90% of the contralateral side), are pain free, and have full motion.

Summary

Meniscal root tears have been shown to induce a rapid progression of knee osteoarthritis given the increased tibiofemoral contact pressure and reduced contact area seen with these lesions. Meniscal root repair is an efficacious treatment option and should be strongly considered in all patients with this pathology. While it is known that knee biomechanics are restored following meniscal root repair, long-term follow-up studies are required to demonstrate that this intervention prevents degenerative joint disease of the knee.

Pearls and Pitfalls
- The position of the anteromedial portal is critical to optimize trajectory to the root and should be placed strategically.
- Liberal use of deep MCL pie-crusting will help for viewing and safe suture passing.
- Robust suture purchase of root tissue is necessary for adequate fixation and to avoid suture cutout.
- Confirm that the cortical button is apposed against cortical bone to assure acceptable fixation.
- Care should be taken to avoid a soft-tissue bridge during suture passage, and, if necessary, small cannulas can be used for assistance.

References

1. Choi CJ, Choi YJ, Lee JJ, Choi CH. Magnetic resonance imaging evidence of meniscal extrusion in medial meniscus posterior root tear. Arthroscopy. 2010;26:1602–6.
2. Padalecki JR, Jansson KS, Smith SD, et al. Biomechanical consequences of a complete radial tear adjacent to the medial meniscus posterior root attachment site: in situ pull-out repair restores derangement of joint mechanics. Am J Sports Med. 2014;42:699–707.
3. Allaire R, Muriuki M, Gilbertson L, Harner CD. Biomechanical consequences of a tear of the posterior root of the medial meniscus. Similar to total meniscectomy. J Bone Joint Surg Am. 2008;90:1922–31.
4. Bin SI, Kim JM, Shin SJ. Radial tears of the posterior horn of the medial meniscus. Arthroscopy. 2004;20:373–8.
5. Ahn JH, Lee YS, Chang JY, Chang MJ, Eun SS, Kim SM. Arthroscopic all inside repair of the lateral meniscus root tear. Knee. 2009;16:77–80.
6. LaPrade RF, Ho CP, James E, Crespo B, LaPrade CM, Matheny LM. Diagnostic accuracy of 3.0 T magnetic resonance imaging for the detection of meniscus posterior root pathology. Knee Surg Sports Traumatol Arthrosc. 2015;23:152–7.
7. Lee BS, Bin SI, Kim JM, Park MH, Lee SM, Bae KH. Partial meniscectomy for degenerative medial meniscal root tears shows favorable outcomes in well-aligned, nonarthritic knees. Am J Sports Med. 2019:363546518819e225.
8. Matheny LM, Ockuly AC, Steadman JR, LaPrade RF. Posterior meniscus root tears: associated pathologies to assist as diagnostic tools. Knee Surg Sports Traumatol Arthrosc. 2015;23:3127–31.
9. LaPrade CM, Smith SD, Rasmussen MT, et al. Consequences of tibial tunnel reaming on the meniscal roots during cruciate ligament reconstruction in a cadaveric model, Part 1: The anterior cruciate ligament. Am J Sports Med. 2015;43:200–6.
10. Ellman MB, James EW, LaPrade CM, LaPrade RF. Anterior meniscus root avulsion following intramedullary nailing for a tibial shaft fracture. Knee Surg Sports Traumatol Arthrosc. 2015;23:1188–91.
11. LaPrade MD, LaPrade CM, Hamming MG, et al. Intramedullary tibial nailing reduces the attachment area and ultimate load of the anterior medial meniscal root: a potential explanation for anterior knee pain in female patients and smaller patients. Am J Sports Med. 2015;43:1670–5.

12. Hoser C, Fink C, Brown C, Reichkendler M, Hackl W, Bartlett J. Long-term results of arthroscopic partial lateral meniscectomy in knees without associated damage. J Bone Joint Surg. 2001;83:513–6.
13. Stein T, Mehling AP, Welsch F, von Eisenhart-Rothe R, Jager A. Long-term outcome after arthroscopic meniscal repair versus arthroscopic partial meniscectomy for traumatic meniscal tears. Am J Sports Med. 2010;38:1542–8.
14. Kaplan DJ, Alaia EF, Dold AP, et al. Increased extrusion and ICRS grades at 2-year follow-up following transtibial medial meniscal root repair evaluated by MRI. Knee Surg Sports Traumatol Arthrosc. 2018;26:2826–34.
15. LaPrade RF, Matheny LM, Moulton SG, James EW, Dean CS. Posterior meniscal root repairs: outcomes of an anatomic transtibial pull-out technique. Am J Sports Med. 2017;45:884–91.
16. Andrews S, Shrive N, Ronsky J. The shocking truth about meniscus. J Biomech. 2011;44:2737–40.
17. Gupta M, Goyal PK, Singh P, Sharma A. Morphology of intra-articular structures and histology of menisci of knee joint. Int J Appl Basic Med Res. 2018;8:96–9.
18. Johannsen AM, Civitarese DM, Padalecki JR, Goldsmith MT, Wijdicks CA, LaPrade RF. Qualitative and quantitative anatomic analysis of the posterior root attachments of the medial and lateral menisci. Am J Sports Med. 2012;40:2342–7.
19. Smigielski R, Becker R, Zdanowicz U, Ciszek B. Medial meniscus anatomy-from basic science to treatment. Knee Surg Sports Traumatol Arthrosc. 2015;23:8–14.
20. Anderson CJ, Ziegler CG, Wijdicks CA, Engebretsen L, LaPrade RF. Arthroscopically pertinent anatomy of the anterolateral and posteromedial bundles of the posterior cruciate ligament. J Bone Joint Surg Am. 2012;94:1936–45.
21. Pagnani MJ, Cooper DE, Warren RF. Extrusion of the medial meniscus. Arthroscopy. 1991;7:297–300.
22. Marzo JM, Gurske-DePerio J. Effects of medial meniscus posterior horn avulsion and repair on tibiofemoral contact area and peak contact pressure with clinical implications. Am J Sports Med. 2009;37:124–9.
23. Bhatia S, LaPrade CM, Ellman MB, LaPrade RF. Meniscal root tears: significance, diagnosis, and treatment. Am J Sports Med. 2014;42:3016–30.
24. Kim YJ, Kim JG, Chang SH, Shim JC, Kim SB, Lee MY. Posterior root tear of the medial meniscus in multiple knee ligament injuries. Knee. 2010;17:324–8.
25. Praz C, Vieira TD, Saithna A, et al. Risk factors for lateral meniscus posterior root tears in the anterior cruciate ligament-injured knee: an epidemiological analysis of 3956 patients from the SANTI study group. Am J Sports Med. 2019:363546518818820.
26. Robertson DD, Armfield DR, Towers JD, Irrgang JJ, Maloney WJ, Harner CD. Meniscal root injury and spontaneous osteonecrosis of the knee: an observation. J Bone Joint Surg. 2009;91:190–5.
27. Kim JH, Chung JH, Lee DH, Lee YS, Kim JR, Ryu KJ. Arthroscopic suture anchor repair versus pullout suture repair in posterior root tear of the medial meniscus: a prospective comparison study. Arthroscopy. 2011;27:1644–53.
28. Seil R, Duck K, Pape D. A clinical sign to detect root avulsions of the posterior horn of the medial meniscus. Knee Surg Sports Traumatol Arthrosc. 2011;19:2072–5.
29. Ahn JH, Jeong HJ, Lee YS, et al. Comparison between conservative treatment and arthroscopic pull-out repair of the medial meniscus root tear and analysis of prognostic factors for the determination of repair indication. Arch Orthop Trauma Surg. 2015;135:1265–76.
30. Ozkoc G, Circi E, Gonc U, Irgit K, Pourbagher A, Tandogan RN. Radial tears in the root of the posterior horn of the medial meniscus. Knee Surg Sports Traumatol Arthrosc. 2008;16:849–54.
31. Lerer DB, Umans HR, Hu MX, Jones MH. The role of meniscal root pathology and radial meniscal tear in medial meniscal extrusion. Skelet Radiol. 2004;33:569–74.
32. Costa CR, Morrison WB, Carrino JA. Medial meniscus extrusion on knee MRI: is extent associated with severity of degeneration or type of tear? Am J Roentgenol. 2004;183:17–23.
33. LaPrade CM, James EW, Cram TR, Feagin JA, Engebretsen L, LaPrade RF. Meniscal root tears: a classification system based on tear morphology. Am J Sports Med. 2015;43:363–9.

34. Krych AJ, Johnson NR, Mohan R, et al. Arthritis progression on serial MRIs following diagnosis of medial meniscal posterior horn root tear. J Knee Surg. 2018;31:698–704.
35. Jones A, Silva PG, Silva AC, et al. Impact of cane use on pain, function, general health and energy expenditure during gait in patients with knee osteoarthritis: a randomised controlled trial. Ann Rheum Dis. 2012;71:172–9.
36. Moe RH, Fernandes L, Osteras N. Daily use of a cane for two months reduced pain and improved function in patients with knee osteoarthritis. J Physiother. 2012;58:128.
37. Kalra M, Bakker R, Tomescu SS, Polak AM, Nicholls M, Chandrashekar N. The effect of unloader knee braces on medial meniscal strain. Prosthetics Orthot Int. 2018:309364618798173.
38. Lamberg EM, Streb R, Werner M, Kremenic I, Penna J. The 2- and 8-week effects of decompressive brace use in people with medial compartment knee osteoarthritis. Prosthetics Orthot Int. 2016;40:447–53.
39. Thorning M, Thorlund JB, Roos EM, Wrigley TV, Hall M. Immediate effect of valgus bracing on knee joint moments in meniscectomised patients: an exploratory study. J Sci Med Sport. 2016;19:964–9.
40. Krych AJ, Johnson NR, Mohan R, Dahm DL, Levy BA, Stuart MJ. Partial meniscectomy provides no benefit for symptomatic degenerative medial meniscus posterior root tears. Knee Surg Sports Traumatol Arthrosc. 2018;26:1117–22.
41. Chung KS, Ha JK, Ra HJ, Kim JG. A meta-analysis of clinical and radiographic outcomes of posterior horn medial meniscus root repairs. Knee Surg Sports Traumatol Arthrosc. 2016;24:1455–68.
42. Chung KS, Ha JK, Yeom CH, et al. Comparison of clinical and radiologic results between partial meniscectomy and refixation of medial meniscus posterior root tears: a minimum 5-year follow-up. Arthroscopy. 2015;31:1941–50.
43. Brophy RH, Wojahn RD, Lillegraven O, Lamplot JD. Outcomes of arthroscopic posterior medial meniscus root repair: association with body mass index. J Am Acad Orthop Surg. 2019;27(3):104–11.
44. Kwak YH, Lee S, Lee MC, Han HS. Large meniscus extrusion ratio is a poor prognostic factor of conservative treatment for medial meniscus posterior root tear. Knee Surg Sports Traumatol Arthrosc. 2018;26:781–6.
45. Krych AJ, Johnson NR, Wu IT, Smith PA, Stuart MJ. A simple cinch is superior to a locking loop for meniscus root repair: a human biomechanical comparison of suture constructs in a transtibial pull-out model. Knee Surg Sports Traumatol Arthrosc. 2018;26:2239–44.
46. Starke C, Kopf S, Grobel KH, Becker R. The effect of a nonanatomic repair of the meniscal horn attachment on meniscal tension: a biomechanical study. Arthroscopy. 2010;26:358–65.
47. Feucht MJ, Kuhle J, Bode G, et al. Arthroscopic transtibial pullout repair for posterior medial meniscus root tears: a systematic review of clinical, radiographic, and second-look arthroscopic results. Arthroscopy. 2015;31:1808–16.
48. Anz AW, Branch EA, Saliman JD. Biomechanical comparison of arthroscopic repair constructs for meniscal root tears. Am J Sports Med. 2014;42:2699–706.
49. Starke C, Kopf S, Lippisch R, Lohmann CH, Becker R. Tensile forces on repaired medial meniscal root tears. Arthroscopy. 2013;29:205–12.
50. LaPrade CM, Foad A, Smith SD, et al. Biomechanical consequences of a nonanatomic posterior medial meniscal root repair. Am J Sports Med. 2015;43:912–20.

Understanding and Treating the Discoid Meniscus

8

Cordelia Carter and Stephen Yu

Introduction

The discoid meniscus is a congenital anatomic variant that is estimated to affect up to 5% of the general US population [1]. In 1889, Young et al. first reported on the morphology of the discoid meniscus, and the associated clinical "snapping knee syndrome" was subsequently described by Middleton et al. in 1936 [2, 3]. As its name implies, the defining feature of the discoid meniscus is its shape, which is that of a circle or a "disk," rather than the characteristic crescent shape of the typical meniscus. The vast majority involve the lateral meniscus, although a handful of cases of medial discoid menisci have been reported [4]. The presence of a discoid meniscus in the knee may simply be an incidental finding discovered either on advanced imaging or at the time of knee arthroscopy performed for other pathology. However, when associated with pain and/or mechanical symptoms, the discoid meniscus may be a clinically significant entity, requiring a methodical approach to its diagnosis and management.

Epidemiology

The vast majority of discoid menisci affect the lateral compartment of the knee. The incidence of lateral discoid meniscus is reported to have a wide range – between 0.4% and 17% – which is largely dependent on the region of the

C. Carter
Joan H & Preston Robert Tisch Center at Essex Crossing, New York, NY, USA
e-mail: Cordelia.Carter@nyumc.org

S. Yu (✉)
NYU Langone Orthopedic Hospital, New York, NY, USA
e-mail: Stephen.Yu@nyumc.org

© Springer Nature Switzerland AG 2020
E. J. Strauss, L. M. Jazrawi (eds.), *The Management of Meniscal Pathology*,
https://doi.org/10.1007/978-3-030-49488-9_8

population [1, 5]. The medial discoid meniscus is much rarer, with an estimated incidence less than 0.3% in the general US population [6, 7]. Estimates of the prevalence of bilateral discoid menisci vary widely, as screening of an asymptomatic contralateral limb is generally not recommended for patients who present with clinical symptoms related to a discoid meniscus in one knee. Cadaver studies investigating the incidence of bilateral discoid meniscus report highly variable results, with an estimated 6% of the US general population having a discoid meniscus present bilaterally, and as many as 97% of the Japanese general population with this finding [4]. Certainly, if a patient requires treatment for a symptomatic unilateral discoid meniscus, there should be high suspicion for a discoid meniscus as a cause for pain and mechanical symptoms that subsequently develop in the contralateral knee.

There is variation in the reported epidemiology of discoid menisci across the globe. The general populations of Japan and Korea seem to have the highest incidence of discoid meniscus, which has been estimated to affect 15% and 13% of the population of each country, respectively [8, 9]. The reported incidence of discoid meniscus in the US population is much lower, estimated to be around 3–5% [1]. This figure may underestimate the actual incidence of discoid meniscus in the US population, as discoid menisci are often incidentally discovered and may presumably remain undetected if they are clinically silent. Interestingly, the presence of discoid meniscus variants has been associated with certain genetic disorders of the musculoskeletal system, such as achondroplasia [10]. An increased incidence of discoid meniscus has also been reported in patients with osteochondritis dissecans lesions of the lateral femoral condyle [11].

Sex-based differences in the incidence and presentation of discoid meniscus have been described, although the data is not robust. In a large-scale observational study performed in China, females were much more likely to have a discoid meniscus and comprised 70% of the study population [12]. By contrast, males consisted of 56% of the study population in a recent study performed in the US [13]. Since screening for discoid meniscus is not typically performed in asymptomatic individuals, the true incidence of discoid meniscus and its relationship to sex is not well understood. That said, a sex-based difference has been described for clinical presentation of the discoid meniscus. Specifically, males may be more likely to present with a traumatic history and report mechanical symptoms, whereas females are generally older at the time of presentation and may be more likely to present with a block to extension on physical examination [12].

Pathoanatomy and Histopathology

The discoid meniscus is a congenital condition whose etiology is poorly understood, although genetics have been postulated to play a role in its manifestation. Interestingly, the appearance of the crescent-shaped meniscus typically found in humans may have been an evolutionary development, as some nonhuman primates have been found to possess menisci that are discoid shaped [14].

In addition to an anomalous disk-like shape when viewed from above, some discoid menisci also have abnormally thickened tissue when viewed from the side – the so-called "block-like" meniscus (Fig. 8.1). Furthermore, discoid menisci have variable degrees of meniscocapsular ligamentous attachments, and in some cases may be grossly unstable or hypermobile. Thus, we use the term "discoid meniscus" to refer to a wide spectrum of pathoanatomy, with some menisci demonstrating minimal pathology and others with more severe involvement. This concept of a spectrum of pathology likely explains why some discoid meniscus variants remain clinically silent over time (e.g., partial, stable menisci) while others (complete, block-like, unstable menisci) present early in life with symptoms.

The histology of a discoid variant is quite different than that of a normal meniscus. Specifically, the collagen matrix in a discoid meniscus has a disorganized

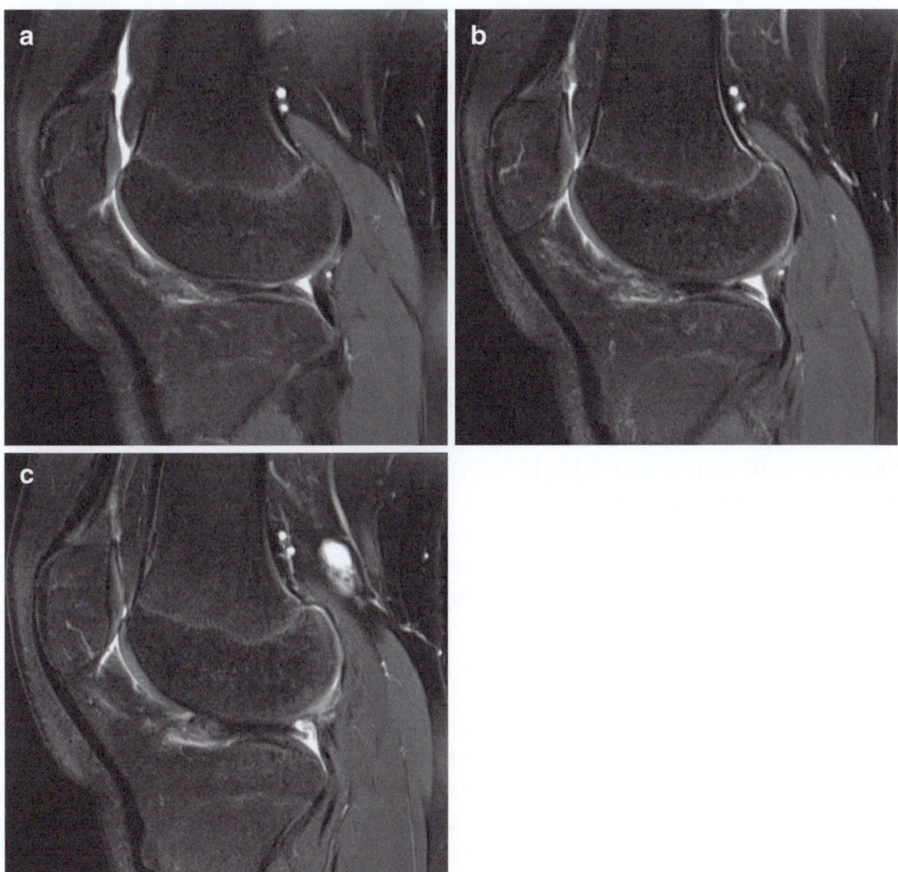

Fig. 8.1 (**a–c**) Three sequential sagittal cuts from a T2-weighted MRI of the knee of a 13-year-old female demonstrating confluence of the anterior and posterior horns with anterior displacement of a thick, amorphous mass of meniscal tissue with complex intrasubstance tearing

orientation and is lower in collagen density than a normal meniscus [15–17]. The inherently weaker ultrastructure of the discoid meniscus renders it more vulnerable to mucoid degeneration and tearing than its normal counterpart [18]. Due to these factors, it is estimated that the discoid meniscus is more than twice as likely to tear than a normal morphology [19].

While in utero, the entire meniscus is richly vascular. After birth, the vascularity slowly recedes to supply primarily the outer and middle third of a developing, semilunar meniscus, and by the second decade of life, the morphology, histology, and vascularity of the meniscus closely approximate those found in an adult. While the shape and underlying histology of the discoid meniscus may differ significantly from those of the normal meniscus, there has not been a demonstrated difference in the vascular pattern and supply of the discoid meniscus.

Classification

The Watanabe classification has traditionally been used to describe the shape of the meniscus and the pattern of its peripheral attachments [20]. A complete type (Watanabe type 1) is a whole disk of meniscus occupying most of the compartment and obscuring the majority of the underlying tibial plateau (greater than 80%). An incomplete type (Watanabe type 2) is more of a semilunar shape, with some redundant central tissue. Both types generally have normal peripheral attachments to the capsule and tibia, conferring normal stability to the abnormally shaped meniscus. By contrast, in the Watanabe type 3 variant, the meniscus lacks a posterior meniscotibial ligament and is contiguous with the Wrisberg ligament; hence its name, the Wrisberg variant (Watanabe type 3). The shape of a type 3 meniscus may be normal; however, it is grossly unstable and hypermobile. Due to a lack of tethering, the Wrisberg type meniscus translates significantly throughout knee range of motion. During extension, it is pulled by the Wrisberg ligament into the intercondylar notch and causes abnormal contact forces across the knee joint due to an incompetent lateral meniscus. This phenomenon usually produces a snapping sensation and may explain the symptoms underlying "snapping knee syndrome."

The Watanabe classification was originally described as an arthroscopically evaluated system, with the meniscus visualized and graded both on appearance (complete, incomplete) and stability (stable, unstable Wrisberg-type). More recently, Klingele et al. further defined the concept of stability by evaluating the discoid meniscus, regardless of morphology, at three anatomical locations [21]. Namely, the stability of the peripheral rim was evaluated using a probe at the anterior horn, the middle body, and the posterior horn; if there was gross detachment in any position from the periphery, it was noted as "unstable." Peripheral rim instability has been found to be present in 28% of the discoid menisci population, most commonly at the anterior horn (47%), then posterior horn (39%), and then middle body (11%). Patients found to have a significant degree of peripheral rim instability tend to be younger at time of presentation, implying that instability plays a large role in symptomatology and predisposition to tearing [21].

The contemporary approach to arthroscopic classification of a discoid meniscus is useful for guiding surgical decision-making: First, the overall morphology (partial or complete discoid shape) is noted. Associated meniscal tears are identified next, followed by assessment of the presence and location of peripheral rim instability.

Diagnosis of a Discoid

The typical age of presentation is between 10 and 16 years, although patients with more severe pathoanatomy may present with knee pain, swelling, and mechanical symptoms in early childhood. Younger patients with block-like and/or hypermobile discoid meniscal variants may complain of intermittent swelling and localized knee pain after participation in sports and physical activities, or they may simply report uncomfortable "snapping" in the knee as it is brought from flexion to extension. Older patients more commonly report mechanical symptoms, including locking, catching, and giving way, that are suggestive of meniscal tearing. Patients that complain about a block to extension tend to be the most symptomatic, and it is reported that up to 50–79% of the patients have an extension block upon first presenting for evaluation [15, 22].

Physical examination of the knee begins with inspection, which may reveal effusion and quadriceps atrophy. Passive range of motion may be limited if the meniscus is so thickened or displaced that it serves as a mechanical block to motion, typically extension. Pain with extremes of passive motion (e.g., terminal extension or hyperflexion may be present, and pain with deep knee bends or squatting that load the meniscus may also be present. While its sensitivity is low (reported to be roughly 40%), the McMurray maneuver is commonly used to detect meniscal pathology [23]. Reproducible snapping of the knee may be elicited in up to 39% of patients [24].

Plain radiographs are typically the first diagnostic study obtained in the evaluation of knee pain, and include lateral, sunrise, tunnel, and a weight-bearing AP view of the affected knee. Although the meniscus itself cannot be visualized on plain films, there are several unique morphologic features that have been described in the setting of discoid lateral meniscus, including increased lateral joint space height and width, lateral femoral condyle hypoplasia or notching, lateral tibia spine hypoplasia, squaring of the lateral tibial plateau, and a high fibular head. Ha et al. aimed to improve our ability to identify a discoid lateral meniscus using plain radiographs alone. These authors described a method for measuring the prominence of each femoral condyle on the tunnel view and calculating the ratio of the lateral condylar prominence measurement to that of the medial condyle. They reported that if the ratio of the lateral to medial condylar prominence was less than 0.8, then the patient likely had a discoid meniscus, with a reported 76% sensitivity, 96% specificity, and 95% positive predictive value. They termed this the "condylar cutoff sign." [25]

Magnetic resonance imaging (MRI) of the knee remains the best study for identification of a discoid meniscus (Fig. 8.1a–c). Traditionally, the diagnosis of discoid lateral meniscus could be made if the anterior and posterior horns are contiguous on three consecutive 5 mm sagittal cuts (the "bow-tie sign"). However, there are other diagnostic criterion on MRI that have more recently been described that have better sensitivity and specificity than the traditional "bow-tie" sign. Samoto et al. described four different parameters: (1) minimum meniscal width on a coronal slice, (2) ratio of minimal coronal meniscal width to maximal coronal tibial width, (3) ratio of the sum of the diameter of the anterior and posterior horn to the total meniscal diameter, (4) the bow-tie sign as described above. They found that the most accurate method was the ratio of the meniscus to the tibia with a cut-off value of at least 20% tibial coverage, or the ratio of the diameters greater than 75%. The sensitive and specificity of this diagnostic criterion were similar for the cut-offs, reported as 95% and 97% respectively [26].

It is important to note that the Wrisberg variant is difficult to diagnose, as the overall shape of the meniscus is essentially normal. The characteristic finding is exactly what makes this variant unique, in that the only posterior attachment of the posterior horn is contiguous with the Wrisberg ligament [27]. The MRI may also note findings of the meniscus extruded into the notch, as this variant is known to be grossly unstable, and may make evaluation even more difficult.

MRI can be a useful tool in not only diagnosing discoid menisci, but also identifying associated injuries contributing to symptoms, specifically meniscal tears and acute cartilaginous injury (ACI). Yilgor et al. report that MRI is very reliable in diagnosing meniscal tears, with a 98% sensitivity and 100% specificity, and a positive predictive value of 100% and negative predictive value of 86% [28]. The authors go on to suggest that although the presence of a tear can be reliably determined using MRI, characterizing the tear remains a challenge and does not correlate reliably with intraoperative findings.

Lau et al. looked at the utility of MRI in detecting ACI and found that MRI alone was not very reliable, with a sensitivity of 60%, specificity of 67%, and a positive predictive value of 55%. However, when combined with positive history and physical exam findings, namely chronic knee pain (>6 months) and a physical block to extension, the reliability of detecting ACI with a discoid meniscus improved to 79% sensitivity, 80% specificity, and 73% positive predictive value [22].

Clinical Management

Patients with an asymptomatic discoid meniscus that is diagnosed incidentally do not typically require treatment. Conversely, patients with mechanical symptoms and/or lateral joint pain and MRI evidence of a discoid lateral meniscus may benefit from surgical treatment.

Surgical indication and timing should be made with knee preservation as the goal of care. As most patients at presentation are young adolescents, management focuses on cartilage preservation. When directly addressing the discoid meniscus, meniscal function and rim preservation are paramount for restoring normal contact stresses in the knee joint, thereby preventing accelerated cartilage wear and progression to early arthritis.

Timing of surgical intervention is also important to consider, since tears of the discoid meniscus have a high probability of propagation. Peripheral rim instability can also progress, and the remaining attachments could be compromised if the instability and intra-meniscal stress persists. Thus, while not an urgent indication, surgery should be performed on a timely basis. From the time the patient is indicated for surgery, a hinged knee brace can be helpful to offer the patient support, while also limiting their activity and potentially preventing further damage. Furthermore, if the patient has a "locked knee" from a bucket-handle tear or gross instability of the meniscus, non-weight-bearing precautions until surgery may be advisable in order to preserve the repairability of the meniscus.

Surgical Techniques

Historically, total meniscectomies were performed for the symptomatic discoid meniscus tear. Similar to the results of normal morphologic menisci treated with subtotal or complete meniscectomies, the majority of the evidence suggests inferior outcomes with this approach compared to more modern surgical techniques and strategies. Manzione et al. reported a rate of 80% of patients developing radiographic evidence of osteoarthritis only 5.5 years post-meniscectomy [29]. In the case of an irreparable discoid meniscus with extensive damage extending to the peripheral rim, a subtotal or total meniscectomy may be indicated [30]. However, understanding the natural history of the knees of young patients who undergo subtotal or complete meniscectomy, this procedure is typically avoided whenever possible.

The goal of surgery is to create a stable, biomechanically functional meniscus (Table 8.1). To address the redundant central tissue that is the hallmark of the discoid meniscus, arthroscopic saucerization is performed. Standard anteromedial and anterolateral portals may be used. Some authors suggest a high portal in the opposite compartment to gain improved access by using a more acute angle to perform the saucerization using an arthroscopic knife. This may be especially important if addressing a medial discoid meniscus [31]. To best access the area of interest, placing the camera in the anteromedial portal and/or making an accessory arthroscopic portal may be useful. Diagnostic arthroscopy is essential for understanding the nature of the discoid meniscus (complete or partial; torn or untorn; unstable or stable; Fig. 8.2a, b).

Saucerization involves resecting the central portion of the discoid and reconstituting the C-shaped rim of meniscal tissue (Fig. 8.2c–e). This may be performed with arthroscopic basket biters or punchers, an arthroscopic shaver, a radiofrequency ablation probe, or a combination of the three. For resection of large amounts of tissue, an arthroscopic knife may be used. Resection should aim to not violate the outer 6–8 mm rim of peripheral meniscal tissue [32, 33]. Margins should be smoothened when possible, and remnants and flaps should be minimized and resected, as

Table 8.1 Special equipment to request for pediatric discoid meniscus surgery

For visualization
Small-joint arthroscope
To improve ease of camera insertion in young children with little knees
For saucerization/partial meniscectomy
Small hand-held shaver
To prevent iatrogenic cartilage injury with multiple instrument passes
Banana blade or beaver blade
To saucerize/contour the anterior horn in the setting of thick, redundant tissue
For meniscal repair
18-gauge spinal needles
For outside-in repair technique, typically of the anterior horn
Zone-specific cannulae with double-armed sutures
For inside-out repair technique, typically for mid-body and/or posterior horn repairs
Absorbable sutures (e.g., PDS) may be useful for younger patients
Nonabsorbable sutures may be used in older patients
All-inside implants
A variety of commercial devices are available, typically for posterior horn repair
Meniscal rasp
To abrade/prepare the capsule for stabilization sutures
For biologic healing environment enhancement
Microfracture picks
To enhance the biologic healing environment following isolated meniscal repair

meniscus following initial saucerization. (**f**) Abrasion of the capsule and meniscal tissue is performed to augment the healing response. (**g**) Sequential inside-out sutures placed in the mid-body assist with meniscal reduction and tensioning. (**h**) Probing the posterior horn following suture placement demonstrates restoration of peripheral rim stability. (**i**) Following saucerization, repair and stabilization using 2 all-inside "hay-baling" sutures in the posterior horn and 5 inside-out sutures placed in the mid-body and mid-body–anterior horn junction. (**j**) Microfracture of the notch

they can be sources for re-tear or propagation of a fragment [32]. The re-tear rate remains high, ranging from 6% to 15.6%, and presents as a late sequalae into adulthood due to the inherent histological difference of the meniscus [32, 34, 35].

Once saucerization is completed, the remainder of the meniscus should be carefully evaluated for residual tears and/or rim instability. Partial meniscectomy should be performed for inner, white–white zone tears that have low rates of healing due to the avascular nature of the tissue. Meniscal repair is performed when a repairable tear – good-quality tissue, good vascular supply – is present in the saucerized meniscus. Common meniscal repair techniques include inside-out repair using zone-specific cannulae, all-inside repair (typically performed in the posterior horn using a commercially available device), or outside-in repair (typically used for tears of the anterior horn). Optimization of the biologic environment for meniscal healing by means of meniscal and/or capsular abrasion using a shaver or rasp instrument may improve healing rates (Fig. 8.2f, i).

Following saucerization and repair, the meniscus is once again evaluated for instability of the peripheral rim at the mensicocapsular junction; often, sutures placed for repair of meniscal tears also serve to stabilize the meniscus to the

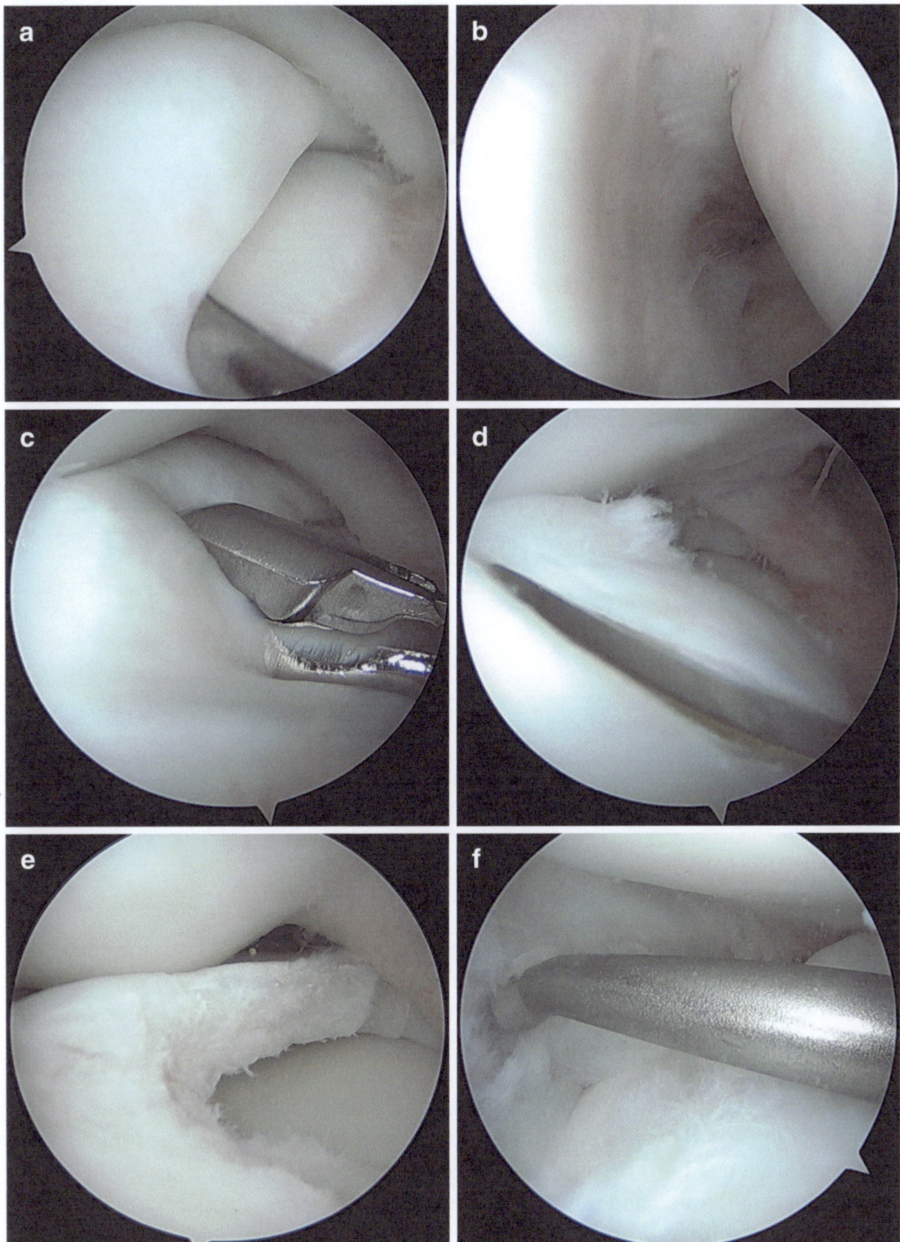

Fig. 8.2 Arthroscopic saucerization, repair, and stabilization of a complete, torn, unstable discoid lateral meniscus in a 12-year-old male. (**a**) Arthroscopic appearance of a complete discoid lateral meniscus with coverage of the entire tibial plateau. (**b**) Arthroscopic view from the lateral gutter demonstrating extensive tearing with displacement of the posterior meniscus with minimal peripheral meniscal tissue remaining. (**c**) Initial saucerization is performed with a meniscal biter. (**d**) Saucerization of the anterior horn is performed using a beaver blade. (**e**) The appearance of the

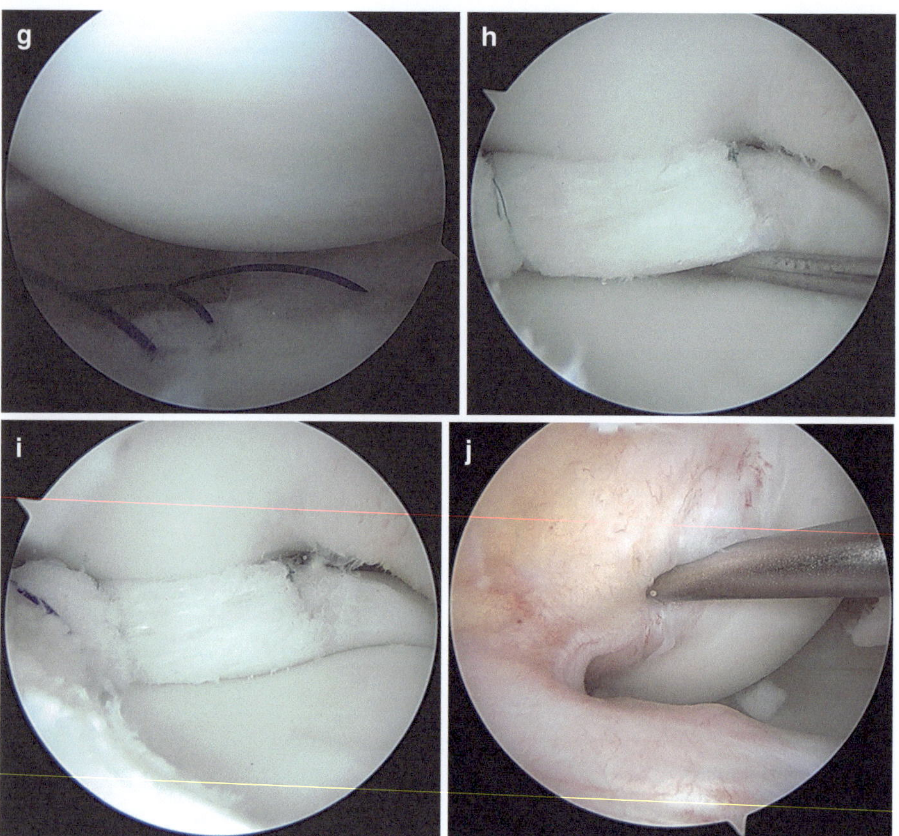

Fig. 8.2 (continued)

capsule. If, however, residual peripheral rim instability is identified, the meniscus can be reattached to capsule using techniques similar to those used for meniscal repair (Fig. 8.2g, h). Technical pearls for surgical treatment of discoid lateral meniscus are summarized in Table 8.2.

Aftercare following surgery may be guided by the nature and extent of surgery. Patients who require only arthroscopic saucerization may be treated in a similar fashion to those who undergo arthroscopic partial meniscectomy; a hinged knee brace and crutches may be used for comfort, but these patients may immediately weight bear as tolerated and range the knee freely. Conversely, patients who undergo repair and/or stabilization are given weight-bearing restrictions and are instructed to use an assistive device (e.g., crutches) and a hinged knee brace–limiting hyperextension and flexion past 90° to avoid overt pressures across the repair in the early phase of healing. The knee brace may be unlocked around 4 weeks and then the weight-bearing status may be advanced between 4 and 6 weeks postoperatively. Physical therapy is an integral component of postoperative rehabilitation to enable patients to regain knee motion, strength, and function.

Table 8.2 Technical pearls for surgical management of the symptomatic discoid meniscus

Identify and treat associated pathology
There is often significant synovitis and fat pad hypertrophy anterior to the discoid lateral meniscus that obscures visualization and is best removed with a hand-held shaver, taking care not to disrupt the intermeniscal ligament and/or the anterior meniscocapsular junction.
OCD of the lateral femoral condyle may be present in as many as 15% of patients with a discoid lateral meniscus and should be treated concurrently.
Understand what you're looking at
Confirm anatomic reduction of the meniscus prior to proceeding with saucerization, repair and/or stabilization.
During saucerization, ensure you know where the peripheral rim is at all times to avoid over-resection and inadvertent subtotal meniscectomy.
With significant peripheral rim instability, a temporary tethering stitch may be placed in the meniscus to assist with tissue tension during saucerization/partial meniscectomy.
Keep moving
It is easy to lose time trying to make a perfect "first pass" at saucerization for complete or near-complete discoid menisci; initial resection should focus on removal of redundant tissue rather than cosmetic appearance of the remaining meniscus. Once a 6–8 mm rim of meniscal tissue remains, this can be meticulously trimmed of rough edges and flaps and smoothed with a shaver.
Be systematic
Perform saucerization first, aiming to leave 6–8 mm of peripheral tissue intact
Following saucerization, inspect the remaining meniscal tissue for tears, and perform meniscal repair as indicated
Residual horizontal cleavage tears are common and may be treated with "hay-baling" repair technique rather than traditional mattress configurations.
Assess the entirety of the meniscus for peripheral rim instability and perform stabilization as indicated. Often, sutures placed for meniscal repair act to stabilize the peripheral rim.
Optimize the environment for healing
Prepare the tissue and adjacent capsule with a rasp
Consider microfracture of the notch

Clinical Outcomes

Reported surgical outcomes of arthroscopic saucerization with or without stabilization are generally favorable. There is a breadth of literature that report short- and long-term outcomes [34, 36–44]. Age at presentation has been implicated in outcome. Ohnishi et al. studied the effect of the age at the time of surgical intervention on outcomes following arthroscopic saucerization [36]. Their study included 52 consecutive patients and had a mean follow-up of 30 months. They reported that younger patients, specifically <13 years old, had significantly better postoperative patient-reported outcome measures (PROMs). The authors suggest that a later presentation and intervention are negative prognostic indicators due to advanced tissue degeneration and inferior remodeling potential. Yoo et al. echoes these results, reporting patients younger than 10 years of age as a positive prognostic factor [43]. Fu et al. also report a higher incidence of articular cartilage lesions in patients with delayed presentation or symptoms >6 months [44]. Regardless of age, timely intervention is warranted to prevent further damage and progression of pathology to both the meniscus and cartilage.

The indication of meniscal stabilization in addition to a saucerization procedure is less elucidated. In general, instability noted on arthroscopic evaluation is generally surgically addressed. Carter et al. reported on the short-term outcomes in a cohort of patients who underwent arthroscopic saucerization and compared those who required stabilization versus saucerization alone [37]. Meniscal saucerization was performed in all 51 patients in study, and a repair/stabilization procedure was performed if instability was present (24 patients). Short-term PROMs and complication rates were equivalent in both groups. This suggests that meniscal instability can be addressed without a negative effect on the outcome. Yoo et al. also reported excellent mid-term outcomes in all patients who were indicated to either saucerization versus saucerization plus stabilization [43]. While there is no study that examines the direct effect of stabilization in unstable menisci, the current standard of care is to fix and stabilize menisci when instability is present.

Associated chondral injury or resultant osteochondritis dissecans (OCD) is a known postoperative sequela. [45] During saucerization, a significant portion of tissue is removed from a compartment that has been influenced by discoid meniscus throughout development. Once removed, the environment is affected, with immature chondrocytes on the femoral condyle and tibial plateau receiving drastically different contact stress patterns and impact. In addition, the alignment of the knee may shift to a more valgus position, as the lateral compartment is no longer overstuffed with meniscus [46]. Clinically significant sequalae of this phenomenon have only been described in case reports, however, and it remains unclear how the newly created surgical environment affects cartilage contact stress and gait mechanics in the long term [47].

Long-term outcomes remain satisfactory. Haskel et al. report a study of 21 patients with an average follow-up of 11 years [38]. They previously reported satisfactory outcomes at 2-year follow-up, but found a 37% reoperation rate and decreased PROMs as follow-up duration increased, with significantly higher knee pain and mechanical/functional limitations. It is unclear whether this is due to the effects of the surgery or the natural progression of the symptomatic discoid meniscus. Ahn et al. similarly report satisfactory clinical outcomes in 38 patients at a long-term follow-up of 10.1 years, but identify progressive degenerative changes in at least 40% of the patients [39]. Smuin et al. performed a systematic review with a meta-analysis on five long-term studies, comparing arthroscopic saucerization, saucerization with repair, and total meniscectomy [40]. The authors concluded that saucerization with and without repair are clinically equivalent in the long term, and that both groups outperform total meniscectomy.

Conclusion

The discoid meniscus is a congenital anomaly that predisposes affected patients to knee pain and dysfunction. Patients with symptomatic discoid menisci should undergo careful and timely evaluation and treatment. Arthroscopic saucerization with or without stabilization is currently the gold standard for surgical intervention, with total meniscectomy reserved for only unsalvageable meniscus pathology. Short- and long-term outcomes are satisfactory, but abnormal cartilage contract stresses may persist despite saucerization, predisposing to early arthritis. More research is needed in this area to determine the best surgical techniques to address discoid meniscus and instability in an effort to enhance long-term knee preservation.

References

1. Jordan MR. Lateral meniscal variants: evaluation and treatment. J Am Acad Orthop Surg. 1996;4(4):191–200.
2. Young RB. The external semilunar cartilage as a complete disc. In: Cleland J, Mackay JY, Young RB, editors. Memoirs and memoranda in anatomy. London: Williams and Norgate; 1889. p. 179. 31(12):2327–34. https://10.0.3.248/j.arthro.2015.06.032. Epub 2015 Aug 28.
3. Middleton DS. Congenital disc-shaped lateral meniscus with snapping knee. Br J Surg. 1936;24:246–55.
4. Liu WX, Zhao JZ, Huangfu XQ, He YH, Yang XG. Prevalence of bilateral involvement in patients with discoid lateral meniscus: a systematic literature review. Acta Orthop Belg. 2016;83(1):153–60.
5. Kim JG, Han SW, Lee DH. Diagnosis and treatment of discoid meniscus. Knee Surg Relat Res. 2016;28(4):255–62. https://doi.org/10.5792/ksrr.16.050.
6. Rao SK, Sripathi Rao P. Clinical, radiologic and arthroscopic assessment and treatment of bilateral discoid lateral meniscus. Knee Surg Sports Traumatol Arthrosc. 2007;15(5):597–601.
7. Kini SG, Walker P, Bruce W. Bilateral symptomatic discoid medial meniscus of the knee: a case report and review of literature. Arch Trauma Res. 2015;4:e27115.
8. Vandermeer RD, Cunningham FK. Arthroscopic treatment of the discoid lateral meniscus: results of long-term follow-up. Arthroscopy. 1989;5(2):101–9.
9. Kim SJ, Lee YT, Kim DW. Intraarticular anatomic variants associated with discoid meniscus in Koreans. Clin Orthop Relat Res. 1998;356:202–7.
10. Atanda A Jr, Wallace M, Bober MB, Mackenzie W. Arthroscopic treatment of discoid lateral meniscus tears in children with achondroplasia. J Pediatr Orthop. 2016;36(5):e55–8. https://doi.org/10.1097/BPO.0000000000000622.
11. Takigami J, Hashimoto Y, Tomihara T, Yamasaki S, Tamai K, Kondo K, Nakamura H. Predictive factors for osteochondritis dissecans of the lateral femoral condyle concurrent with a discoid lateral meniscus. Knee Surg Sports Traumatol Arthrosc. 2018;26(3):799–805. https://doi.org/10.1007/s00167-017-4451-8. Epub 2017 Feb 14.
12. Chen G, Zhang Z, Li J. Symptomatic discoid lateral meniscus: a clinical and arthroscopic study in a Chinese population. BMC Musculoskelet Disord. 2016;17:329. https://doi.org/10.1186/s12891-016-1188-3.
13. Sabbag OD, Hevesi M, Sanders TL, Camp CL, Dahm DL, Levy BA, Stuart MJ, Krych AJ. Incidence and treatment trends of symptomatic discoid lateral menisci: an 18-year population-based study. Orthop J Sports Med. 2018;6(9):2325967118797886. https://doi.org/10.1177/2325967118797886. eCollection 2018 Sep.
14. Le Minor JM. Comparative morphology of the lateral meniscus of the knee in primates. J Anat. 1990;170:161–71.
15. Atay OA, Pekmezci M, Doral MN, et al. Discoid meniscus: an ultrastructural study with transmission electron microscopy. Am J Sports Med. 2007;35:475–8.
16. Bisicchia S, Botti F, Tudisco C. Discoid lateral meniscus in children and adolescents: a histological study. J Exp Orthop. 2018;5(1):39. https://doi.org/10.1186/s40634-018-0153-5.
17. Nathan PA, Cole SC. Discoid meniscus: a clinical and pathological study. Clin Orthop Relat Res. 1969;64:107–13.

18. Papadopoulos A, Kirkos JM, Kapetanos GA. Histomorphologic study of discoid meniscus. Arthroscopy. 2009;25(3):262–8.
19. Rohren EM, Kosarek FJ, Helms CA. Discoid lateral meniscus and the frequency of meniscal tears. Skelet Radiol. 2001;30:316–20.
20. Watanabe M, Takeda SJ, Ikeuchi HJ. Atlas of arthroscopy. 2nd ed. Igaku-Shoin Ltd: Tokyo; 1969.
21. Klingele KE, Kocher MS, Hresko MT, Gerbino P, Micheli LJ. Discoid lateral meniscus: prevalence of peripheral rim instability. J Pediatr Orthop. 2004;24(1):79–82.
22. Lau BC, Vashon T, Janghala A, Pandya NK. The sensitivity and specificity of preoperative history, physical examination, and magnetic resonance imaging to predict articular cartilage injuries in symptomatic discoid lateral meniscus. J Pediatr Orthop. 2018;38(9):e501–6. https://doi.org/10.1097/BPO.0000000000001221.
23. Kim SJ, Hwang BY, Choi DH, et al. The paradoxical McMurray test for the detection of meniscal tears: an arthroscopic of mechanisms, types, and accuracy. J Bone Joint Surg Am. 2012;94:1181–7.
24. Aichroth PM, Patel DV, Marx CL. Congenital discoid lateral meniscus in children. A follow-up study and evolution of management. Bone Joint J. 1991;73:932–6.
25. Ha CW, Lee YS, Park JC. The condylar cutoff sign: quantifying lateral femoral condylar hypoplasia in a complete discoid meniscus. Clin Orthop Relat Res. 2009;467(5):1365–9. https://doi.org/10.1007/s11999-008-0447-5. Epub 2008 Aug 20.
26. Samoto N, Kozuma M, Tokuhisa T, Kobayashi K. Diagnosis of discoid lateral meniscus of the knee on MR imaging. Magn Reson Imaging. 2002;20(1):59–64.
27. Singh K, Helms CA, Jacobs MT, Higgins LD. MRI appearance of Wrisberg variant of discoid lateral meniscus. AJR Am J Roentgenol. 2006;187(2):384–7.
28. Yilgor C, Atay OA, Ergen B, Doral MN. Comparison of magnetic resonance imaging findings with arthroscopic findings in discoid meniscus. Knee Surg Sports Traumatol Arthrosc. 2014;22(2):268–73. https://doi.org/10.1007/s00167-013-2371-9. Epub 2013 Jan 22.
29. Manzione M, Pizzutillo PD, Peoples AB, Schweizer PA. Meniscectomy in children: a long-term follow-up study. Am J Sports Med. 1983;11(3):111–5.
30. Räber DA, Friederich NF, Hefti F. Discoid lateral meniscus in children. Long-term follow-up after total meniscectomy. J Bone Joint Surg Am. 1998;80(11):1579–86.
31. Song IS, Kim JB, Lee JK, Park BS. Discoid medial meniscus tear, with a literature review of treatments. Knee Surg Relat Res. 2017;29(3):237–42. https://doi.org/10.5792/ksrr.15.054.
32. Hayashi LK, Yamaga H, Ida K, Miura T. Arthroscopic meniscectomy for discoid lateral meniscus in children. J Bone Joint Surg Am. 1988;70(10):1495–500.
33. Kocher MS, Logan CA, Kramer DE. Discoid lateral meniscus in children: diagnosis, management, and outcomes. J Am Acad Orthop Surg. 2017;25(11):736–43. https://doi.org/10.5435/JAAOS-D-15-00491.
34. Wong T, Wang CJ. Functional analysis on the treatment of torn discoid lateral meniscus. Knee. 2011;18(6):369–72. https://doi.org/10.1016/j.knee.2010.07.002. Epub 2010 Aug 8.
35. Sugawara O, Miyatsu M, Yamashita I, Takemitsu Y, Onozawa T. Problems with repeated arthroscopic surgery in the discoid meniscus. Arthroscopy. 1991;7(1):68–71.
36. Ohnishi Y, Nakashima H, Suzuki H, Nakamura E, Sakai A, Uchida S. Arthroscopic treatment for symptomatic lateral discoid meniscus: the effects of different ages, groups and procedures on surgical outcomes. Knee. 2018;5(6):1083–90. https://doi.org/10.1016/j.knee.2018.06.003.
37. Carter CW, Hoellwarth J, Weiss JM. Clinical outcomes as a function of meniscal stability in the discoid meniscus: a preliminary report. J Pediatr Orthop. 2012;32(1):9–14. https://doi.org/10.1097/BPO.0b013e31823d8338.
38. Haskel JD, Uppstrom TJ, Dare DM, Rodeo SA, Green DW. Decline in clinical scores at long-term follow-up of arthroscopically treated discoid lateral meniscus in children. Knee Surg Sports Traumatol Arthrosc. 2018;26(10):2906–11. https://doi.org/10.1007/s00167-017-4825-y. Epub 2018 Jan 5.
39. Ahn JH, Kim KI, Wang JH, Jeon JW, Cho YC, Lee SH. Long-term results of arthroscopic reshaping for symptomatic discoid lateral meniscus in children. Arthroscopy. 2015;31(5):867–73.

40. Smuin DM, Swenson RD, Dhawan A. Saucerization versus complete resection of a symptomatic discoid lateral meniscus at short- and long-term follow-up: a systematic review. Arthroscopy. 2017;33(9):1733–42. https://doi.org/10.1016/j.arthro.2017.03.028.
41. Good CR, Green DW, Griffith MH, Valen AW, Widmann RF, Rodeo SA. Arthroscopic treatment of symptomatic discoid meniscus in children: classification, technique, and results. Arthroscopy. 2007;23(2):157–63.
42. Lee CR, Bin SI, Kim JM, Lee BS, Kim NK. Arthroscopic partial meniscectomy in young patients with symptomatic discoid lateral meniscus: an average 10-year follow-up study. Arch Orthop Trauma Surg. 2018;138(3):369–76. https://doi.org/10.1007/s00402-017-2853-1. Epub 2017 Nov 29.
43. Yoo WJ, Jang WY, Park MS, Chung CY, Cheon JE, Cho TJ, Choi IH. Arthroscopic treatment for symptomatic discoid meniscus in children: midterm outcomes and prognostic factors. Arthroscopy. 2015;31(12):2327–34.
44. Fu D, Guo L, Yang L, et al. Discoid lateral meniscus tears and concomitant articular cartilage lesions in the knee. Arthroscopy. 2014;30:311–8.
45. Stanitski CL, Bee J. Juvenile osteochondritis dissecans of the lateral femoral condyle after lateral discoid meniscal surgery. Am J Sports Med. 2004;32:797–801. https://doi.org/10.1177/0363546503261728.
46. Zhang P, Zhao Q, Shang X, Wang Y. Effect of arthroscopic resection for discoid lateral meniscus on the axial alignment of the lower limb. Int Orthop. 2018;42(8):1897–903. https://doi.org/10.1007/s00264-018-3944-5.
47. Harato K, Sakurai A, Kudo Y, Nagura T, Masumoto K, Otani T, Niki Y. Three-dimensional knee kinematics in patients with a discoid lateral meniscus during gait. Knee. 2016;23(4):622–6. https://doi.org/10.1016/j.knee.2015.10.007. Epub 2016 Mar 12.

Meniscal Allograft Transplantation: Indications, Techniques, and Outcomes

Matthew T. Kingery and Eric J. Strauss

Introduction

I. S. Smillie, the Scottish surgeon who pioneered the operative treatment of meniscus injuries, wrote that "treatment consists of excision of the meniscus; and the sooner the torn degenerate structure is removed, the better is the immediate and long-term result." [1] Yet, well before Smillie performed his 6500th total meniscectomy in 1965, T. J. Fairbank's radiographic analysis of meniscectomized patients revealed evidence that removing the meniscus leads to unintended consequences [2]. Fairbank described flattening of the femoral condyle, formation of a ridge on the femoral condyle, and joint space narrowing, suggesting that meniscectomy alters the biomechanics of the knee in such a way that the articular surfaces are overloaded [2]. The early progression of arthritic changes observed in early meniscus-deficient patients were then supported by long-term studies that showed unsatisfactory functional outcomes and a high risk of eventual total knee arthroplasty [3–5].

Although patients often report good clinical outcomes following surgery, meniscectomy leads to degeneration of the cartilage and subchondral bone in as little as 5 years, due to the disruption of normal knee kinematics [6–9]. As increasingly large amounts of meniscus are removed from the knee, the contact area between the tibia and femur decreases, causing a subsequent increase in tibiofemoral contact stress [10]. Biomechanical studies have demonstrated that intra-articular contact stresses double following medial meniscectomy and triple following lateral meniscectomy [11–15]. Peak contact pressure increases proportionally to the percentage of meniscus removed and damage to articular cartilage occurs at the area of peak

M. T. Kingery (✉) · E. J. Strauss
Division of Sports Medicine, Department of Orthopaedic Surgery, NYU Langone Health, New York, NY, USA
e-mail: Matthew.Kingery@nyulangone.org; Eric.Strauss@nyulangone.org

© Springer Nature Switzerland AG 2020
E. J. Strauss, L. M. Jazrawi (eds.), *The Management of Meniscal Pathology*,
https://doi.org/10.1007/978-3-030-49488-9_9

contact pressure, illustrating the impaired ability of meniscus deficient knees to accommodate stress [10, 16, 17].

The intact meniscus plays several roles related to the overall health and function of the knee. Removing the meniscus in whole or part weakens the ability of the meniscus to perform each of these roles optimally. In addition to increasing the contact area of the tibiofemoral joint and diminishing the intra-articular shock absorption [10], meniscectomy destabilizes the knee joint. The native meniscus acts an important secondary stabilizer to protect against anterior–posterior motion of the joint, and medial meniscectomy yields a significant increase in anterior tibial translation, especially in ACL-deficient knees [18]. The meniscus also assists with lubrication of the knee joint and contains mechanoreceptors that provide proprioception, both of which are compromised following meniscectomy [19, 20].

The end result of altered knee mechanics, excessive contact forces, and impaired joint stability is a significantly increased risk of osteoarthritis in meniscus deficient knees [21]. Forty years after undergoing total meniscectomy with Dr. Smillie, a cohort of 53 of his patients were evaluated in what is the longest available follow-up duration of meniscus-deficient patients to date. Clinical and radiographic evaluation revealed that meniscectomy was associated with a fourfold increase in risk of developing osteoarthritis and a 132-fold increase in the rate of total knee arthroplasty compared to a matched cohort [5].

Despite the deleterious effects of meniscectomy, the procedure clearly continues to play an important role in the treatment of symptomatic meniscus injuries. While the management of meniscus injuries has shifted away from total meniscectomy in favor of preserving tissue or repairing tears whenever possible, there are situations in which meniscectomy is warranted. For patients with symptomatic meniscus tears that are poor candidates for repair, meniscectomy remains the best option. However, given the association between meniscus deficiency and osteoarthritis, there is an obvious role for a procedure that protects the articular cartilage from future degradation.

Several of the first recorded attempts to replace an injured meniscus occurred in 1916 and 1933 by several surgeons who performed autologous fat flap interpositional arthroplasties [22]. In the early 1900s, complete knee transplantations included meniscal allografts [23]. In the 1980s, surgeons attempted to repair tibial plateau fractures with large osteochondral allografts that included the meniscus [24]. The first meniscal allograft transplants (MAT) resembling modern techniques were reported by Milachowski in 1989. The author concluded that MAT is a safe and effective procedure for restoring stability and function to meniscus deficient knees [22].

Roughly 30 years after Milachowski presented his cohort of successful MATs, the procedure has become an established method of optimizing knee function and protecting against the long-term consequences of meniscectomy. Animal models have demonstrated that MAT, whether performed immediately after meniscectomy or in delayed fashion, slows the rate of degenerative chondral changes but does not cease articular degeneration completely [25, 26]. The same chondroprotective benefits have yet to be definitively demonstrated in humans. However, for young patients with irreparable meniscal tears or who have previously undergone meniscectomy in the setting of maintained articular surfaces, MAT can be used to successfully increase the tibiofemoral contact area, decrease contract stress, and restore the physiologic mechanics of the knee [13, 27–29].

Indications and Contraindications

Indications

In general, meniscal allograft transplantations are performed in young patients who present with symptomatic meniscal deficiency [30, 31]. The deficiency in this patient population is typically the result of a recurrent tear, failed attempt at repair, or a complex meniscal injury leading to total or subtotal meniscectomy. Patients will often present with a history of multiple ipsilateral knee injuries with associated ligament or cartilage pathology, as well as a failed trial of nonoperative management. MAT is most often performed in patients that are deemed too young for unicondylar or total knee arthroplasty who want to restore normal knee mechanics.

The indications for the procedure include an absent or nonfunctioning meniscus causing activity-related pain in nonobese patients less than 50 years of age. Although ideally patients selected for MAT have Outerbridge grade II articular changes or less in the affected compartment, there is evidence to suggest that patients with advanced articular cartilage degradation should not be excluded from MAT [32, 33]. While MAT is thought to be chondroprotective, prophylactic transplantation in asymptomatic meniscus-deficient patients is not currently an accepted indication.

Contraindications

Contraindications for MAT include age greater than 50 years, flattening of the femoral condyle or tibial plateau (Fairbank changes on plain radiographs), osteophytes or other architectural changes, inflammatory arthritis, synovial disease, preoperative loss of knee extension greater than 5°, preoperative flexion less than 125°, and obesity due to concern that the elevated level of stress would increase risk of graft failure [30, 31, 34–37]. As discussed above, advanced articular disease with Outerbridge grade III or IV changes has typically been used as a contraindication to MAT, although this may not be necessary, as concomitant cartilage repair procedures can be performed [32, 33]. It should be noted that many of the generally accepted contraindications for MAT are theoretical and there is no objective data demonstrating inferior outcomes with these comorbidities.

Although intact ligaments, normal lower extremity alignment, and pristine cartilage make preoperative planning for the MAT more straightforward, combinations of associated knee pathology do not exclude patients from transplantation. However, these associated injuries must be addressed either concurrently with MAT or in a staged fashion. When malalignment, ligamentous instability, and focal chondral defects are not corrected, the success of the MAT is limited. When these pathologies are addressed simultaneously, clinical outcomes are not different than performing the procedures in isolation [38–47].

Patients with meniscus deficiency and abnormal lower extremity alignment should have corrective osteotomy performed at the time of meniscus transplant or in a staged fashion with osteotomy preceding the MAT by several months [48, 49]. Similarly, patients with injuries of both the meniscus and one or more ligaments should undergo simultaneous meniscal transplant and ligament reconstruction [50]. An isolated chondral lesion is also not a contraindication for surgery, provided that a cartilage-restoring procedure, such as an osteochondral allograft transplantation or autologous chondrocyte implantation, is also performed [45, 51, 52].

Graft Preparation

Processing and Preservation

There are a variety of methods for processing and preserving meniscal allografts prior to implantation. As MAT becomes more common, optimizing this process will become critical in order to ensure that allografts are readily available in a variety of sizes that can be matched with the recipient's anatomy.

There are four methods currently available for preservation of meniscal allografts. Lyophilization, in which grafts are dehydrated and frozen in a vacuum, has been associated with a greater risk of effusion and synovitis compared to alternative methods of graft preservation [22, 53]. The process destroys the viable cell population, and after implantation these grafts undergo remodeling which causes the meniscus to shrink [54–56]. This process is no longer recommended for MAT.

Cryopreservation involves freezing the grafts using dimethyl sulfide or glycerol. This process preserves viable chondrocytes, but metabolic activity of the cells decreases with longer storage times [57]. In vitro studies have demonstrated that the process of cryopreservation does not affect the ultrastructure of the meniscus and likely does not alter the biomechanical properties, but the population of viable cells is highly variable and unpredictable at the time of implantation [58]. Further studies of cryopreservation have shown that the preservation process induces an apoptosis-mediated decreased in the cell population [59]. The clinical implications of these findings are not currently well understood.

Fresh allografts must be harvested within 12 hours of cold ischemia time, and can then be stored at 4 °C for 7 days before there is loss of viable cells. These grafts contain the greatest number of viable cells, which is thought to help maintain the mechanical integrity of the graft [23, 56].

The most easily available, and generally most cost-effective, type of graft is the fresh-frozen allograft [60, 61]. These menisci are harvested and stored at −80 °C. Animal models have shown that at 4 weeks after implantation, there are no appreciable donor fibrochondrocytes remaining in fresh-frozen allografts, but host cells have populated the graft by this time point [62].

Irradiation of the graft was previously recommended, but is no longer performed due to studies demonstrating deleterious effects on the mechanical properties of the graft [40, 63–66]. Furthermore, immune-matching of the donor and recipient was originally performed in early cases of MAT, but was eventually found to provide no additional benefit, and is therefore no longer required [18, 67]. Rejection of the allograft is rare, as the meniscus is believed to be immune-privileged, perhaps because the chondrocytes are embedded in a dense proteoglycan network and less accessible to host immune cells [23, 68].

Sizing

Graft sizing is one of the most critical aspects of MAT because the size of the graft is closely associated with the resulting biomechanics, and suboptimal contact forces can negatively affect functional outcomes. The meniscus allograft should be sized to closely match the native meniscus, with meniscus width being the most important dimension. A study of lateral meniscus allografts demonstrated that oversized grafts prevent compressive forces from being appropriately distributed across the joint and may lead to excessive stress on the cartilage. Conversely, undersized grafts lead to excessive forces across the meniscus allograft itself, increasing the risk of postoperative tearing and failure [69]. Most studies conclude that mismatches of graft size within 10% of the native meniscus size are acceptable [69].

Until recently, the most common method of preoperative allograft sizing was performed using plain radiographs and the Pollard technique, originally described by Matthew Pollard in 1995 [70]. With this technique, the medial meniscus width is determined from the AP radiograph as the distance between one vertical line that runs tangent to the most medial aspect of the tibial metaphysis and another vertical line that runs through the peak of the medial tibial spine. Lateral meniscus width is measured using corresponding points on the lateral tibial metaphysis and lateral tibial spine (Fig. 9.1). The lines used for width sizing should be perpendicular to the joint line and parallel to each other. Basing meniscal width on the edge of the metaphysis, rather than the joint space, helps to avoid measurement errors associated with osteophytes in patients with arthritis [70].

Meniscus length is determined on a lateral radiograph as the distance between most anterior point of the tibia superior to the tuberosity and a line tangent to the posterior aspect of the tibia at the level of the joint line. These lines should be parallel and, if the knees are extended, posteriorly tilted approximately 7° to align with the normal anatomic orientation of the tibial joint surface in the sagittal plane. Because the true length of the meniscus does not extend to these bony landmarks, the measured distance is then multiplied by 0.8 for medial meniscus sizing or 0.7 for lateral meniscus sizing [70].

While the method outlined by Pollard continues to be a useful technique for graft sizing in situations where the surgeon must rely on radiographs, follow-up

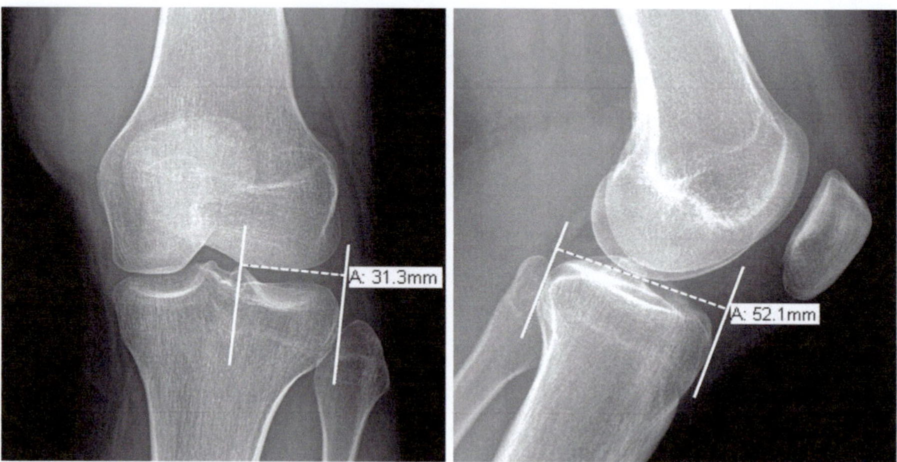

Fig. 9.1 Pollard technique of lateral meniscus sizing. The width of the lateral meniscus is measured as 31.3 mm in this patient. The measured length of 52.1 mm is multiplied by a factor of 0.7 for lateral menisci, which gives a corrected length of 36.5 mm. (*Source*: Kingery, Matthew. 2019)

studies have often failed to reproduce the reported level of accuracy originally associated with this technique [71, 72]. As a result, MRI sizing has become more common and is now generally regarded as the gold standard due to its superior accuracy [73–76]. In a direct comparison of several meniscal allograft–sizing techniques, the Pollard technique was found to significantly overestimate the width and length of the lateral meniscus. The Pollard technique is therefore not recommended for lateral meniscus sizing. If a plain radiograph must be used (e.g., MRI is not available), a mathematical correction to the Pollard technique has been developed and found to yield more accurate measurements [77, 78]. For the medial meniscus, the Pollard technique was found to be comparable to MRI sizing [77]. However, it is important to note that deviation from true AP and lateral views on the radiograph significantly decreases the accuracy of measurements [76].

Regardless of the method used to size the allograft, each dimension should be measured independently as length cannot be used to accurately predict width of the meniscus [79]. If a patient has already undergone meniscectomy and the native ipsilateral meniscus cannot be measured, the size can be approximated using the contralateral meniscus, although there are often differences between meniscus sizes within individuals [80]. One group developed a formula based on patient height, weight, and gender to mathematically predict meniscus dimensions. Although likely less reliable than MRI measurements, this remains an option for patients with bilateral meniscal deficiency, making imaging-based measurements difficult [81]. Measurements are sent to the tissue bank and an offer for a size-matched allograft is returned to the physician (Fig. 9.2).

FRESH FROZEN CRYOPRESERVED (FFC) ALLOGRAFT
OFFER FORM

Physician: Strauss, Eric	Patient: ▮▮▮▮▮▮
Graft Type Requested: Lateral Meniscus w/ Bone Block, Right	
Graft Type Offered: Lateral Meniscus w/ Bone Block, Right	
ID#: ▮▮▮▮▮▮	Graft Expiration Date:12/22/2016

Patient Size: TW= N/A, W= 3.50cm, L= 3.40cm, (This size is based on the patient's films or other provided)

Donor Size: TW=N/A, W= 3.40cm, L= 3.30cm (This is the offered graft's size)

Comments: NA

JRF Representative: ▮▮▮▮▮▮▮▮   Offer Date: 2/5/2014

Fig. 9.2 Size-matched meniscal allograft offer from the tissue bank. (*Source*: Strauss, Eric. 2014)

Surgical Technique

When first introduced, MAT was performed through an arthrotomy and involved splitting the collateral ligament. In 1994, Shelton first described the arthroscopic approach that eventually replaced the open approach and remains in use today [82]. Following the approach and introduction of the graft into the joint, the meniscus is fixated using one of several techniques. The method used to fixate the meniscal allograft is thought to be closely associated with the resultant biomechanical alterations and postoperative outcomes [29, 83].

Historically, stabilization of the graft was often achieved by suturing the donor meniscus to the recipient meniscal remnant without fixation of the anterior and posterior horns, or with stabilization of the horns with suture tied over a button or bone bridge [56, 84]. The soft tissue fixation technique, however, is no longer recommended as studies have demonstrated that securing both meniscal horns is required to achieve intra-articular contact pressures that most closely approximate the load-bearing function of an intact meniscus [85]. Without any form of bony fixation, the load transmission profile of the knee after MAT resembles the meniscus-deficient knee, and any biomechanical advantage provided by meniscus transplant is lost [29]. Cadaveric studies have also suggested that bone plug fixation provides greater strength than soft-tissue fixation [29, 86].

Bony fixation of the allograft, therefore, is thought to be an essential component of a successful MAT. There are currently two techniques that are used to achieve bony, anatomic fixation of the horns. In the bridge-in-slot technique, the meniscal horns remain attached to a single bone block. This allows the original anatomic orientation of the meniscal horns to be maintained during implantation, which is believed to optimize the ability of the meniscus to accommodate hoop stresses [15]. The bone plug technique involves bone tunnels drilled in the proximal tibia to accept bone plugs attached to the anterior and posterior meniscal horns. This technique is more technically demanding given the additional challenge of achieving proper tunnel placement. The bridge-in-slot technique is most commonly used for isolated lateral MATs. Although the bridge-in-slot can also be used for isolated medial

MATs and has been shown to yield the same biomechanical results as the bone plug technique [13], the proximity of the ACL insertion often requires debridement of ACL fibers to achieve bridge-in-slot fixation. Therefore, bony fixation using bone plugs is often preferred for medial MATs.

As discussed previously, when meniscus insufficiency is accompanied by an associated ligament or focal chondral injury, both pathologies should be addressed appropriately. When meniscal transplantation is performed with a concomitant ACL reconstruction, the bone plug technique is preferred for both medial and lateral allografts in order to avoid interference between the bone bridge and the tibial ACL tunnel. For patients that require an alignment-correcting osteotomy, the operation is typically performed in a staged fashion. The surgeon should first correct the valgus or varus deformity and allow the patient to recover for 4 to 6 months before returning to the operating room for the MAT. Patients presenting with both meniscal deficiency and focal osteochondral defects should undergo concomitant MAT and cartilage restoration procedure. Autologous chondrocyte implantation and osteochondral allograft implantation can be performed simultaneously with the MAT and do not dictate which method of bony fixation is used.

Bridge-in-Slot Technique for Lateral MAT

Positioning

With the patient in the supine position on the table, the operative leg is placed in a circumferential leg holder and the foot of the table is dropped (Fig. 9.3). This allows the leg to be maneuvered during the procedure to provide unobstructed access to the

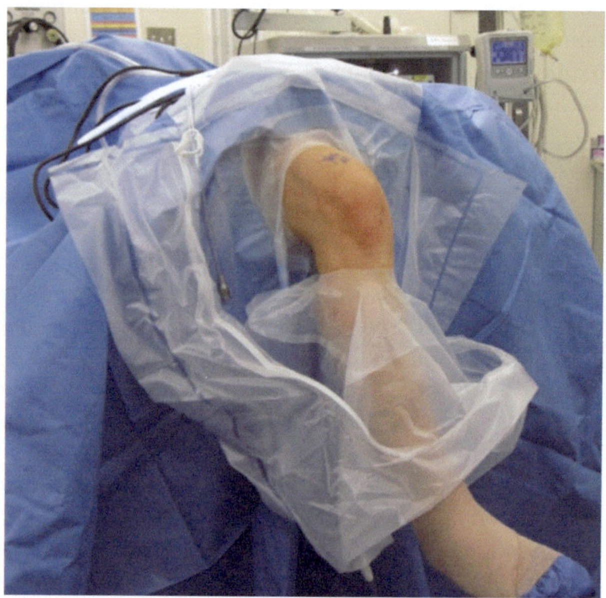

Fig. 9.3 The patient is positioned with the foot of the table dropped to allow access to the posteromedial and posterolateral aspects of the knee. (*Source*: Jazrawi, Laith. 2014)

posteromedial and posterolateral aspects of the knee for the allograft repair portion of the procedure. A folded blanket is placed under the proximal thigh of the contralateral leg to bring the hip into slight flexion and prevent any tension on the femoral nerve. A tourniquet is placed on the thigh of the operative leg, which is prepped and draped in a sterile fashion. Appropriate anatomic landmarks are then marked on the operative knee, including the site of the posterolateral incision.

Diagnostic Arthroscopy and Meniscus Debridement

Using anterolateral and anteromedial portal sites, a diagnostic arthroscopy is performed. For lateral meniscal transplantations, the anteromedial portal site should be 1 mm to 2 mm superior to the standard anteromedial portal site to facilitate access to the lateral compartment over the tibial spines. The meniscal deficiency is confirmed and the condition of the articular cartilage is assessed before proceeding.

If the diagnostic arthroscopy reveals the presence of meniscus remnant, an arthroscopic biter and standard 4.5 mm shaver are used to debride the native meniscus down to a 1 mm to 2 mm peripheral rim until punctate bleeding occurs (Fig. 9.4). In cases where there is no remnant meniscus, a rasp is used to abrade the capsule until a bleeding bed is created to encourage tissue healing.

Graft Preparation

As the arthroscopy and debridement are being performed, the allograft is prepared on the back table (Fig. 9.5). The attachment sites of the meniscus graft to the bone block are first identified. A cutting block, bridge-sizing guide, and sagittal saw are used to create a bone bridge that measures 7 mm in width by 10 mm in depth and connects the anterior and posterior meniscal horns. The lateral tibial spine is removed using a saw or rongeur. A #2 nonabsorbable suture is then passed through

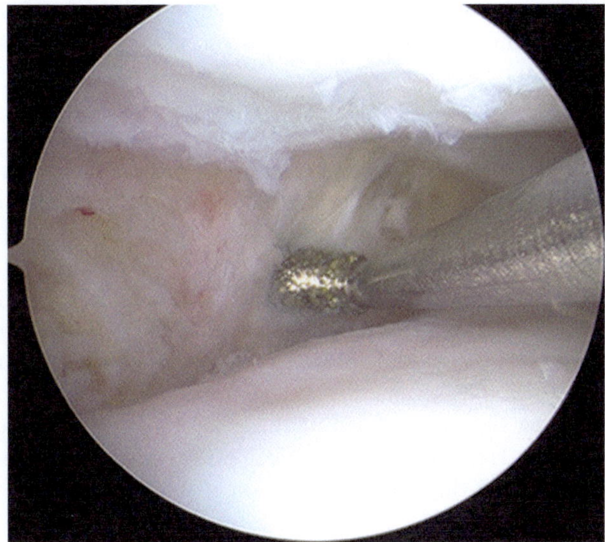

Fig. 9.4 The meniscal remnant is debrided, leaving a 1–2 mm peripheral rim to aid in fixation of the allograft. (*Source*: Jazrawi, Laith. 2014)

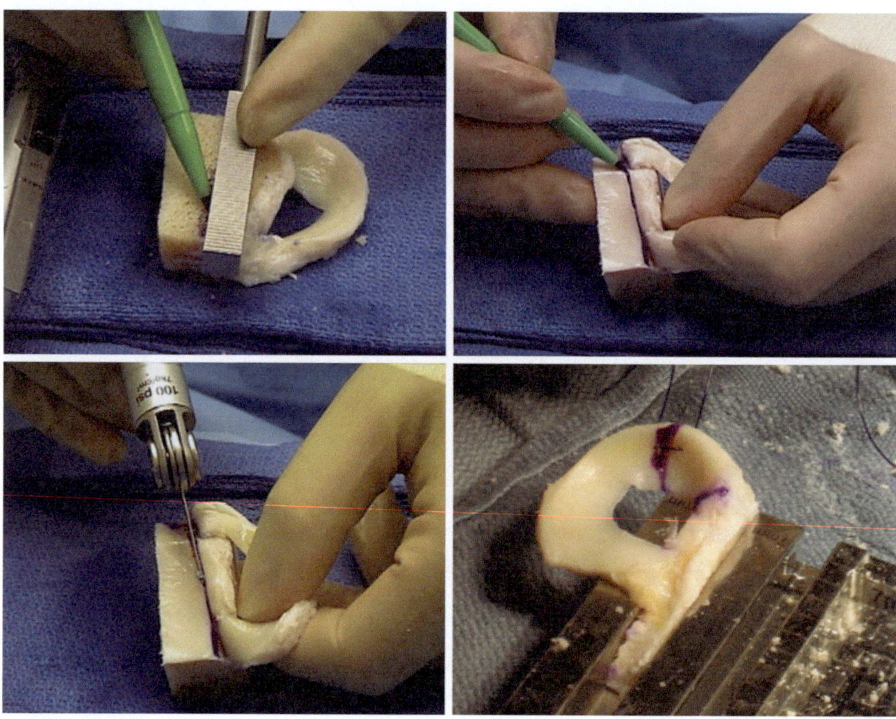

Fig. 9.5 Preparation of the meniscal allograft. The bone bridge is measured, marked, and cut before placing a suture through the graft to facilitate passage into the joint. (*Source*: Jazrawi, Laith. 2014)

the meniscus at the point where the body of the allograft meets the posterior horn. This suture will be used to facilitate introduction of the meniscus into the knee. After being prepared, the allograft is placed in a basin with wet gauze until it is ready to be inserted.

Approach

The biceps femoris tendon is palpated and a posterolateral incision is made anterior to the tendon insertion to prevent injuring the common peroneal nerve (Fig. 9.6). The incision should be 3 inches in length with one-third of the incision above the joint line and two-thirds of the incision below the joint line. The interval between the posterior aspect of the iliotibial band and the biceps femoris tendon is identified with dissection. Through the identified interval, the lateral head of the gastrocnemius is palpated while plantarflexing and dorsiflexing the foot to confirm appropriate positioning. A space is created deep to the gastrocnemius to allow for an interval between the lateral head of the gastrocnemius and the posterolateral capsule. A spoon or Henning retractor is then inserted to protect the neighboring neurovascular structures during the repair portion of the procedure.

Fig. 9.6 Incision for the posterolateral approach is made anterior to the biceps femoris insertion to protect the common peroneal nerve. (*Source*: Jazrawi, Laith. 2014)

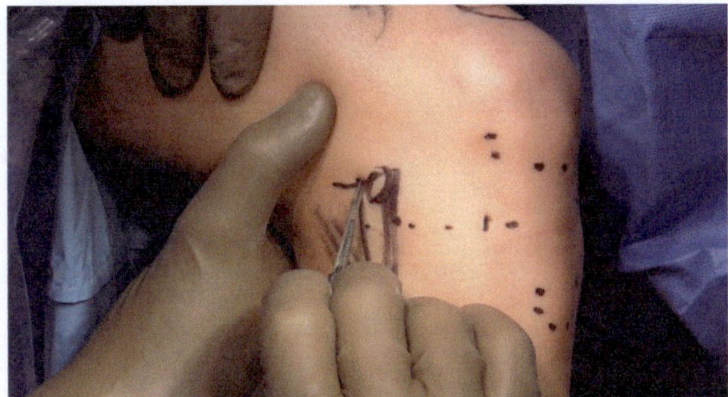

Fig. 9.7 Diagnostic arthroscopy and meniscus debridement is performed through the medial and lateral portal sites (1 and 2). An accessory anterolateral portal is created for slot preparation and eventual graft introduction (3). (*Source*: Jazrawi, Laith. 2014)

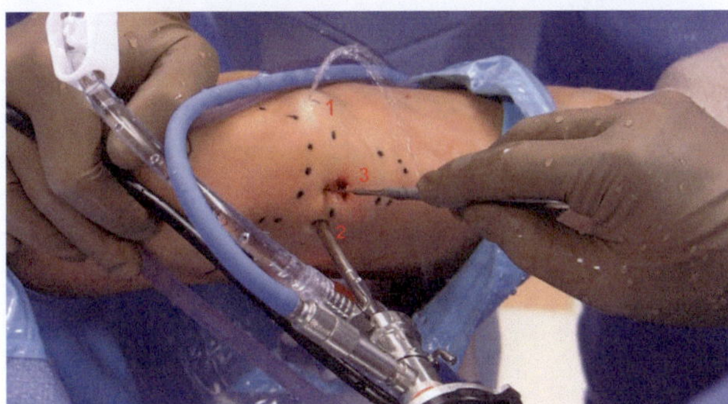

Slot Preparation

The bridge-in-slot technique aims to create a tibial slot based on the native meniscal attachment sites. Using a spinal needle to aid with localization, an anterolateral accessory portal is created in line with the anterior and posterior root insertions of the lateral meniscus (Fig. 9.7). A 4 mm bone-cutting shaver is inserted through the anterolateral accessory portal and used to create a superficial preliminary reference slot that connects the centers of the anterior and posterior horn attachment sites (Fig. 9.8). The reference slot should run parallel to the sagittal slope of the tibial plateau and reach a depth of 4 mm.

A hooked depth gauge is inserted through the anterolateral accessory portal and placed into the reference slot (Fig. 9.9). The hooked tip of the gauge should engage the posterior tibial cortex. A guide pin is inserted through the drill guide into the posterior tibial cortex, ensuring that the pin does not over-penetrate the cortex. Proper depth can be confirmed with direct palpation of the cortex through the posterolateral portal. Although not required, intraoperative fluoroscopy can also be used to confirm appropriate drill depth. The drill guide is removed and the pin is over-reamed with an 8 mm cannulated reamer. The drill bit and guide pin are then removed. Any remaining debris can be removed using an arthroscopic shaver or basket.

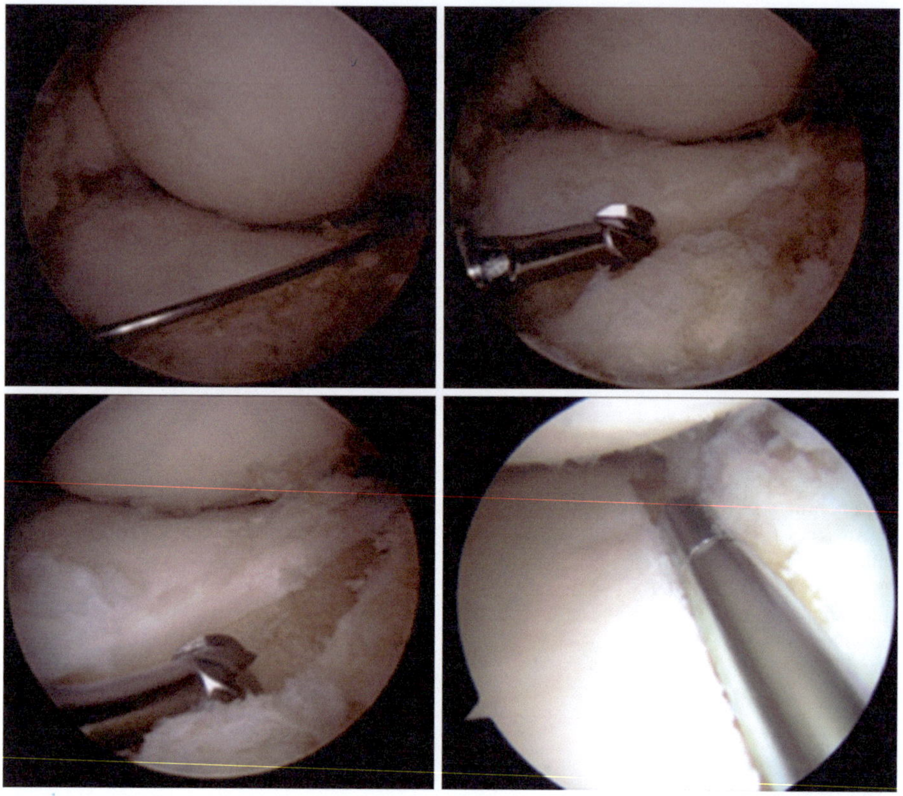

Fig. 9.8 A spinal needle is used to align the accessory anterolateral portal with the horns of the meniscus (top left). Creation of the superficial reference slot using a 4 mm burr to connect the sites of the anterior and posterior horns (top right and bottom). (*Source*: Jazrawi, Laith. 2014)

Fig. 9.9 A depth gauge is used to measure the anterior–posterior dimension of the plateau to prevent overpenetration of the pin. (*Source*: Jazrawi, Laith. 2014)

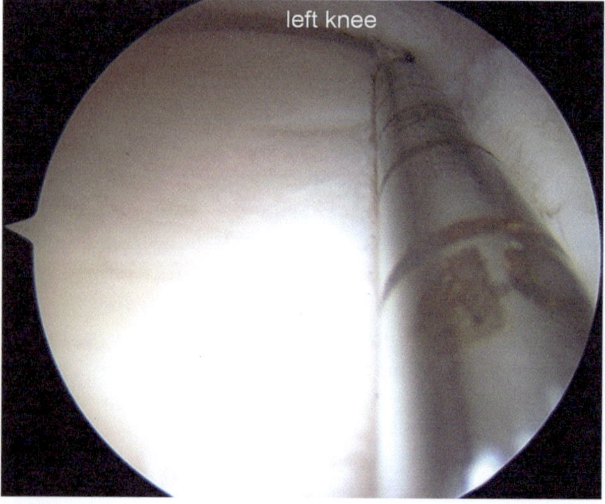

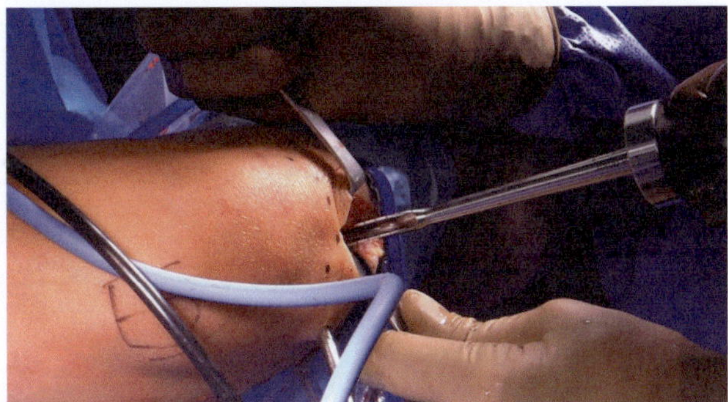

Fig. 9.10 The box chisel is inserted through the accessory anterolateral arthrotomy to create the final tibial slot. (*Source*: Jazrawi, Laith. 2014)

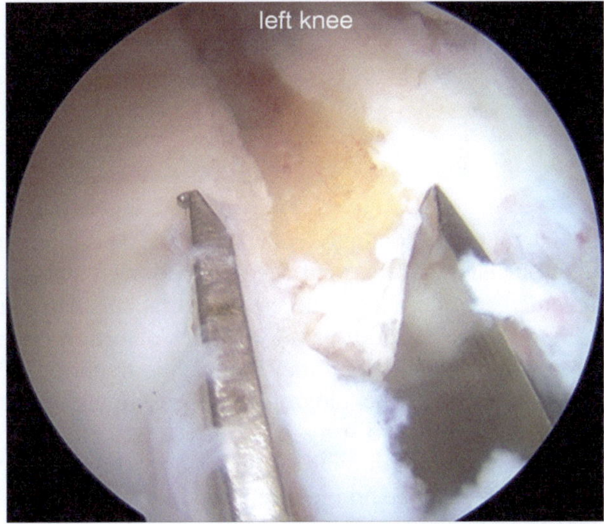

Fig. 9.11 Continuous arthroscopic visualization should be maintained as the box chisel is inserted into reamed tunnel. Care should be taken to avoid injuring the articular surface of the condyle. (*Source*: Jazrawi, Laith. 2014)

The final tibial slot is created using an 8 mm slot-cutting chisel (Fig. 9.10). The box chisel is gently impacted with a mallet along the course of the premade tunnel to the level of the posterior tibial cortex. The tines of the box chisel should be continuously visualized arthroscopically to ensure no damage to the surrounding tissue or opposing femoral articular cartilage (Fig. 9.11). The box chisel creates a rectangular slot measuring 8 mm in width and 10 mm in depth, matching the prepared bone bridge. To facilitate easy placement of the bone bridge, 7 and 8 mm rasps are used to enlarge the recipient slot until the 8 mm rasp sits flush with the tibial plateau (Fig. 9.12). The recipient slot is now complete.

Graft Introduction and Fixation

To prepare for introduction of the graft into the knee, the anterolateral accessory portal should first be extended into an arthrotomy large enough to permit passage of the graft. A zone-specific cannula is then placed into the medial portal. A meniscal repair needle is passed through the remnant of the native meniscus slightly anterior

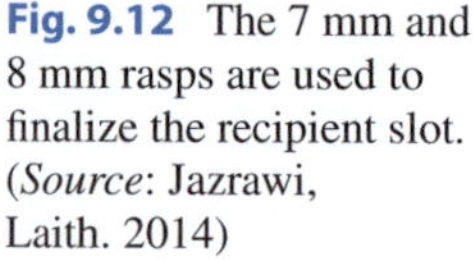

Fig. 9.12 The 7 mm and 8 mm rasps are used to finalize the recipient slot. (*Source*: Jazrawi, Laith. 2014)

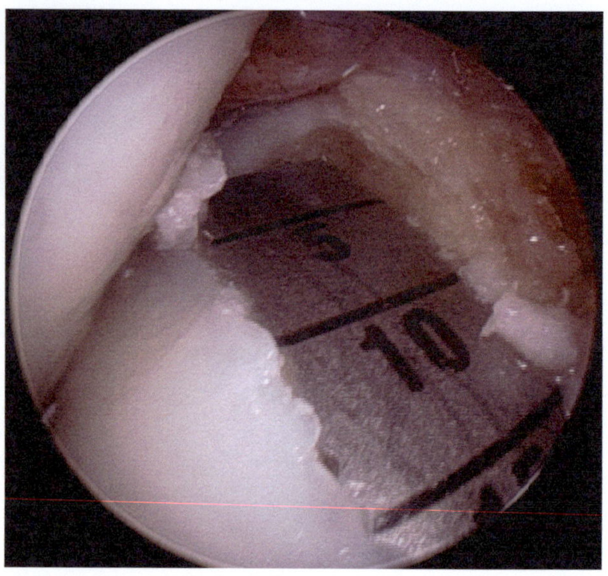

and lateral to the popliteus tendon. The needle is then retrieved through the posterolateral incision. The second needle is removed and the suture is retrieved through the enlarged anterolateral accessory portal site. This suture is tied into a loop and used to shuttle the graft passage sutures placed in the prepared meniscus allograft through the posterolateral incision. Gentle traction is maintained on the graft passage sutures while the allograft is passed through the arthrotomy and aligned with the recipient slot. Two army–navy retractors are used to maintain clear visualization of the recipient slot through the arthrotomy (Fig. 9.13). While applying varus stress to the knee, the bone bridge is reduced into the slot using gentle digital pressure and traction on the passage sutures. The knee can be cycled to aid with proper placement of the meniscus between the tibiofemoral articulation.

Once the allograft is in position, the meniscus is secured peripherally with 2–0 nonabsorbable sutures using multiple inside-out vertical mattress sutures (Fig. 9.14). Placing sutures on both the superior and inferior aspects of the meniscus allows the periphery of the graft to be closely approximated to the capsule in a balanced fashion. As the periphery is being secured, the sutures are retrieved through the posterolateral incision. An all-inside technique is then used to secure the graft directly posterior to the popliteus tendon and for fixation of the posterior horn.

After confirming that the periphery of the meniscus has been secured, the bone bridge is stabilized in the slot. A nitinol guide wire is first placed central to the bone bridge, and then a 7 × 23 mm bioabsorbable interference screw is used to achieve the final fixation of the bridge in the slot (Fig. 9.15).

The knee is placed in full extension and the meniscus repair sutures are tied. Maintaining visualization of the meniscus arthroscopically ensures that the sutures are placed directly on the capsule. Fixation of the most anterior aspect of the

Fig. 9.13 Graft introduction into the knee joint using passage sutures. (*Source*: Jazrawi, Laith. 2014)

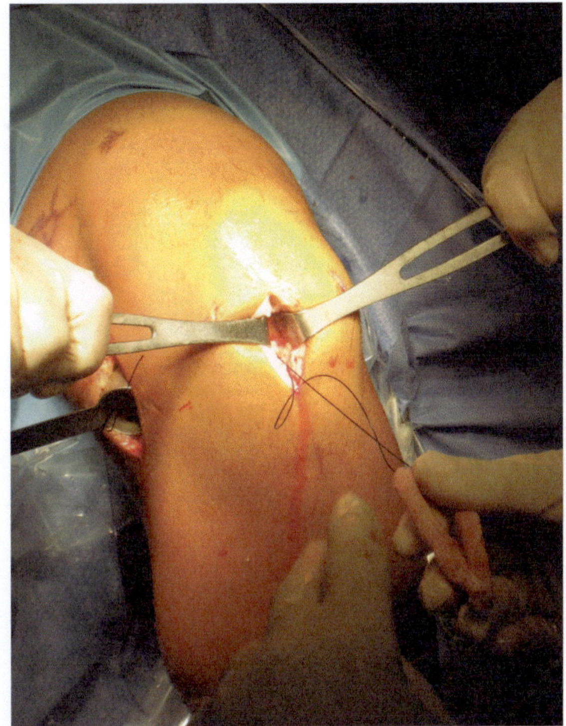

Fig. 9.14 Peripheral meniscal fixation using vertical mattress sutures through an open posterolateral approach. (*Source*: Jazrawi, Laith. 2014)

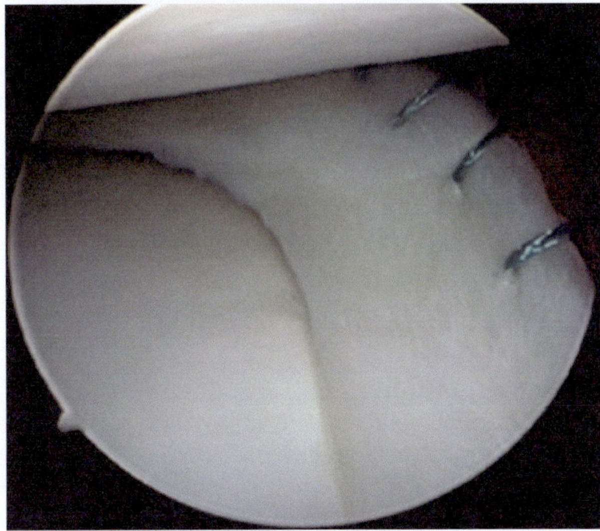

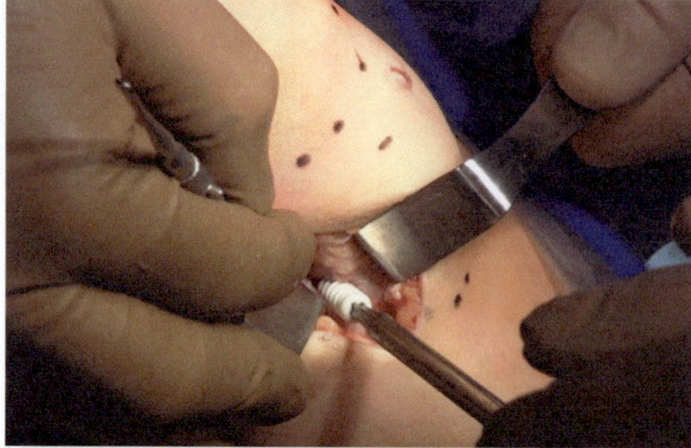
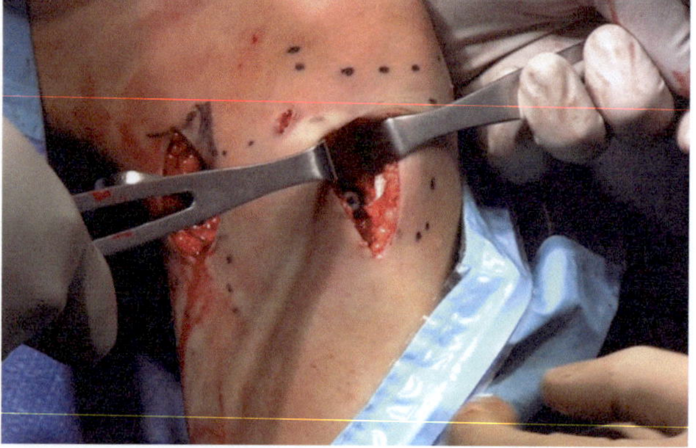

Fig. 9.15 Allograft fixation using 7 × 23 mm interference screw placed central to the bone bridge. (*Source*: Jazrawi, Laith. 2014)

meniscus is performed with 2–0 sutures placed through the anterolateral arthrotomy. The graft is then probed to confirm adequate stabilization.

The posterolateral approach and anterolateral arthrotomy are irrigated and closed in layers. The portals are closed subcuticularly, skin adhesive is applied to the incisions, and sterile dressings are applied. The knee is then placed in hinged brace that is locked in extension.

Bone Plug Technique for Medial MAT

Graft Preparation

Patient positioning, diagnostic arthroscopy, and meniscal debridement are first performed using the methods described for the bridge-in-slot technique. As the arthroscopy and debridement are being performed, the allograft is prepared on the back table (Fig. 9.16). Any excess soft tissue is dissected away and the anterior and posterior horn insertion sites are isolated. A 2.4 mm guide pin is placed in the center of each horn attachment site. A collared reamer is placed over the guide pins and used to create the bone plugs, which are then sized to 8 mm in width by 10–12 mm in

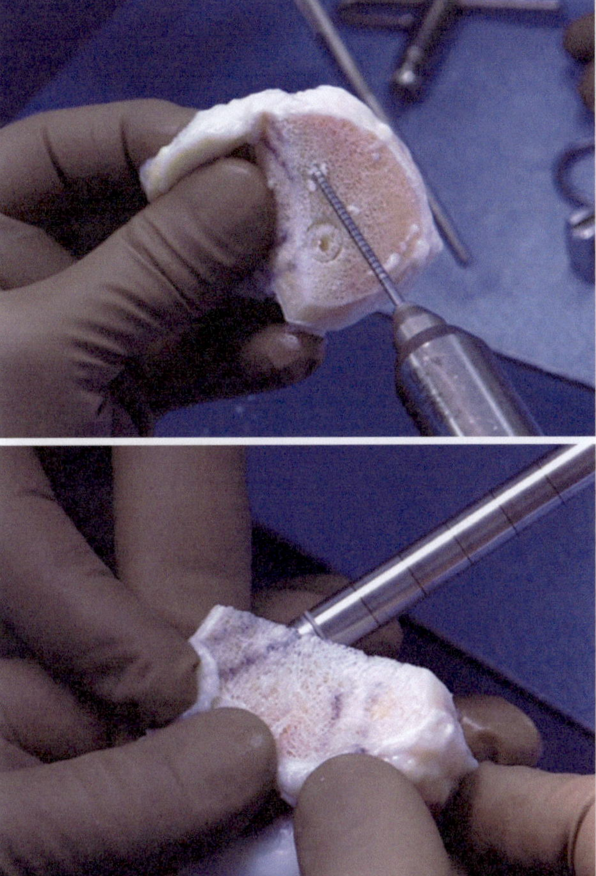

Fig. 9.16 Bone plug preparation for medial meniscal allograft transplantation. A guide pin is inserted into the center of the meniscal horn attachment site (top). A collared reamer placed over the guide pin is used to create the bone plugs (bottom). (*Source*: Jazrawi, Laith. 2014)

depth. Sutures are passed through each bone plug, first incorporating the horn attachment site, and then exiting through the central hole of the plug (Fig. 9.17). These sutures will be used to seat the donor plugs into the recipient tunnels. An additional suture is passed through junction of the meniscal body and the posterior horn to facilitate graft passage and reduction (Fig. 9.18). After being prepared, the allograft is placed in a basin with wet gauze to prevent drying.

Approach

The approach for a medial MAT utilizes a posteromedial incision similar to the approach for an inside-out meniscus repair. The MCL is palpated and the incision is made just posterior to the ligament, with one-third of the incision above the joint line and two-thirds of the incision below the joint line. The interval between the medial head of the gastrocnemius and the semimembranosus is identified. Palpating the gastrocnemius while plantarflexing and dorsiflexing the foot will confirm the appropriate positioning. Blunt dissection is then used to create an interval between

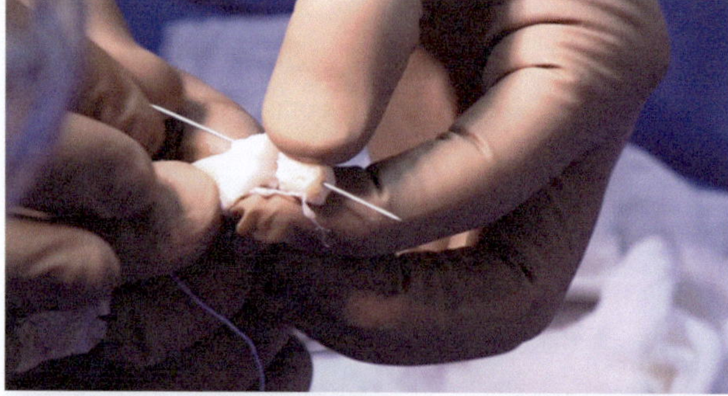

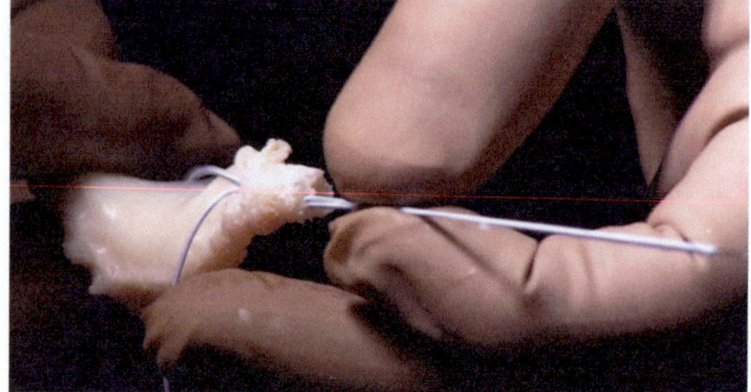

Fig. 9.17 Sutures are inserted through the meniscus attachment sites, exiting through the bone plugs. (*Source*: Jazrawi, Laith. 2014)

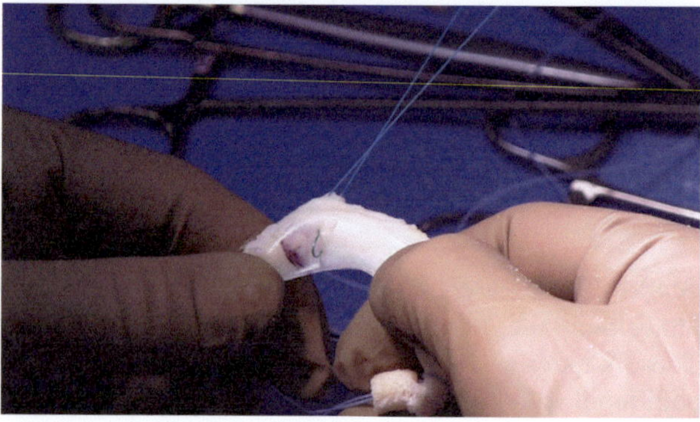

Fig. 9.18 A passing suture is placed to facilitate graft introduction and placement. (*Source*: Jazrawi, Laith. 2014)

the medial head of the gastrocnemius and the posteromedial capsule. A spoon or Henning retractor can be inserted into this space to protect the surrounding neurovascular structures during the remainder of the procedure.

Tunnel Preparation, Graft Introduction, and Fixation

The posterior tunnel is created first. An ACL tibial drill guide is used to pass a retrograde reamer into the location of the native meniscal posterior insertion site. An 8.5 mm diameter tunnel is reamed to a depth of 12–15 mm. A looped passing suture is then placed through the posterior tunnel and retrieved through the anteromedial portal (Fig. 9.19). This will be used to facilitate passing of the posterior bone plug.

Fig. 9.19 The guide wire is drilled through the posterior horn insertion site and reamed to an appropriate depth (top). A passing suture is placed through the tunnel and brought out through the anteromedial portal (bottom). (*Source*: Jazrawi, Laith. 2014)

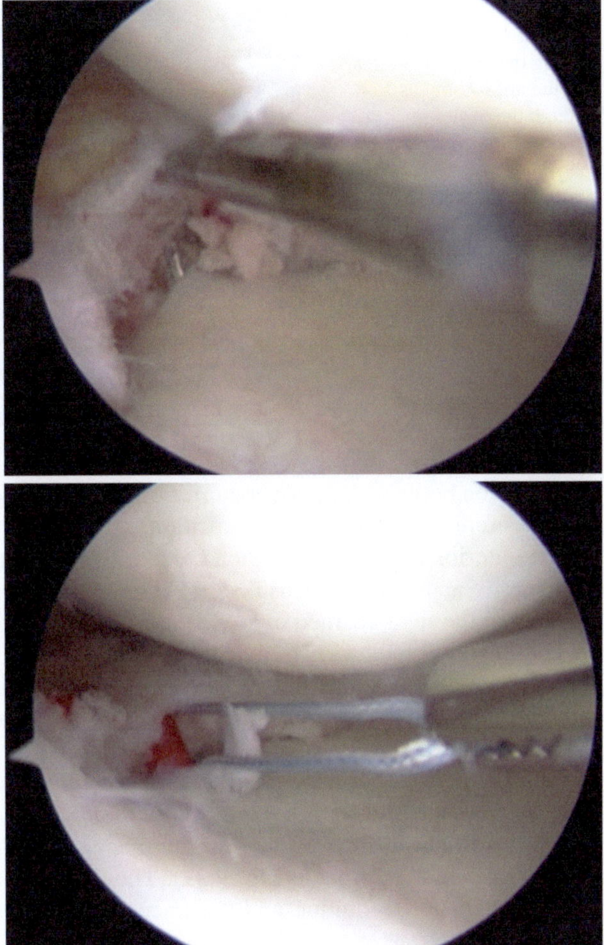

The anteromedial portal is extended to create an arthrotomy large enough to pass the allograft. The graft passage sutures placed in the donor meniscus during preparation are passed through the arthrotomy and retrieved through the posteromedial incision (Fig. 9.20). The posterior bone plug sutures are placed through the posterior tunnel passing suture placed previously. After the posterior bone plug sutures are passed through the posterior tunnel, gentle traction on the sutures is used to reduce the bone plug into the tunnel. A Freer elevator or another blunt instrument can be used to guide the bone plug into place. The meniscus graft is then reduced under the medial femoral condyle. Arthroscopic visualization is used to confirm appropriate placement of the posterior bone plug and the meniscus allograft.

Following placement of the posterior bone plug, the meniscal repair portion of the procedure is performed. Zone-specific cannulas are used for an inside-out medial meniscus repair with sutures passed in the vertical mattress fashion. Sutures

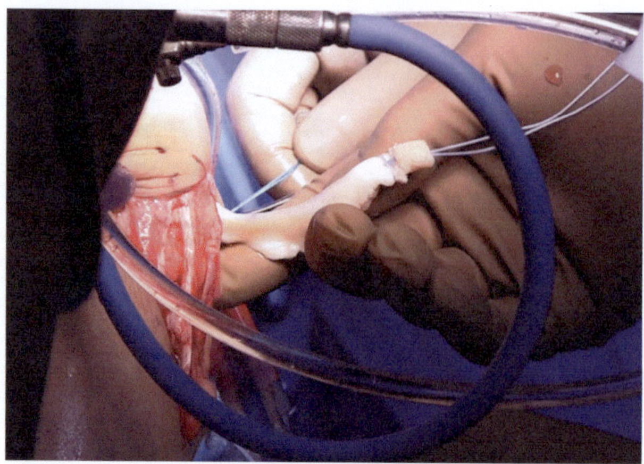

Fig. 9.20 The allograft is introduced into the knee by feeding the passing sutures into the arthrotomy and through the posteromedial incision. Note: This image was obtained during a combined medial MAT and bone–patellar tendon–bone ACL reconstruction, explaining the large anterior incision. (*Source*: Jazrawi, Laith. 2014)

are placed on both the superior and inferior aspects of the allograft to ensure that the meniscus remains in an anatomic position.

The anterior bone tunnel is then created by first placing a guide pin at the site of the native anterior meniscus insertion site through the anteromedial arthrotomy. An 8.5 mm tunnel is reamed over the guide pin to a depth of 15 mm. Starting 2 cm distal to the joint line, a 2.5 mm drill bit is used to drill superiorly into the anterior tunnel. A Hewson suture passer is then used to shuttle the anterior bone plug sutures through the anterior tunnel. The anterior bone plug is then reduced into the tunnel.

With the periphery of the meniscus secured and the bone plugs seated in their tunnels, the bone plugs are fixed by tying their sutures over cortical buttons. The knee is placed in full extension and the meniscal repair sutures are tied through the posteromedial approach (Fig. 9.21). The incisions are closed as described for the bridge-in-slot technique and the knee is placed in a hinged brace locked in extension.

Postoperative Rehabilitation

To date, there is no well-established postoperative rehabilitation protocol that has been shown to provide superior outcomes compared to other protocols. Most studies that describe the postoperative rehabilitation involve bracing, restricted range of motion, and limited weight-bearing following surgery. A hinged brace should be used for 6–8 weeks following the procedure to protect against flexion of the knee past 90° and prevent excessive translation of the meniscus relative to the tibia. Tibial rotation should also be avoided for 8 weeks. Early joint exercises and progressive advancement of weight-bearing are typically recommended with the goal of achieving full range of motion within 2–3 months, use of a stationary bike at 2 months, light jogging at 3–4 months, and athletic activity at 6–9 months postoperatively [44, 50, 87, 88].

Fig. 9.21 The meniscus repair sutures are tied through the posteromedial approach. (*Source*: Jazrawi, Laith. 2014)

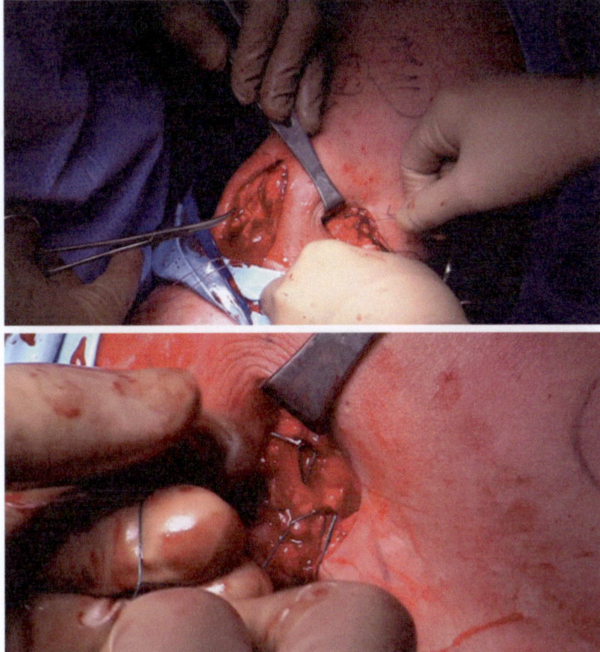

During the first 2 weeks following MAT, the patient is typically encouraged to proceed with toe-touch weightbearing with the knee locked in full extension. Carefully controlled stress placed on recently transplanted allografts is believed to stimulate collagen synthesis and enhance graft strength [89]. After 2 weeks, the patient can progress to weight-bearing as tolerated with the use of crutches [90–92]. However, weight-bearing with the knee flexed greater than 90° should be avoided until 8 weeks after surgery. Although one study found no difference in outcomes after MAT between a rehabilitation protocol involving restricted weight-bearing and range of motion and another protocol without any restrictions, further studies are needed to determine the optimal protocol that will allow patients to return to work or sport as quickly and safely as possible [93]. A recommended postoperative rehabilitation protocol is provided in Table 9.1.

Outcomes

As meniscal transplantation has become a more common solution for young patients with symptomatic meniscal deficiency, there have been a large number of studies that have shown MAT to be a safe and effective procedure with satisfactory outcomes. However, the conclusions that can be drawn from the existing outcomes studies are limited by heterogeneity in graft preservation technique, surgical technique, bony fixation method, and the rehabilitation protocol utilized. Additionally, surgical technique has evolved since meniscus transplants were first introduced,

Table 9.1 Recommended postoperative rehabilitation protocol for MAT

Phase 1 (weeks 0–8)	
Weight-bearing	
Toe-touch weight-bearing	Weeks 0–2
Weight-bearing as tolerated with crutches	Weeks 2–4
Weight-bearing as tolerated, discontinue crutches if gait is normalized	Weeks 4–8
No weight-bearing with flexion >90° during weeks 0–8	
Hinged knee brace	
Locked in full extension for ambulation and sleeping, remove for hygiene	Weeks 0–2
Set to range from 0° to 90° for ambulation, remove for sleeping and hygiene	Weeks 2–6
Discontinue brace	Week 6
Range of motion (ROM)	
0°	Weeks 0–2
0–90°	Weeks 2–6
Full non-weight-bearing ROM as tolerated	Weeks 6–8
Therapeutic exercises	
Heel slides, straight leg raises, patellar mobilizations (with brace)	Weeks 0–2
Add heel raises, terminal knee extensions (with brace)	Weeks 2–6
Continue exercises without brace	Weeks 6–8
Avoid tibial rotation during weeks 0–8	
Phase 2 (weeks 8–12)	
Weight-bearing	
As tolerated	Weeks 8–12
Range of motion	
Full active ROM	Weeks 8–12
Therapeutic exercises	
Progress to closed chain extension exercises, begin hamstring strengthening	Weeks 8–12
Lunges (0–90°), leg press (0–90°)	Weeks 8–12
Proprioception exercises	Weeks 8–12
Stationary bike	Weeks 8–12
Phase 3 (months 3–6)	
Weight-bearing	
Full weight-bearing with normal gait patterns	Months 3–6
Range of motion	
Full ROM	Months 3–6
Therapeutic exercises	
Continue quadriceps and hamstring strengthening	Months 3–6
Focus on single-leg strength	Months 3–6
Sport-specific drills	Months 4–6
Begin maintenance program for strength and endurance	Month 6
Activity goals	
Begin jogging	Month 3
Return to sport	Months 6–9

Source: Kingery M. T., Jazrawi L., Strauss E. J. (2019)

making it difficult to compare studies over time. Nevertheless, the overall positive outcomes demonstrated by the literature have helped solidify MAT as beneficial treatment for appropriately selected patients (Table 9.2).

The initial evidence that helped establish MAT as an effective treatment option was provided by a series of small cohort studies. In 2001, Rath et al. reported the outcomes of 22 cryopreserved meniscal allografts implanted in 18 patients [87]. At

Table 9.2 Summary of selected studies regarding MAT outcomes

Author (year)	Level of evidence	Follow-up, mean (range)	Patients (grafts)	Graft preservation	Fixation technique	Isolated MAT	Combined MAT	Findings
Rath (2001)	IV	54 months (24–97)	18 (22)	Cryopreserved	Medial: bone plug Lateral: bridge-in-slot	3 patients	15 patients	Improvement in pain and function Continued functional limitations based on IKDC
Noyes (2004)	IV	40 months (24–69)	38 (40)	Cryopreserved	Medial: bone plug Lateral: bridge-in-slot	13 patients	25 patients	Improvement in pain and function 89% of patients reported improvement in condition 76% of patients returned to light low-impact sports
Verdonk (2005)	IV	7.2 years (0.5–14.5)	95 (100)	Fresh	Soft tissue	69 allografts	31 allografts	Improvement in pain and function 28% of medial MATs and 16% of lateral MATs failed Cumulative allograft survival time of 11.6 years 10 year survival rates were 74.2% for medial MATs and 69.8% for lateral MATs
Cole (2006)	IV	33.5 months (24–57)	36 (40)	> 80% cryopreserved, < 20% fresh-frozen	Medial: bone plug Lateral: keyhole	21 allografts	19 allografts	Improvement in pain and function 77.5% of patients reported being mostly or completely satisfied

(continued)

Table 9.2 (continued)

Author (year)	Level of evidence	Follow-up, mean (range)	Patients (grafts)	Graft preservation	Fixation technique	Isolated MAT	Combined MAT	Findings
Sekiya (2006)	IV	3.3 years (2–6)	25 (25)	Cryopreserved	Lateral: 5 bone plug, 12 bridge-in-slot, 8 soft tissue	25 patients	0 patients	96% of patients reported improvement in overall function No difference in joint space narrowing compared to contralateral lateral compartment Bony fixation was associated with greater range of motion compared to soft tissue fixation
Verdonk (2006)	IV	12.1 years (10.0–14.8)	41 (42)	Fresh	Soft tissue	31 allografts	11 allografts	Improvement in pain and function Combined medial MAT and HTO was associated with greater improvement compared to isolated medial MAT 41% of patients had no change in joint space narrowing Overall failure rate was 18%
Lee (2010)	III	5.1 years (3.5–8.3)	43 (43)	Fresh-frozen	Medial: bone plug Lateral: keyhole	NR	NR	At 1 year postoperatively, 40% of allografts were classified as extruded Extrusion did not affect functional outcomes or joint space width

Elattar (2011)	IV (Meta-analysis)	4.6 years (0.67–20)	1068 (1136)	40% cryopreserved, 36.2% fresh-frozen, 11.2% fresh, 1.5% lyophilized, 3.5% unknown	Soft tissue, bone plug, bone bridge	352 allografts	617 allografts	All studies reported satisfactory outcomes Overall complication rate of 21.3%
Kim (2012)	IV	49.4 months (24–164)	106 (110)	5 cryopreserved, 105 fresh-frozen	Medial: 3 trough, 9 keyhole, 15 bone plug Lateral: 2 trough, 81 keyhole	82 knees	28 knees	Improvement in pain and function On MRI, mean extrusion was 3.7 mm
Lee (2012)	III	2 years	31 (31)	Fresh-frozen	Medial: bone plug Lateral: keyhole	29 patients	2 patients	Over 1 year, 19.4% of patients had mild meniscal shrinkage, 16.1% had moderate shrinkage, and 0% had severe shrinkage Morphological changes did not correlate with clinical outcomes
Saltzman (2012)	IV	8.5 years (6.8–11.2)	22 (22)	Fresh-frozen	Medial: 12 bone plug, 1 bridge-in-slot Lateral: 5 keyhole, 4 bridge-in-slot	8 allografts	14 allografts	Improvement in pain and function Average satisfaction was 8.8 out of 10 Overall success rate of 88%
Abat (2012)	II	40 months (36–48)	88 (88)	Fresh-frozen	33 soft tissue, 55 bone plug	88 allografts	0 allografts	Mean percentage of meniscal tissue extruded was greater in soft tissue fixation group No association between degree of extrusion and functional outcomes

(continued)

Table 9.2 (continued)

Author (year)	Level of evidence	Follow-up, mean (range)	Patients (grafts)	Graft preservation	Fixation technique	Isolated MAT	Combined MAT	Findings
Koh (2012)	IV	32 months (24–59)	99 (99)	Fresh-frozen	Medial: bone plug Lateral: keyhole	75 patients	24 patients	Lateral menisci extruded more significantly than medial menisci Extrusion did not affect functional outcomes
Chalmers (2013)	IV	3.3 years (1.9–5.7)	13 (13)	Fresh-frozen	10 bridge-in-slot, 3 bone plug	6 patients	7 patients	77% of high school or higher level athletes returned to sport after MAT
McCormick (2014)	IV	59 months (24–118)	200 (202)	Fresh-frozen	Bridge-in-slot (modified for concomitant ACL reconstruction)	81 patients	119 patients	32% of patients required reoperation, most commonly arthroscopic debridement (59% of reoperation patients) Mean time to reoperation of 21 months 4.7% of patients required revision MAT or TKA
Jauregui (2018)	IV (Meta-analysis)	60 months (25–168)	NR (1637)	NR	485 soft tissue, 489 bony fixation	NR	NR	Improvement in pain and function Overall graft tear rate of 9% and failure rate of 12.6% No difference in outcomes between soft tissue fixation and bony fixation

| Bin (2018) | IV (Meta-analysis) | > 5 years | NR (694) | Cryopreserved, fresh, fresh-frozen | Bone plug, soft tissue | NR | NR | Lateral MAT was associated with greater improvements in pain and function compared to medial MAT
No difference in midterm and long-term survival rates between medial and lateral MATs |
| Grassi (2019) | IV (Meta-analysis) | 3.4 years (NR) | 467 (NR) | Fresh-frozen (6 studies), unknown (3 studies) | Soft tissue, bone plug, bone bridge | NR | ≥ 301 patients | 77% of patients returned to sport, with 67% returning to the same sport or physical activity level
Mean time to return to sport was 9.2 months |

NR not recorded, *IKDC* International Knee Documentation Committee a mean follow-up of 4.5 years following surgery, there was an overall improvement in both pain and function. Repeat radiographs taken at the latest follow-up time demonstrated no significant difference in the joint space compared to preoperative radiographs. Eight of the 22 transplanted menisci tore during the study period requiring repeat meniscectomy. Histologic examination of the removed meniscal tissue revealed revascularization of the periphery, consistent with prior studies [39, 53, 94]. However, the torn allografts contained fewer fibrochondrocytes and lower levels of growth factors compared to torn native menisci. The authors postulated that reduced biologic activity of the allograft may be associated with the increased rate of tears [87].

Further studies demonstrated clinical improvements similar to those reported by Rath et al. [88, 95–98] In an evaluation of 40 cryopreserved allografts, the percentage of patients experiencing pain with daily activities decreased from 79% preoperatively to 11% at 3.3 years after MAT [88]. In another cohort, 77.5% of patients were mostly satisfied or completely satisfied with the outcomes of the procedure [95]. In addition to improved pain and function, analysis of 32 allografts found no significant difference in joint space loss between involved and uninvolved knees [98]. Kim et al. presented a group of 110 MAT cases with improved function in 94.5% of patients at a minimum of 2 years after surgery [97]. Despite the low level of evidence provided by these initial investigations, they served as an early description of the short- and intermediate-term efficacy of MAT.

Verdonk evaluated a cohort of 100 allografts preserved in culture, transplanted either in isolation or with concomitant high tibial osteotomy, with a mean follow-up time of 7.2 years [99]. Overall, MAT resulted in significant improvements in both pain and function. Failure, defined as moderate or severe occasional pain, persistent pain, or poor knee function, occurred in 28% of medial allografts at a mean of 6 years and 16% of lateral allografts at a mean of 4.8 years. For medial meniscal allografts, mean survival rate was 86.2% at 5 years, 74.2% at 10 years, and 52.8% at 14.5 years. For lateral allografts, mean survival rate was 90.2% at 5 years, 69.8% at 10 years, and 69.8% at 14 years. There was no difference in survival between medial and lateral grafts. The level of cartilage degeneration at the time of surgery did not affect the risk of failure, in contrast to previous studies which have suggested that failure rate is higher with advanced degeneration [36, 40]. The difference can perhaps be due to the study's utilization of nonirradiated, fresh allografts, which may be more resistant to failure in patients with moderate or severe preexisting cartilage damage compared to the irradiated, cryopreserved allografts used in contradicting studies.

An additional study of graft survival was carried out by McCormick et al. [100] This cohort consisted of 172 patients who received fresh-frozen, nonirradiated allografts using the bridge-in-slot technique or, if concomitant ACL reconstruction was performed, a modified bridge technique. At a mean follow-up of 4.9 years, 4.7% of patients had experienced graft failure requiring revision MAT or TKA. Despite a greater than 95% graft survival rate, 32% of the cohort required re-operation during the study period. The most common reason for re-operation was arthroscopic debridement of scar tissue, with an average time to reoperation of

21 months. Patients requiring reoperation had graft survival rate of 88%, although they were at an increased risk of failure compared to patients who did not require reoperation [100]. This investigation suggests that although roughly one in three MAT patients will undergo reoperation, there is still a high likelihood of graft survival.

Verdonk also reported on a cohort of patients consisting of 39 culture-maintained allografts in 38 patients with a mean follow-up time of 12.1 years [101]. Like this group's earlier results, pain and function improved significantly for both medial and lateral allografts. Despite the noted improvements, patients continued to experience functional impairment and symptoms at the time of follow-up. Eighteen percent of the study group had undergone total knee arthroplasty after a mean of 6.5 years due to progression of pain and functional limitation. There was no additional change in joint space narrowing in 41% of the patients at the time of follow-up, suggesting that MAT may attenuate progression of cartilage degradation and provide a chondroprotective effect. Similar to other existing studies [102, 103], MRI outcomes (including femoral and tibial cartilage degeneration, meniscus signal intensity, meniscus position, extrusion, and tears) did not correlate with subjective clinical outcomes. The authors conclude that the evaluation of patient outcomes should rely primarily on clinical measures rather than radiographic measures [101]. This is consistent with a later study which found that although significant meniscus shrinkage occurred by 1 year postoperatively, the morphologic changes were not associated with clinical outcomes [104].

Saltzman performed a longitudinal study of patient satisfaction following MAT with the most recent update consisting of 22 allografts at a mean follow-up time of 8.5 years [105]. There were significant improvements in pain, functional outcomes, and quality of life with no difference between medial allografts and lateral allografts. At the time of follow-up, the patients reported an average satisfaction score of 8.8 out of 10. Eight of the 22 patients were completely satisfied with the results of the procedure, and the remaining 14 patients reported being mostly satisfied. This same cohort of patients was evaluated at 2 and 4 years postoperatively, and it was found that that pain, severity of symptoms, and function were generally consistent from the earlier follow-up times to the most recent evaluation [105]. This suggests that the benefits achieved shortly after rehabilitation are maintained for at least 8 years following MAT.

A 2011 meta-analysis examined 44 trials consisting of 1136 total grafts in 1068 patients with a mean age of 34.8 years [106]. Although the included studies differed in their outcome measures, they consistently demonstrated an improvement in clinical outcomes with MAT. Of the studies that specified, only 36% of MATs were isolated, while the remainder were performed with another procedure. Among all included studies, 84% of patients described their knee function as normal or nearly normal, and 89% were satisfied with their results. The overall complication rate was 21.3%, with the most common adverse events being tearing of the graft and adhesions requiring MUA. There was a failure rate of 10.6% when defined as destruction or removal of the graft with or without conversion to arthroplasty. Of the studies that included radiographic or MRI follow-up, most noted little to no progression of joint space narrowing at last follow-up. The chondroprotective effect of MAT has been demonstrated in animal models [107], and while this analysis provides additional support for a similar effect in humans, definitive evidence is still lacking. Despite the unknown efficacy in terms of cartilage preservation, the consistent clinical improvement and low rate of serious complications found in this analysis suggest that MAT is a safe and effective procedure in carefully selected patients.

A similarly large 2018 meta-analysis included 38 studies consisting of 1637 MATs with a mean age of 34 years [108]. There was overall tear rate of 9% and a failure rate of 12.6%, when defined as requiring revision, removal of the graft, or persistent knee pain. Interestingly, there was no difference in graft tears, failure rates, functional improvement, or pain improvement between bony fixation and soft tissue fixation. This contrasts the biomechanical studies which have largely concluded that bony fixation is superior to soft tissue fixation [29, 86]. In another study comparing suture-only MAT and bone plug MAT, there was similarly no difference in functional outcomes, although the suture-only technique was associated with higher risk of extruded meniscal body at 40 months postoperatively [83]. While the measured functional outcomes may be similar between the two different methods of securing the meniscus, soft-tissue fixation has largely fallen out of favor among surgeons.

Bin et al. performed a meta-analysis comparing the mid-term and long-term outcomes of medial MAT versus lateral MAT [109]. The analysis included nine studies consisting of 287 medial MATs and 407 lateral MATs. At 5 to 10 years postoperatively, the graft survival rate was 85.8% for medial allografts and 89.2% for lateral allografts. Greater than 10 years following transplantation, the graft survival rate was 52.6% for medial allografts and 56.6% for lateral allografts. At both mid-term follow-up and long-term follow-up, there was no significant difference in graft survival rate between medial and lateral MATs. However, lateral MAT was found to be associated with greater improvement in pain and function. The authors suggested that lateral MAT may be more successful because patients with lateral meniscus injuries tend to have shorter intervals between meniscectomy and transplantation, perhaps leading to less cartilage damage accumulation [99]. Further studies are needed to explain this difference.

Early studies initially suggested that meniscal extrusion was associated with poorer outcomes [110]. However, subsequent studies found that graft extrusion did not affect the progression of joint space narrowing at 5 years [64]. Additionally, although lateral menisci tend to extrude to a greater extent than medial menisci, neither was associated with clinical outcomes [64, 111].

A 2019 systematic review and meta-analysis examined the rate of return to physical activity following MAT [112]. Based on the nine included studies, 77% of patients were able to return to any level of sport or physical activity at minimum 2-year follow-up, with 67% returning to the same level of preinjury activity. One of the included studies specifically analyzed 13 high-level athletes (nine collegiate athletes, three high school varsity athletes, and one professional athlete) who had undergone prior partial or total meniscectomies and had been undeniable to return to their preinjury level of play [113]. In this study, 10 athletes (77%) returned to their previous level of play after a mean of 16.5 months and nine (70%) returned to their desired level of play after MAT. The existing data regarding return to sport after MAT is generally low-level, making it difficult to draw conclusions, especially related to high-impact sports and activities.

Conclusion

Within the relatively short history of meniscal allograft transplantation, the techniques used to preserve and implant the grafts have advanced dramatically. While the procedure in its current state is not capable of entirely eliminating the sequelae associated with the meniscectomized knee, MAT does represent an opportunity to restore the mechanics of the knee joint, improve function, and alleviate pain. As the body of data surrounding meniscal transplantation grows, the surgical techniques will continue to be refined and the lifespan of the allografts will likely improve, offering even greater benefits for patients with symptoms related to meniscus insufficiency.

References

1. Smillie IS. The current pattern of internal derangements of the knee joint relative to the menisci. Clin Orthop Relat Res. 1967;51:117–22.
2. Fairbank TJ. Knee joint changes after meniscectomy. J Bone Joint Surg. 1948;30b(4):664–70.
3. Tapper EM, Hoover NW. Late results after meniscectomy. J Bone Joint Surg Am. 1969;51(3):517–526 passim.
4. Johnson RJ, Kettelkamp DB, Clark W, Leaverton P. Factors effecting late results after meniscectomy. J Bone Joint Surg Am. 1974;56(4):719–29.
5. Pengas IP, Assiotis A, Nash W, Hatcher J, Banks J, McNicholas MJ. Total meniscectomy in adolescents: a 40-year follow-up. J Bone Joint Surg. 2012;94(12):1649–54.
6. Bolano LE, Grana WA. Isolated arthroscopic partial meniscectomy. Functional radiographic evaluation at five years. Am J Sports Med. 1993;21(3):432–7.
7. Burks RT, Metcalf MH, Metcalf RW. Fifteen-year follow-up of arthroscopic partial meniscectomy. Arthroscopy. 1997;13(6):673–9.
8. Salata MJ, Gibbs AE, Sekiya JK. A systematic review of clinical outcomes in patients undergoing meniscectomy. Am J Sports Med. 2010;38(9):1907–16.
9. Williams RJ 3rd, Warner KK, Petrigliano FA, Potter HG, Hatch J, Cordasco FA. MRI evaluation of isolated arthroscopic partial meniscectomy patients at a minimum five-year follow-up. HSS J. 2007;3(1):35–43.
10. Lee SJ, Aadalen KJ, Malaviya P, et al. Tibiofemoral contact mechanics after serial medial meniscectomies in the human cadaveric knee. Am J Sports Med. 2006;34(8):1334–44.
11. Bai B, Shun H, Yin ZX, Liao ZW, Chen N. Changes of contact pressure and area in patellofemoral joint after different meniscectomies. Int Orthop. 2012;36(5):987–91.
12. McDermott ID, Amis AA. The consequences of meniscectomy. J Bone Joint Surg. 2006;88(12):1549–56.
13. Verma NN, Kolb E, Cole BJ, et al. The effects of medial meniscal transplantation techniques on intra-articular contact pressures. J Knee Surg. 2008;21(1):20–6.
14. Van Thiel GS, Frank RM, Gupta A, et al. Biomechanical evaluation of a high tibial osteotomy with a meniscal transplant. J Knee Surg. 2011;24(1):45–53.

15. Baratz ME, Fu FH, Mengato R. Meniscal tears: the effect of meniscectomy and of repair on intraarticular contact areas and stress in the human knee. A preliminary report. Am J Sports Med. 1986;14(4):270–5.
16. Bullough P, Goodfellow J. The significance of the fine structure of articular cartilage. J Bone Joint Surg. 1968;50(4):852–7.
17. Korkala O, Karaharju E, Gronblad M, Aalto K. Articular cartilage after meniscectomy. Rabbit knees studied with the scanning electron microscope. Acta Orthop Scand. 1984;55(3):273–7.
18. Levy IM, Torzilli PA, Warren RF. The effect of medial meniscectomy on anterior-posterior motion of the knee. J Bone Joint Surg Am. 1982;64(6):883–8.
19. Mac CM. The movements of bones and joints; the synovial fluid and its assistants. J Bone Joint Surg. 1950;32-b(2):244–52.
20. Aagaard H, Verdonk R. Function of the normal meniscus and consequences of meniscal resection. Scand J Med Sci Sports. 1999;9(3):134–40.
21. Englund M, Lohmander LS. Risk factors for symptomatic knee osteoarthritis fifteen to twenty-two years after meniscectomy. Arthritis Rheum. 2004;50(9):2811–9.
22. Milachowski KA, Weismeier K, Wirth CJ. Homologous meniscus transplantation. Experimental and clinical results. Int Orthop. 1989;13(1):1–11.
23. Rijk PC. Meniscal allograft transplantation--part I: background, results, graft selection and preservation, and surgical considerations. Arthroscopy. 2004;20(7):728–43.
24. Locht RC, Gross AE, Langer F. Late osteochondral allograft resurfacing for tibial plateau fractures. J Bone Joint Surg Am. 1984;66(3):328–35.
25. Cummins JF, Mansour JN, Howe Z, Allan DG. Meniscal transplantation and degenerative articular change: an experimental study in the rabbit. Arthroscopy. 1997;13(4):485–91.
26. Aagaard H, Jorgensen U, Bojsen-Moller F. Reduced degenerative articular cartilage changes after meniscal allograft transplantation in sheep. Knee Surg Sports Traumatol Arthrosc. 1999;7(3):184–91.
27. Andrish JT, Kambic HE, Valdevit ADC, et al. Selected knee osteotomies and meniscal replacement: effects on dynamic intra-joint loading. J Bone Joint Surg Am. 2001;83-A Suppl 2 Pt 2:142–50.
28. Alhalki MM, Hull ML, Howell SM. Contact mechanics of the medial tibial plateau after implantation of a medial meniscal allograft. A human cadaveric study. Am J Sports Med. 2000;28(3):370–6.
29. Paletta GA Jr, Manning T, Snell E, Parker R, Bergfeld J. The effect of allograft meniscal replacement on intraarticular contact area and pressures in the human knee. A biomechanical study. Am J Sports Med. 1997;25(5):692–8.
30. Sekiya JK, Ellingson CI. Meniscal allograft transplantation. J Am Acad Orthop Surg. 2006;14(3):164–74.
31. Trentacosta N, Graham WC, Gersoff WK. Meniscal allograft transplantation: state of the art. Sports Med Arthrosc Rev. 2016;24(2):e23–33.
32. Kempshall PJ, Parkinson B, Thomas M, et al. Outcome of meniscal allograft transplantation related to articular cartilage status: advanced chondral damage should not be a contraindication. Knee Surg Sports Traumatol Arthrosc. 2015;23(1):280–9.
33. Stone KR, Pelsis JR, Surrette ST, Walgenbach AW, Turek TJ. Meniscus transplantation in an active population with moderate to severe cartilage damage. Knee Surg Sports Traumatol Arthrosc. 2015;23(1):251–7.
34. Lee AS, Kang RW, Kroin E, Verma NN, Cole BJ. Allograft meniscus transplantation. Sports Med Arthrosc Rev. 2012;20(2):106–14.
35. Jarit GJ, Bosco JA 3rd. Meniscal repair and reconstruction. Bull NYU Hosp Jt Dis. 2010;68(2):84–90.
36. de Boer HH, Koudstaal J. Failed meniscus transplantation. A report of three cases. Clin Orthop Relat Res. 1994;306:155–62.
37. Mascarenhas R, Yanke AB, Frank RM, Butty DC, Cole BJ. Meniscal allograft transplantation: preoperative assessment, surgical considerations, and clinical outcomes. J Knee Surg. 2014;27(6):443–58.

38. Harris JD, Cavo M, Brophy R, Siston R, Flanigan D. Biological knee reconstruction: a systematic review of combined meniscal allograft transplantation and cartilage repair or restoration. Arthroscopy. 2011;27(3):409–18.
39. van Arkel ER, de Boer HH. Human meniscal transplantation. Preliminary results at 2 to 5-year follow-up. J Bone Joint Surg. 1995;77(4):589–95.
40. Cameron JC, Saha S. Meniscal allograft transplantation for unicompartmental arthritis of the knee. Clin Orthop Relat Res. 1997;337:164–71.
41. Getgood A, Gelber J, Gortz S, De Young A, Bugbee W. Combined osteochondral allograft and meniscal allograft transplantation: a survivorship analysis. Knee Surg Sports Traumatol Arthrosc. 2015;23(4):946–53.
42. Lee BS, Kim HJ, Lee CR, et al. Clinical outcomes of meniscal allograft transplantation with or without other procedures: a systematic review and meta-analysis. Am J Sports Med. 2018;46(12):3047–56.
43. Sekiya JK, Giffin JR, Irrgang JJ, Fu FH, Harner CD. Clinical outcomes after combined meniscal allograft transplantation and anterior cruciate ligament reconstruction. Am J Sports Med. 2003;31(6):896–906.
44. Ryu RK, Dunbar VW, Morse GG. Meniscal allograft replacement: a 1-year to 6-year experience. Arthroscopy. 2002;18(9):989–94.
45. Abrams GD, Hussey KE, Harris JD, Cole BJ. Clinical results of combined meniscus and femoral osteochondral allograft transplantation: minimum 2-year follow-up. Arthroscopy. 2014;30(8):964–970.e961.
46. Farr J, Rawal A, Marberry KM. Concomitant meniscal allograft transplantation and autologous chondrocyte implantation: minimum 2-year follow-up. Am J Sports Med. 2007;35(9):1459–66.
47. Kazi HA, Abdel-Rahman W, Brady PA, Cameron JC. Meniscal allograft with or without osteotomy: a 15-year follow-up study. Knee Surg Sports Traumatol Arthrosc. 2015;23(1):303–9.
48. Bonasia DE, Amendola A. Combined medial meniscal transplantation and high tibial osteotomy. Knee Surg Sports Traumatol Arthrosc. 2010;18(7):870–3.
49. Amendola A. Knee osteotomy and meniscal transplantation: indications, technical considerations, and results. Sports Med Arthrosc Rev. 2007;15(1):32–8.
50. Graf KW Jr, Sekiya JK, Wojtys EM. Long-term results after combined medial meniscal allograft transplantation and anterior cruciate ligament reconstruction: minimum 8.5-year follow-up study. Arthroscopy. 2004;20(2):129–40.
51. Rue JP, Yanke AB, Busam ML, McNickle AG, Cole BJ. Prospective evaluation of concurrent meniscus transplantation and articular cartilage repair: minimum 2-year follow-up. Am J Sports Med. 2008;36(9):1770–8.
52. Gomoll AH, Kang RW, Chen AL, Cole BJ. Triad of cartilage restoration for unicompartmental arthritis treatment in young patients: meniscus allograft transplantation, cartilage repair and osteotomy. J Knee Surg. 2009;22(2):137–41.
53. Garrett JC, Steensen RN. Meniscal transplantation in the human knee: a preliminary report. Arthroscopy. 1991;7(1):57–62.
54. Milachowski KA, Kohn D, Wirth CJ. [Transplantation of allogeneic menisci]. Der Orthopade. 1994;23(2):160–3.
55. Weismeier K, Wirth CJ, Milachowski KA. [Transplantation of the meniscus. Experimental study]. Revue de chirurgie orthopedique et reparatrice de l'appareil moteur. 1988;74(2):155–9.
56. Siegel MG, Roberts CS. Meniscal allografts. Clin Sports Med. 1993;12(1):59–80.
57. Arnoczky SP, McDevitt CA, Schmidt MB, Mow VC, Warren RF. The effect of cryopreservation on canine menisci: a biochemical, morphologic, and biomechanical evaluation. J Orthop Res. 1988;6(1):1–12.
58. Gelber PE, Gonzalez G, Torres R, Garcia Giralt N, Caceres E, Monllau JC. Cryopreservation does not alter the ultrastructure of the meniscus. Knee Surg Sports Traumatol Arthrosc. 2009;17(6):639–44.
59. Villalba R, Pena J, Navarro P, et al. Cryopreservation increases apoptosis in human menisci. Knee Surg Sports Traumatol Arthrosc. 2012;20(2):298–303.

60. Lubowitz JH, Verdonk PC, Reid JB 3rd, Verdonk R. Meniscus allograft transplantation: a current concepts review. Knee Surg Sports Traumatol Arthrosc. 2007;15(5):476–92.
61. Rodeo SA. Meniscal allografts–where do we stand? Am J Sports Med. 2001;29(2):246–61.
62. Jackson DW, Whelan J, Simon TM. Cell survival after transplantation of fresh meniscal allografts. DNA probe analysis in a goat model. Am J Sports Med. 1993;21(4):540–50.
63. Wirth CJ, Peters G, Milachowski KA, Weismeier KG, Kohn D. Long-term results of meniscal allograft transplantation. Am J Sports Med. 2002;30(2):174–81.
64. Lee DH, Kim SB, Kim TH, Cha EJ, Bin SI. Midterm outcomes after meniscal allograft transplantation: comparison of cases with extrusion versus without extrusion. Am J Sports Med. 2010;38(2):247–54.
65. Noyes F. Irradiated meniscus allografts in the human knee: a two to five years follow-up study. Revue de chirurgie orthopedique et reparatrice de l'appareil moteur. 1995;81(2):207–8.
66. Yahia L, Zukor D. Irradiated meniscal allotransplants of rabbits: study of the mechanical properties at six months postoperation. Acta Orthop Belg. 1994;60(2):210–5.
67. von Lewinski G, Milachowski KA, Weismeier K, Kohn D, Wirth CJ. Twenty-year results of combined meniscal allograft transplantation, anterior cruciate ligament reconstruction and advancement of the medial collateral ligament. Knee Surg Sports Traumatol Arthrosc. 2007;15(9):1072–82.
68. Goble EM, Kohn D, Verdonk R, Kane SM. Meniscal substitutes--human experience. Scand J Med Sci Sports. 1999;9(3):146–57.
69. Dienst M, Greis PE, Ellis BJ, Bachus KN, Burks RT. Effect of lateral meniscal allograft sizing on contact mechanics of the lateral tibial plateau: an experimental study in human cadaveric knee joints. Am J Sports Med. 2007;35(1):34–42.
70. Pollard ME, Kang Q, Berg EE. Radiographic sizing for meniscal transplantation. Arthroscopy. 1995;11(6):684–7.
71. Wilmes P, Pape D, Kohn D, Seil R. The reproducibility of radiographic measurement of lateral meniscus horn position. Arthroscopy. 2007;23(10):1079–86.
72. Wilmes P, Anagnostakos K, Weth C, Kohn D, Seil R. The reproducibility of radiographic measurement of medial meniscus horn position. Arthroscopy. 2008;24(6):660–8.
73. Haut TL, Hull ML, Howell SM. Use of roentgenography and magnetic resonance imaging to predict meniscal geometry determined with a three-dimensional coordinate digitizing system. J Orthop Res. 2000;18(2):228–37.
74. Prodromos CC, Joyce BT, Keller BL, Murphy BJ, Shi K. Magnetic resonance imaging measurement of the contralateral normal meniscus is a more accurate method of determining meniscal allograft size than radiographic measurement of the recipient tibial plateau. Arthroscopy. 2007;23(11):1174–1179.e1171.
75. Huang A, Hull ML, Howell SM, Haut DT. Identification of cross-sectional parameters of lateral meniscal allografts that predict tibial contact pressure in human cadaveric knees. J Biomech Eng. 2002;124(5):481–9.
76. Shaffer B, Kennedy S, Klimkiewicz J, Yao L. Preoperative sizing of meniscal allografts in meniscus transplantation. Am J Sports Med. 2000;28(4):524–33.
77. Kaleka CC, Netto AS, Silva JC, et al. Which are the most reliable methods of predicting the meniscal size for transplantation? Am J Sports Med. 2016;44(11):2876–83.
78. Yoon JR, Kim TS, Lim HC, Lim HT, Yang JH. Is radiographic measurement of bony landmarks reliable for lateral meniscal sizing? Am J Sports Med. 2011;39(3):582–9.
79. Yoon JR, Kim TS, Wang JH, Yun HH, Lim H, Yang JH. Importance of independent measurement of width and length of lateral meniscus during preoperative sizing for meniscal allograft transplantation. Am J Sports Med. 2011;39(7):1541–7.
80. Johnson DL, Swenson TM, Livesay GA, Aizawa H, Fu FH, Harner CD. Insertion-site anatomy of the human menisci: gross, arthroscopic, and topographical anatomy as a basis for meniscal transplantation. Arthroscopy. 1995;11(4):386–94.
81. Van Thiel GS, Verma N, Yanke A, Basu S, Farr J, Cole B. Meniscal allograft size can be predicted by height, weight, and gender. Arthroscopy. 2009;25(7):722–7.

82. Shelton WR, Dukes AD. Meniscus replacement with bone anchors: a surgical technique. Arthroscopy. 1994;10(3):324–7.
83. Abat F, Gelber PE, Erquicia JI, Pelfort X, Gonzalez-Lucena G, Monllau JC. Suture-only fixation technique leads to a higher degree of extrusion than bony fixation in meniscal allograft transplantation. Am J Sports Med. 2012;40(7):1591–6.
84. Stone KR, Rosenberg T. Surgical technique of meniscal replacement. Arthroscopy. 1993;9(2):234–7.
85. Chen MI, Branch TP, Hutton WC. Is it important to secure the horns during lateral meniscal transplantation? A cadaveric study. Arthroscopy. 1996;12(2):174–81.
86. Alhalki MM, Howell SM, Hull ML. How three methods for fixing a medial meniscal autograft affect tibial contact mechanics. Am J Sports Med. 1999;27(3):320–8.
87. Rath E, Richmond JC, Yassir W, Albright JD, Gundogan F. Meniscal allograft transplantation. Two- to eight-year results. Am J Sports Med. 2001;29(4):410–4.
88. Noyes FR, Barber-Westin SD, Rankin M. Meniscal transplantation in symptomatic patients less than fifty years old. J Bone Joint Surg Am. 2004;86-a(7):1392–404.
89. Krippaehne WW, Hunt TK, Jackson DS, Dunphy JE. Studies on the effect of stress on transplants of autologous and homologous connective tissue. Am J Surg. 1962;104:267–72.
90. Hannon MG, Ryan MK, Strauss EJ. Meniscal allograft transplantation a comprehensive historical and current review. Bull Hosp Jt Dis (2013). 2015;73(2):100–8.
91. Fritz JM, Irrgang JJ, Harner CD. Rehabilitation following allograft meniscal transplantation: a review of the literature and case study. J Orthop Sports Phys Ther. 1996;24(2):98–106.
92. Kohn D, Aagaard H, Verdonk R, Dienst M, Seil R. Postoperative follow-up and rehabilitation after meniscus replacement. Scand J Med Sci Sports. 1999;9(3):177–80.
93. Barber FA. Accelerated rehabilitation for meniscus repairs. Arthroscopy. 1994;10(2):206–10.
94. Arnoczky SP, Warren RF, McDevitt CA. Meniscal replacement using a cryopreserved allograft. An experimental study in the dog. Clin Orthop Relat Res. 1990;252:121–8.
95. Cole BJ, Dennis MG, Lee SJ, et al. Prospective evaluation of allograft meniscus transplantation: a minimum 2-year follow-up. Am J Sports Med. 2006;34(6):919–27.
96. Vundelinckx B, Bellemans J, Vanlauwe J. Arthroscopically assisted meniscal allograft transplantation in the knee: a medium-term subjective, clinical, and radiographical outcome evaluation. Am J Sports Med. 2010;38(11):2240–7.
97. Kim JM, Lee BS, Kim KH, Kim KA, Bin SI. Results of meniscus allograft transplantation using bone fixation: 110 cases with objective evaluation. Am J Sports Med. 2012;40(5):1027–34.
98. Sekiya JK, West RV, Groff YJ, Irrgang JJ, Fu FH, Harner CD. Clinical outcomes following isolated lateral meniscal allograft transplantation. Arthroscopy. 2006;22(7):771–80.
99. Verdonk PC, Demurie A, Almqvist KF, Veys EM, Verbruggen G, Verdonk R. Transplantation of viable meniscal allograft. Survivorship analysis and clinical outcome of one hundred cases. J Bone Joint Surg Am. 2005;87(4):715–24.
100. McCormick F, Harris JD, Abrams GD, et al. Survival and reoperation rates after meniscal allograft transplantation: analysis of failures for 172 consecutive transplants at a minimum 2-year follow-up. Am J Sports Med. 2014;42(4):892–7.
101. Verdonk PC, Verstraete KL, Almqvist KF, et al. Meniscal allograft transplantation: long-term clinical results with radiological and magnetic resonance imaging correlations. Knee Surg Sports Traumatol Arthrosc. 2006;14(8):694–706.
102. Verstraete KL, Verdonk R, Lootens T, Verstraete P, De Rooy J, Kunnen M. Current status and imaging of allograft meniscal transplantation. Eur J Radiol. 1997;26(1):16–22.
103. van Arkel ER, Goei R, de Ploeg I, de Boer HH. Meniscal allografts: evaluation with magnetic resonance imaging and correlation with arthroscopy. Arthroscopy. 2000;16(5):517–21.
104. Lee BS, Chung JW, Kim JM, Cho WJ, Kim KA, Bin SI. Morphologic changes in fresh-frozen meniscus allografts over 1 year: a prospective magnetic resonance imaging study on the width and thickness of transplants. Am J Sports Med. 2012;40(6):1384–91.
105. Saltzman BM, Bajaj S, Salata M, et al. Prospective long-term evaluation of meniscal allograft transplantation procedure: a minimum of 7-year follow-up. J Knee Surg. 2012;25(2):165–75.

106. Elattar M, Dhollander A, Verdonk R, Almqvist KF, Verdonk P. Twenty-six years of meniscal allograft transplantation: is it still experimental? A meta-analysis of 44 trials. Knee Surg Sports Traumatol Arthrosc. 2011;19(2):147–57.
107. Kelly BT, Potter HG, Deng XH, et al. Meniscal allograft transplantation in the sheep knee: evaluation of chondroprotective effects. Am J Sports Med. 2006;34(9):1464–77.
108. Jauregui JJ, Wu ZD, Meredith S, Griffith C, Packer JD, Henn RF 3rd. How should we secure our transplanted meniscus? A meta-analysis. Am J Sports Med. 2018;46(9):2285–90.
109. Bin SI, Nha KW, Cheong JY, Shin YS. Midterm and long-term results of medial versus lateral meniscal allograft transplantation: a meta-analysis. Am J Sports Med. 2018;46(5):1243–50.
110. Potter HG, Rodeo SA, Wickiewicz TL, Warren RF. MR imaging of meniscal allografts: correlation with clinical and arthroscopic outcomes. Radiology. 1996;198(2):509–14.
111. Koh YG, Moon HK, Kim YC, Park YS, Jo SB, Kwon SK. Comparison of medial and lateral meniscal transplantation with regard to extrusion of the allograft, and its correlation with clinical outcome. J Bone Joint Surg. 2012;94(2):190–3.
112. Grassi A, Bailey JR, Filardo G, Samuelsson K, Zaffagnini S, Amendola A. Return to sport activity after meniscal allograft transplantation: at what level and at what cost? A systematic review and meta-analysis. Sports Health. 2019;1941738118819723
113. Chalmers PN, Karas V, Sherman SL, Cole BJ. Return to high-level sport after meniscal allograft transplantation. Arthroscopy. 2013;29(3):539–44.

Future Treatment Modalities

10

Berkcan Akpinar and Philip A. Davidson

Abbreviations

AC	Articular chondrocyte
ACMEM	Acellular meniscus extracellular matrix
ADSC	Adipocyte-derived stem cell
BMP-2	Bone morphogenic protein-2
BMSC	Bone marrow-derived mesenchymal stem cell
CMI	Collagen meniscus implant
CTGF	Connective tissue growth factor
DCB	Demineralized cancellous bone
ECM	Extracellular matrix
ET-1	Endothelin-1
FGF-2	Fibroblast growth factor-2
GAG	Glycosaminoglycan
HCT	Horizontal cleavage tear
HGF	Hepatocyte growth factor
HIF-1alpha	Hypoxia inducible factor-1alpha
ICRS	International Cartilage Repair Society
IKDC	International Knee Documentation Committee Score
KOOS	Knee Injury and Osteoarthritis Outcome Scores
MDC	Meniscus-derived cell
MMSC	Meniscus-derived mesenchymal stem cell
MPC	Meniscus progenitor cell

B. Akpinar
Department of Orthopedic Surgery, New York University Langone Orthopedic Hospital, New York, NY, USA

P. A. Davidson (✉)
Davidson Orthopedics, Salt Lake City, UT, USA

E. J. Strauss, L. M. Jazrawi (eds.), *The Management of Meniscal Pathology*,
https://doi.org/10.1007/978-3-030-49488-9_10

MSC	Mesenchymal stem cell
MStC	Mesenchymal stromal cell
PDGF-AB	Platelet-derived growth factor-AB
PRP	Platelet-rich plasma
rAAV	Recombinant adeno-associated virus
SDF-1/CXCR4	Stromal cell–derived factor 1/chemokine receptor type 4
SPIO	Superparamagnetic iron oxide
TDMSC	Tonsil-derived mesenchymal stem cell
TGF beta-3	Transforming growth factor beta-3
VAS	Visual analog scale
VEGF	Vascular endothelial growth factor

Introduction: Regenerative Potential of the Meniscus

Management of meniscus tears has evolved significantly since the advent of arthroscopy. In order to understand the future direction of treatment, the pathophysiology of meniscus tearing must be briefly considered. The meniscus is a complex structure under constant stresses with an array of dynamic loading forces. Furthermore, the meniscus has a heterogeneous, hypocellular tissue makeup with a limited nutrient supply. These factors combine to make healing a meniscus tear or repair intrinsically difficult. Biomechanically, the meniscus is a dynamic structure undergoing substantial shape and force alterations during tibiofemoral joint articulation and loading [1–3]. Thus, a meniscus tear is under a variety of deforming forces potentially resulting in meniscal gapping at a repair or healing site [4]. From a tissue biology standpoint, relatively recent developments have further elucidated the regenerative potential of the meniscus.

Historically, the meniscus was generally considered to be a largely fibrocartilaginous structure with fibroblasts, chondrocytes, fibrochondrocytes, and a unique meniscal cell population with limited regenerative potential [5–9]. Histologically, the natural progression of a tear has been studied in multiple animal models [10–12]. In the context of the synovial fluid environment bathing the meniscus, many tears simply do not heal. In those where some healing takes place, there is significant early infiltration of the injured area with phagocytic cells in the acute phase after a tear [10]. This initial inflammatory response may be accompanied by subsequent synovial hyperplasia and an abundance of fibroblasts and fibrochondrocytes. These cells deposit new meniscocartilage into the damaged region with the assistance of various progenitor cells [10–14]. The obvious challenge moving forward is to promote or facilitate this healing response in the mechanically and histologically hostile environment in which the meniscus resides.

The cellular constituency of the meniscus and its surrounding tissue have been specifically elucidated in recent studies [15, 16]. The surrounding tissues, as compared to the relatively acellular central collagenous tissue, principally contribute to the biological response observed after a meniscus injury. The meniscal fibrochondrocyte cell population, in particular, has been shown to be critical in the regenerative response of the meniscus after a large meniscus defect [10, 15]. Evidence suggests these cells not only possess strong chondrogenic regenerative potential directly applicable to meniscus healing, but also a variable capacity for adipogenic and osteogenic differentiation based on proximity of isolation in reference to the outer rim of the meniscus [15]. Recent investigations also demonstrate that progenitor cells exist within the meniscus itself – meniscus-derived mesenchymal stem cells (MMSC). MMSCs have properties common to other mesenchymal stem cell (MSC) lineages such as clonogenicity, self-renewal, and multipotency. However, unlike a tendency toward osteogenic differentiation as seen in bone marrow–derived MSCs (BMSC), MMSCs exhibit a preference toward chondrogenic differentiation in smaller colonies in vitro at a slower rate of growth [17, 18]. This intrinsic tendency for chondrogenic differentiation may be further augmented through paracrine factors in the meniscus microenvironment, given evidence demonstrating the influence of coculturing MSCs with mature meniscus-derived cells (MDC) also promotes meniscal phenotype differentiation [6]. Further evidence suggests that MDCs isolated from human meniscus tissue have the capacity to de-differentiate under in vitro culture and subsequently re-differentiate into tissue resembling meniscus in scaffolds such as polyglycolic acid–hyaluronan. These dynamic characteristics demonstrate the versatility of this cell population [19]. Promoting and optimizing the selective differentiation of MDCs is a key goal to facilitate enhanced meniscal healing. In terms of actual cell marker expression, the meniscus contributes significantly to cell phenotype. All MDCs express higher amounts of CD14, CD26, CD49c, and CD49f compared to articular chondrocytes, while MDCs isolated from the outer region of the meniscus expressed more CD90, CD166, and CD271 in comparison with MDCs isolated from the inner, relatively avascular meniscus region [16]. Seol et al. describe a similar meniscus progenitor cell (MPC) population isolated from the peripheral vascular region of the meniscus that exhibits capacity to regenerate meniscus tissue in the setting of a tear both in the vascular and avascular region of the meniscus with gene expression profiles similar to other previously discovered progenitor cell populations [20]. Relevant to the stated goal of enhanced healing, as opposed to MSCs which can be stimulated toward chondrogenic differentiation in vitro, the MPCs described above only demonstrated enhanced meniscus fibrocartilage formation in the presence of extracellular matrix (ECM) in situ [20].

The microenvironment adjacent to the meniscus readily contributes to the progenitor cell pool after an acute injury. Matsukura et al. showed a dramatic increase in human MSCs as evidenced by cell phenotype and marker expression (CD44, CD73, CD90, and CD105) after isolated meniscus injury, suggesting that there is a distinct population of regenerative cells present at the time of injury, which can be utilized or promoted from a therapeutic clinical perspective [14]. Tarafder et al. demonstrate controlled application of connective tissue growth factor (CTGF) followed by transforming growth factor beta-3 (TGF beta-3) allowed synovial MSCs released at the time of meniscus injury to functionally regenerate, or heal, avascular meniscus tears in human subjects. This was facilitated through an initial fibrous matrix formation which remodeled with TGF beta-3 application into a fibrocartilaginous matrix bridging the tears, allowing for functional recovery [21]. Thus, recent developments demonstrate that the cell populations are much more complex than previously described. Furthermore, by understanding the microcellular environment, biologic modalities can be harnessed to promote healing, potentially with or without surgical repair. Progenitor cells certainly exist within the meniscus and the adjacent tissue potentially capable of providing regeneration after a meniscus tear, contrary to historical beliefs regarding absent intrinsic meniscal healing capability.

The vascularity of the meniscus has been extensively studied and described as a trait which governs and limits the healing potential of various meniscus tears. Given the avascular nature of the inner region of the meniscus, early studies performed with continuous passive motion have demonstrated access to low molecular weight nutrients, such as sulfate, are incorporated into this meniscus tissue and the limited cell population of this region through diffusion [22]. The meniscus has differential vascularity, with studies demonstrating as little as the outer 10% having vascularity in the mature knee of adults. There are many studies evaluating whether this reduction in direct nutrient supply plays a direct role in the altered healing response seen in the inner, avascular regions of the meniscus [23–26]. Hennerbichler et al. demonstrated that in the absence of variable nutrients restrictions generated in vivo meniscal explant tissue from the avascular versus vascular regions demonstrate similar healing properties in vitro [23].

In addition to differential access to nutrients, the limited vascular supply of the meniscus alters the regional access to paracrine signals necessary for tissue homeostasis and regeneration in the setting of an injury. The important stimulatory effect of various cytokines on meniscus cells derived from the outer, intermediate, and inner regions of the meniscus has been studied. These cells populations all increase protein synthesis and migratory activity levels upon exposure to human platelet–derived growth factor-AB (PDGF-AB), hepatocyte growth factor (HGF), and bone morphogenic protein-2 (BMP-2) [27, 28]. The specific location of a tear determines the cellular response to cytokines in the presence of a tear in vivo. Lu et al. demonstrate that dependent on the proximity to the red zone (periphery) of the meniscus, the expression of vascular endothelial growth factor (VEGF) and hypoxia inducible factor-1alpha (HIF-1alpha) both vary, even in the presence of injury, with greater baseline levels being expressed in the outer region of the meniscus, allowing for increased paracrine signaling after a tear [29]. Further, the secretion of endothelin-1 (ET-1) expressed predominantly in vessels throughout the meniscus outer rim acts as a strong chemotaxis signal to MSCs in the presence of a meniscus tear, which is much more robust in the outer region as compared to the inner [30]. Lastly, the blood vessels in the periphery of the meniscus provide access to various cell populations in the setting of a tear, which may not be present in the inner meniscus. The presence of multipotent stem cells existing within blood vessels is well known and was recently shown to be present in the vascular region of the meniscus as well, capable of differentiating into meniscus fibrochondrocytes both in vitro and in vivo during meniscus injury [31–33].

Aside from the unique cellular and vascular composition of the meniscus, the makeup and orientation of the macromolecules within which it exists pose difficulty when repairing and attempting to replicate meniscus tissue during larger repairs. Macroscopically, the collagen fibril orientation of the meniscus splays out radially with circumferential orientation in the superficial and deep layers. Thus, these fibers contribute significantly to distribution of hoop stresses during dynamic loading moments with native knee motion [34]. It is considerably challenging to replicate this network of fibrils in the setting of a meniscus repair while simultaneously preserving the interspersed cellularity of the meniscus without stimulating an immune response from the native surrounding tissue as well [35].

Although there is theoretical potential for meniscus self-regeneration after a tear or meniscectomy, the reality is the aforementioned regenerative cell populations are sparse, bridging tissue for allowing sufficient engraftment of regenerative cells is often lacking, and necessary growth factors are not intrinsically present without external stimuli in the form of scaffolds or biologic augmentation. Further, a substantial amount of the regenerative potential witnessed in the above reports are in animal studies with limited translation to the natural history of human meniscus tears.

Current Treatment Strategy Limitations

Historically, meniscal repair has principally been directed toward vertically oriented tears in the vascular, or peripheral, zone of the meniscus. In recent years, newer techniques have demonstrated favorable repair outcomes in other types of tears. Nonetheless, meniscectomy remains a very common procedure. The incidence of meniscal repair has been increasing over recent decades as newer, safer repair methods and implants have been introduced. In addition, overwhelming data continues to demonstrate the negative consequences of meniscal resection, with increased rates of osteoarthritis and cartilage degeneration after this procedure [36]. Guidelines for management of some meniscal tears, particularly degenerative ones, still remain controversial, given that the benefits of invasive procedures may not necessarily be superior to those of conservative measures. There has been high-quality data demonstrating that symptomatic, nonobstructive meniscus tears treated with physical therapy may provide equal clinical benefits compared to patients receiving meniscectomy [37, 38]. While meniscectomy demonstrates early functional benefits at timepoints of 6 months, it has not shown benefit when compared to physical therapy for degenerative meniscal tears in the long term, which raises concern regarding the utility of this procedure [39]. However, for tears currently deemed irreparable and symptomatic, meniscectomy is one of the few surgical treatment options available for many patients [40, 41].

In recent years, further studies have clarified the feasibility and success of repairing previously "irreparable" tears such as white–white tears, horizontal cleavage tears (HCT), tears in "older" patients, and revision meniscus repair tears. Regarding the avascular white–white zone, Rubman et al. demonstrated in a 198-patient series a reoperation rate of 20%, with only 25% of patients in having healed completely [42]. Similarly, Kimura et al. propose avascularity of tears as a major hurdle in achieving tear healing without other sources of biological stimulation, such as ligamentous tear involvement or use of a synovial flap during meniscus repair [43]. These results are conflicting with other reports in that they suggest better rates of recovery following repairs of meniscus tears extending into the avascular zone, which may be due to the degree of extension into the avascular region, surgical technique, and patient factors [44, 45]. In addition to repairs, surgeons currently employ marrow stimulation to further the healing process in these hypovascular tears, which studies have shown to be of some benefit [46]. HCTs have also been historically viewed as irreparable given their degenerative nature; however, certain studies suggest favorable outcomes, especially with concurrent marrow-stimulating techniques as described [40, 47, 48]. Repair re-tears may have significant degenerative components on repeat arthroscopy, frequently requiring debridement and salvage meniscectomy rather than revision repair to ameliorate patient symptoms [49]. Lastly, patient-related factors, such as body mass, health status, smoking, and lifestyle have traditionally contributed to relative indications for meniscus repair [50]. The overall composition of the meniscus undergoes age-related changes: cell regenerative potential diminishes, central degenerative micro-tears evolve, and cartilaginous macrostructure deformities begin to occur, resulting in reduced native meniscus function [50–52]. In fact, a significant amount of the middle-aged population already has subclinical micro-tears in their menisci that result in degenerative changes and render the meniscus potentially resistant to surgical repair if symptoms develop [52]. As a result of these limitations, many new treatments are being developed, some of which are already in clinical use. The most clinically utilized modality for meniscal deficiency is meniscus allograft transplantation [53]. However, concerns related to size-matched donor availability, cost, and potential immunogenic response creates ample room for the development of novel alternative technologies, as will be discussed here.

Overview of Future Treatment Modalities

There are multiple avenues within the realm of regenerative medicine being considered as viable options for future treatments in the setting of meniscus tears and resection. These include tissue substrates such as scaffolds, with composition varying in cellular, polymeric, and graft nature. In addition, biologic modalities that facilitate healing absenting or in conjunction with a formal repair have been proposed and utilized [54]. In the setting of post-meniscectomy degeneration, prosthetic spacers and implants are being trialed and indicated.

Various biological constructs have been developed in the recent years to improve tibiofemoral joint force mechanics and minimize osteoarthritic changes encountered in the aftermath of meniscectomy [41]. The theory behind the use of biomaterials in the setting of these tears is that once enough meniscal tissue has been removed to disrupt its ability to resist hoop stresses, alterations in load-bearing biomechanics and long-term risks for cartilage degeneration occur. Meniscal grafting seeks to restore native biomechanics and avoid or minimize degenerative changes [55]. In addition to collagenous and polymeric scaffolds [55], there have been recent developments in this area using biological fascia [56], demineralized bone [57], autologous grafts [58], xenografts [59], and augmentation of these with biologics, including a variety of cell populations [60].

In addition to implant-based constructs and scaffolds, there are also a series of nonstructural biological materials utilized in tandem with traditional repairs, or in lieu of repairs, for a variety of meniscus tears, which have been under investigation in recent years. In the setting of minimal tissue defects [requiring biomaterial gap filling], these biological augmentations are used with the intent of both enhancing the native tissue regenerative response, as well as introducing cell populations, growth factors, and other biomaterials known to stimulate meniscus repair [61]. These biological augmentation strategies involve the use of acellular [62] and cellular blood products [63], gene therapies [64], growth factor concentrates [65], and small molecule drugs [66].

Meniscus Implants

The overarching goal behind segmental meniscal implants (as compared to meniscal replacement) is to restore arthroprotective meniscal tissue in a durable fashion with appropriate tissue-implant interface healing. Generally, the indications for these implants include subjects with considerable, segmental meniscal defects as a result of large tears or meniscectomy. From a technical standpoint, the implant region requires intact anterior and posterior meniscal remnants and an intact outer meniscal rim for successful implant fixation [67, 68]. The two most studied and clinically applied meniscal implants to date are the collagen-based CMI™ (previously MenaFlex™, Stryker; Mahwah, NJ) and the polymeric synthetic ActiFit™ (Orteq; New York, NY) implants (Fig. 10.1) [69, 70].

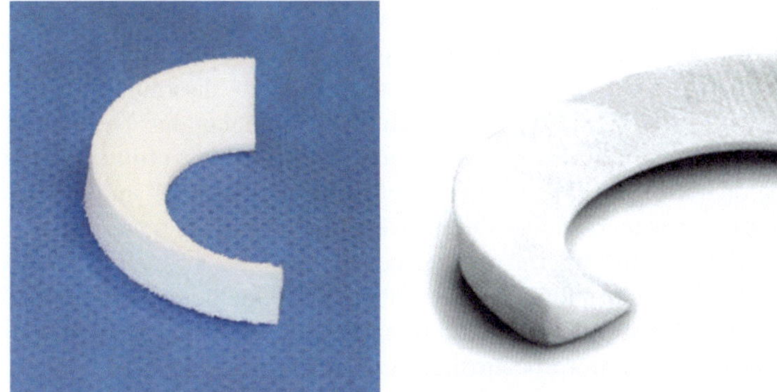

Fig. 10.1 Actifit™ (left) and CMI™ (right) implants. (Images used with permission of Orteq Sports Medicine Ltd. and © Springer International Publishing AG)

CMI™ and ActiFit™

The CMI™ was the first of its kind to be used in clinical practice [68]. Rodkey et al. described combining purified type I collagen fibers from bovine Achilles tendon, stoichiometric amounts of hyaluronic acid, chondroitin sulfate, and glycosamino-glycans (GAG) to achieve appropriate scaffold composition. Subsequently, the tissue was molded and the macromolecules cross-linked with formaldehyde once adequate tissue hydration levels and tissue molding were finished to resemble a meniscus in morphology and molecular consistency [68]. In their initial eight-subject trial, Rodkey et al. fixed the implants using a standard inside-out technique. Subjects, of whom seven had prior meniscectomies, were followed for 24–32 months and demonstrated clinical, radiological, and histological healing in their knees [68]. However, given a limited population with prior surgical interventions confounding cohort analysis, broad conclusions could not be made from the initial trial. Rodkey et al. followed up their initial study with a much larger population ($n = 311$) comparing CMI™ application to partial meniscectomy in subjects with acute and chronic meniscus tears. They conducted subsequent arthroscopic, histological, and clinical follow-up at a mean of 59 months [71]. As expected from their prior study, there was histological filling of the meniscus implants with fibrocartilaginous tissue resembling meniscus in both acute and chronic meniscectomy cohorts receiving the CMI™. There was also more tissue coverage of the joint surfaces in the intervention group. Interestingly, only the chronic tear cohort receiving CMI™ implantation demonstrated clinical improvements in visual analog scale (VAS) pain, Lysholm, and patient self-assessment scores, despite there being evidence of tissue regeneration in both acute and chronic cohorts [71].

Since the development of this implant, multiple long-term studies with a mean follow-up ranging from 5 to 11.1 years have demonstrated the potential utility of CMI™ as a reliable long-term treatment that may be superior to partial meniscectomy for irreparable meniscus tears [67]. In most studies, there was MRI imaging showing an intact meniscus implant with preservation of periarticular cartilage, radiographic preservation of joint space, and improved clinical pain levels at short- (3-month) and long-term follow-up [67, 72]. However, these studies also reported a portion of subjects experiencing chronic low-level pain at the implant site, evidence of myxoid degeneration throughout the implants, and complete dissolution of the CMI™ in some cases [67, 69, 72, 73]. The durability of the implant has been studied at length. Studies suggest it may not have the longevity needed to fully convey lasting arthroprotecion uniformly [74]. Lastly, the efficacy of the CMI™ implant for patients with acute meniscus tears remains controversial [73].

A biosynthetic meniscal scaffold graft was introduced to address perceived challenges with the CMI™. Potential shortcomings of the CMI™ include risk of immunogenicity [75], reports of myxoid degeneration, and residual chronic pain. While initial clinical trials of CMI™ were occurring, synthetic meniscal implants were being developed in the preclinical setting. De Groot et al. described a porous polyurethane structure consisting of 50/50 copoly(l-lactide/ε-caprolactone) with an appropriate compression modulus capable of allowing successful fibrocartilage ingrowth as demonstrated in canine preclinical trials [76, 77]. Unlike prior polyurethane constructs being studied at the time, this molecular composition did not subject the receiving host to toxic degradation products with in vivo metabolism [76, 78, 79] and was deemed safe in humans [77, 80].

Initial investigation of the Actifit™ implant [74] was conducted on a small cohort of patients ($n = 10$), validating patient safety and implant viability in vivo. The findings were encouraging, with a general absence of significant joint inflammation or synovitis, reflecting the general tolerability and biocompatibility of the polyurethane polymeric structure at 1-year follow-up [81]. The ActiFit Group subsequently reported their initial proof-of-concept results in 52 patients with irreparable partial meniscus defects. Clinical efficacy of the ActiFit implant was reported, with global improvements in the International Knee Documentation Committee (IKDC), Knee Injury and Osteoarthritis Outcome Score (KOOS), Lysholm, and VAS scores [82]. Tissue ingrowth was witnessed at 3 months in 81% of patients, as determined by dynamic contrast-enhanced MRI, with improvement to 97% at 12 months [74]. There was also no histological evidence of cell necrosis at 12 months, with complete tissue viability seen [74]. In a similar fashion to the native meniscus, three layers were also observed histologically, varying in vascularity, cellularity, and fibrocartilage composition [74]. However, of significant note, the study did have implant failures in nine subjects, including one postoperative deep infection, one conversion to knee unicompartmental arthroplasty, three scaffold dislocations, one incidence of chondromalacia requiring microfracture, one incidence of painful suture requiring removal, and one scaffold non-integration [82].

A follow-up implant investigation on 54 subjects who had lateral meniscus defects diagnosed with post-meniscectomy syndrome was conducted with close clinical assessment at 3, 6 12, and 24 months [83]. Bouyarmane et al. reported an all-around incremental clinical improvement with each consecutive follow-up in terms of the VAS, IKDC, and KOOS scores [83]. In their series, the rate of reoperation was less than that of Veronk et al. [74], with only three patients requiring intervention for implant-related complications (one medial femoral osteochondritis dissecans, and two partial scaffold removals) [83]. At 5-year follow-up, KOOS, VAS, and IKDC scores remained improved from initial preoperative scores, as measured in the remaining 25 subjects in the trial. However, certain sub-scores (sports, stiffness) had diminished, as compared to the 2-year interval follow-up results [84]. With regards to cartilage preservation, 7 of 15 subjects with cartilage assessments at the preoperative 2-, and 5-year interval assessments demonstrated preservation, while the rest demonstrated worsening International Cartilage Repair Society (ICRS) scores. Out of the 44 subjects that were followed to the 5-year mark, 14 were deemed to have failed implants, of which 3 required implant removal, 5 required meniscal allograft transplant, 4 required unicompartmental knee replacement, and 2 required total knee replacement [84].

In the context of these mixed clinical results for the ActiFit™ synthetic implant, recent investigations have suggested that the implant, in its studied form, may not yet be optimal for clinical use [85–87] despite relatively acceptable outcomes at short-term follow-up [88]. While functional scores (KOOS, IKDC, VAS) improved and remained stable, with acceptable degrees of meniscus extrusion, studies with long-term follow-up using advanced imaging demonstrate that the ActiFit™ scaffolds fail to stimulate substantial meniscal tissue regeneration and ingrowth. Further, there are abnormal signal enhancements within the remaining implant tissue, suggestive of chronic degeneration, and the failure rates requiring reoperation still remain high [85–87]. In general, polyurethane scaffolds improve functional and patient-reported measures in the majority of subjects over the near-term, but fail to prevent the deterioration objective factors such as the status of articular cartilage and degree of meniscal extrusion [89]. While the degree of preoperative meniscal morphology and extrusion may play a role the success of polyurethane scaffolds, the pathologic changes known to occur in the knee after long-term follow-up of these implants are not yet understood [89, 90].

Overall, the CMI™ and ActiFit™ implants both appear to demonstrate acceptable short-term results, but their durability and effects on adjacent structures have been the major concerns with long-term clinical follow-up [70, 87, 91]. These implants demonstrate failure in up to approximately one-third of subjects according to the trials cited. Furthermore, these grafts also display significant MRI signal intensity abnormalities, along with in vivo dissolution without successful long-term generation of new meniscal tissue [91]. Interestingly, at short-term follow-up, these implants have had the most success when paired with ligament reconstructions and high tibial osteotomies, which suggests that a potential marrow-stimulated environment may facilitate better implant incorporation and new meniscal ingrowth [69, 84, 87, 91].

NUsurface™

Interpositional meniscal substitution has been developed in light of the challenges seen with the use of meniscus scaffolds and allografts. The NUsurface™ (Active Implants; Memphis, TN) is a total medial meniscus replacement possessing a biomechanical profile similar to native meniscus tissue (Fig. 10.2) [92, 93]. The implant does not require surgical fixation unlike the MenaFlex™ and ActiFit™ implants. The implant, in theory, provides immediate restoration of meniscal-type function

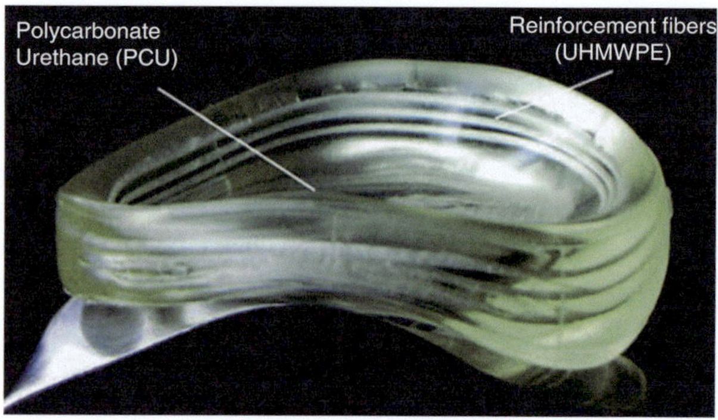

Fig. 10.2 NUsurface™ prosthetic. (Image used with permission of © Springer International Publishing AG)

without requiring biologic incorporation or healing. This meniscal replacement may have a role as a joint-preserving procedure in patients with a blunted biological healing response, in whom prosthetic meniscal implantation may delay the need for arthroplasty. Currently, the NUsurface™ implant is being assessed in two randomized clinical trials in the USA – the VENUS (Verification of the Effectiveness of the NUsurface™ System) and SUN (Safety Utilizing NUsurface™) trials.

Other Acellular Implants

Other acellular meniscal implants are presently being developed with an array of characteristics that may be of potential clinical benefit. A meniscus implant composed of novel silk fibroin protein has been studied in bovine knees, assessing biomechanical, histological, and tissue ingrowth outcomes at 6- to 8-month follow-up. The silk fibroin implants display in vivo biomechanical properties resembling that of a native meniscus; they appear to be chondroprotective and display a significant capacity for tissue ingrowth. However, the long-term risks of using this technology needs to be elucidated in light of the limitations seen thus far with CMI™ and ActiFit™ implants [94, 95]. A hybrid of the silk fibroin protein and CMI™ scaffold has also been studied in rabbits. This consists of a silk sponge containing an external collagen coating that theoretically enhances the biomechanical and tissue ingrowth properties of the material, while also reducing the degree of adjacent cartilage degeneration [96].

Acellular meniscus extracellular matrix (ACMEM) has also been studied independently and in tandem with demineralized cancellous bone (DCB) in an effort to develop an optimal scaffold for meniscus grafting [97]. Given the affinity of meniscus fibrochondrocytes for DCB in vitro, it may serve as a useful adjuvant to meniscal scaffold healing [57]. Alone, ACMEM or DCB matrices do not possess the optimal biomechanical properties necessary for meniscus replacement. However, a combined ACMEM/DCB scaffold is capable of withstanding appropriate joint mechanics [in rabbits], protecting articular cartilage, and allowing for successful ingrowth [though glycosaminoglycan (GAG) content was still lacking upon further analysis] [97].

The most promising acellular meniscus implant studied in animals to date is the poly-ε-caprolactone-based scaffold generated using 3D biomaterial printing. This is morphologically and biomechanically similar to meniscus tissue [98]. This constructed implant has microchannels lined with CTGF and TGF beta-3, which are spatiotemporally released. Upon implantation, the CTGF is released initially followed by gradual TGF beta-3 release in vivo stimulating a sequence of biological responses in sheep. While other implants cause myxoid degeneration, this implant stimulates endogenous MPC migration and ingrowth into the acellular scaffold matrix. It also stimulates selective MPC collagen type I and type II deposition resembling that of the native meniscus [98]. Given this apparent favorable tissue and cellular response [21], this scaffold design may progress to human trials in the near future.

Additional acellular scaffolds include electrospun nanofiber assemblies, which may have a role in meniscus repair and grafting [99]. The utility of these scaffolds is likely to be enhanced when cell-seeding is applied. Lastly, hydrogels are also under investigation in the treatment of meniscus defects. The hydrogel formed after treating polyvinyl alcohol with sodium sulfate has comparable compressive structure to a native human meniscus and displayed no cytotoxicity during preliminary in vitro testing, suggesting potential biocompatibility [100].

Cell-Augmented Implants

Though the above prosthetic strategies have demonstrated significant promise and short-term success, a proven, viable, long-term biologic option has yet to be developed for significant meniscus defects. Despite successful surgical implantation, initially functional biomechanics, and early tissue ingrowth, acellular scaffolds appear to undergo degenerative changes in the long-term in the limited human trials to date [72, 85, 87]. Thus, research and investigative efforts have shifted toward developing scaffolds with inbuilt cellular populations to augment the biological response and healing process after implantation.

MDCs have been successfully used to seed polymeric scaffolds in efforts to regenerate whole meniscus defects in rabbit models [101, 102]. Kang et al. seeded MDCs on a polyglycolic acid scaffold, while Lu et al. seeded MDCs on a poly-(3-hydroxybutyrate-co-3-hydroxyvalerate) scaffold for whole meniscus regeneration [101, 102]. The polyglycolic scaffolds displayed a significant increase in collagen and proteoglycan levels at 10 weeks post-implantation. However, there were ultimate differences in macromolecule content and biomechanical functionalities between the neomenisci and meniscal controls [101]. The poly-(3- hydroxybutyrate-co-3-hydroxyvalerate total meniscus implants demonstrated type I collagen formation at 8-week follow-up post-implantation, but early adjacent cartilage degeneration was noted, albeit less than in the total meniscectomy controls [102]. The neomeniscus generation of these scaffold provides further evidence regarding regenerative potential of MDCs [16, 103]. Both polymeric and electrospun collagen-based scaffolds seeded with human meniscus cells have also been shown to provide tissue regeneration superior to acellular grafts. They have shown a significant potential to reorganize and strengthen collagen fiber macrostructure, while also retaining long-term cell viability [19, 104].

Recent investigations have provided evidence highlighting the importance of adjacent knee structures in scaffold healing. Oda et al. incorporated infrapatellar fat pad tissue into collagen scaffolds and implanted them into rabbit meniscal defects [105]. The implant stimulated new tissue regeneration, while also reducing interleukin-1beta expression as compared to controls. This demonstrates the immunomodulatory role provided by fat pad augmentation [105]. In tandem with human chondrocyte seeding, Kwak et al. also explored pretreatment of poly-lactic-co-glycolic acid scaffolds with platelet-rich plasma (PRP) in efforts to stimulate further meniscus formation in a mouse meniscus defect model [106]. When pretreated with

PRP, the chondrocyte-seeded scaffolds healed fully and/or partially in the majority of cases ($n = 16$), whereas controls without PRP treatment did not display any healing at 6-week follow-up [106].

There has been a significant interest in combining scaffolds with stem cells. Given the observed difficulty in achieving tissue integration and durability of regenerated menisci in vivo, augmentation of ActiFit™ with mesenchymal stromal cells (MStC) has been studied in rabbits [107]. As compared to acellular controls, the polyurethane scaffold seeded with MStCs demonstrated increased signs of meniscus healing, including increased vascularity, proteoglycan content, and histological integration. Furthermore, MStC-seeded grafts integrated earlier than their acellular counterparts [107]. Investigations on stem cell augmentation for scaffolds are currently underway given the known regenerative potential, multipotency, and self-renewal capacity of these cell populations. In rabbits, a polyvinyl alcohol/chitosan scaffold seeded with either articular chondrocytes (AC), adipocyte-derived stem cells (ADSC), or an AC–ADSC combination was assessed to evaluate meniscus regeneration and articular cartilage preservation after meniscal replacement. The scaffold groups with AC performed best with regard to meniscus regeneration and articular cartilage preservation, while the ADSCs did not contribute significantly at 7 months post-implantation [108]. This can be at least partially explained by the superiority of AC in forming articular cartilage versus ADSCs. The differentiation and maturation of stem cells into successful meniscus fibrocartilaginous tissue in vivo is complex and requires specific paracrine cell signaling [109, 110]. However, the robust proliferative capacity of stem cells is of tremendous value in implant design. For example, meniscus fibrochondrocytes have a propensity for greater fibrocartilage fiber and GAG generation when seeded in scaffolds versus stem cells, but the higher metabolic rate and proliferative capacity of stem cells offers greater viability when seeded in implants in vivo [59]. Ideally, a combination of native MDCs and stem cells may be used to stimulate optimal meniscal tissue formation [59].

Evidence suggests that seeding scaffolds with a multipotent cell population is of benefit versus acellular controls [111]. In rabbits, seeding poly(ε-caprolactone) scaffolds with BMSCs allowed greater ingrowth and meniscus mechanical function in rabbits at 2 years post-implantation [111]. In vitro studies have demonstrated that stem cell augmentation significantly strengthens scaffold mechanics and fiber organization when compared with acellular scaffolds [112]. In addition to ADSCs and BMSCs, synovial stem cells have been used to augment Achilles tendon–derived meniscus grafts in rats with success when pretreating the graft prior to implantation [13]. Stem cell pretreatment of grafts may also have significant translational capacity intraoperatively given a clinically convenient short pretreatment time of only 10 minutes [13]. Koh et al. utilized hydrogel grafts seeded with tonsil-derived mesenchymal stem cells (TDMSC) in a rabbit model for meniscus regeneration with marked success, providing further evidence of the versatility of stem cells in the setting of meniscal defects [113]. After exposing TDMSCs to a conditioned medium from meniscal fibrochondrocytes and TGF beta-3, these cells expressed increased levels of meniscus-related genes and produced extracellular matrix components resembling meniscus macromolecules. When employed in a rabbit meniscus defect model, the graft was also successful in generating in vivo meniscus tissue with a biocompatible hydrogel crosslinking riboflavin-mediated reaction for graft maturation [113].

In the setting of hydrogel graft use, ADSCs alongside TGF beta-3 treatment have displayed robust capacity for in vitro meniscus tissue formation and a potential for tear repair [114]. As is the case with TDMSCs and synovial stem cells, proper conditioning of stem cells appears to have significant efficacy in promoting meniscus formation after graft deployment [114]. Hydrogel technology has also been used to develop methods of recycling meniscus tissue and incorporating it into new graft generation. In rats, the meniscus was explanted, processed into a meniscal ECM hydrogel, augmented with human MSCs, and subsequently reinjected into the rat meniscus-deficient knees as a vehicle for meniscus regeneration with favorable results [115]. Recently, synovial stem cells have been used in rabbits in tandem with an electrospun bioengineered tissue construct consisting of nanofibers. This new graft is composed of the ECM generated by the grafted synovial stem cells combined with tissue-engineered electrospun nanofibers. This imparts both mechanical and biological stability to the meniscus tear repair [60]. While the electrospun nanofiber construct alone provides an excellent restoration of structural meniscus properties capable of withstanding native hoop stresses, the added stem cell biological component facilitates tissue ingrowth and subsequent preservation of articular cartilage [60]. Whitehouse et al. recently conducted the first human in vivo assessment of cell-augmented scaffolds for meniscus tears. Using iliac crest–derived BMSCs, they seeded a collagen-based scaffold and implanted it into five patients [116]. At 2-year follow-up, three patients had clinical and radiographic improvements with evidence of meniscus healing, while two patients required subsequent meniscectomy for re-tear or failure of graft healing.

Presently, meniscus implants remain at the early stages of clinical application, with mixed results to date. While implants such as the CMI™, ActiFit™, and NUsurface™ have demonstrated promising results at short- to mid-term follow-up, the long-term durability of such acellular implants remains suboptimal. Current development of biocomposite implants is focused on determining the ideal cell–scaffold combination to facilitate long-term scaffold durability, tissue ingrowth, arthroprotection, and biocompatibility. Current animal and in vitro investigations combining biosynthetic tissues with cellular components are encouraging and will form the basis for future study.

Biologics

Biologics are being investigated and used in many orthopedic injuries with the goal of mitigating inflammatory and/or degenerative changes, especially in conditions with impaired healing due to a limited vascular or cell supply [54, 117–119]. Particular to meniscus lesions, a variety of different biologics ranging from cell-based injections, PRP [62], gene therapy [120], growth factors [21], and drugs [66] have been investigated.

Blood Products

Various blood products have been used in efforts to stimulate meniscus healing in the presence of a tear, especially if it extends into the central rim. PRP is in wide clinical use as a biological augment in orthopedics. Depending upon the specific preparation of PRP, it is rich in numerous cytokines and growth factors, including platelet factor 4, VEGF, PDGF, TGF beta-1, TGF beta-2, HGF, and insulin-like growth factor-1 [117]. PRP as an augment to scaffolds for meniscus repair has yielded promising results. Isolated PRP and platelet-rich fibrin matrix is more preliminary at this stage for treatment of meniscus tears and defects [106]. Compared with human serum, PRP is inferior in stimulating meniscus cells in vitro to form adequate meniscus tissue [61, 62]. Human serum may be of more use in stimulating meniscus cell migration toward tears, inducing meniscus-forming gene expression and promoting cell proliferation. Although PRP is able to stimulate better chemotaxis compared to strictly growth factor controls, cell populations appear to possess better chemotaxis-stimulating properties [61, 121]. Given that PRP possesses the cytokines necessary for meniscus tissue formation and stimulation of meniscus fibrochondrocytes, investigations regarding its use in meniscus lesions are ongoing [27]. However, to date, the various clinical trials assessing PRP have demonstrated minimal to no differences in clinical, pain-related, and radiographic outcomes comparing it to saline controls in the setting of meniscus repair augmentation [122–125].

Application of fibrin clots have also been described in the literature as a potential technique to augment meniscus suture repairs, especially for tears in the avascular zone [126, 127]. The literature suggests there may be an added clinical benefit to the use of fibrin clots during tear repair, but evidence of efficacy on the basis of healing at the time of second-look arthroscopy remains limited [128–130].

Given the known effects of various growth factors on meniscus cell behavior, efforts have also been directed at calculated cytokine and growth factor use for meniscus repair [9, 27, 131]. In vitro, the effects of both PRP and BMP-7 stimulate collagen II deposition and MSC proliferation. However, these augments were unsuccessful in regenerating meniscus tissue in a rabbit model in tandem with a hydrogel-based scaffold [54]. BMP-7 remains more promising, as other investigations have proven its utility as an augment to Achilles tendon–based grafts in a rat meniscectomy model of regenerating meniscus tissue [56]. The chondrogenic properties of BMP-7 stimulate increased cartilage formation within the tendinous grafts, creating meniscus-like tissue, while also preventing articular cartilage degeneration in the joint [56]. Recent investigations with human meniscus fibrochondrocytes in vitro have shown that when cultured with adequate exposure to TGF beta-1 and fibroblast growth factor-2 (FGF-2), ECM resembling that of avascular meniscus was generated, suggesting these factors may have potential for clinical use [103]. When oxygen tension was varied, hypoxic conditions seemed more conducive to meniscus ECM generation. This suggests that the avascular environment of the knee joint may present a suitable environment for the use of these growth factors. The importance of TGF on meniscus development has been described, but the clinical combination, quantity, and temporal order of use of these factors has been difficult to optimize [132]. To date, one study has successfully regenerated meniscus tissue in a rabbit meniscus defect model using strictly growth factor–based biologics (CTGF and TGF beta-3) [21]. These investigators used a temporary fibrous matrix as a scaffold within the meniscus defect. CTGF and TGF beta-3 are released in a temporally specific manner; CTGF is first released and acts as a profibrinogenic cue, while the delayed TGF beta-3 acts as a chondrogenic stimulant. Together, both factors allow for proper collagen deposition and meniscus tissue formation with excellent tissue integration in the avascular meniscus region [21]. Thus, a combination of CTGF and TGF beta-3, along with FGF-2 and BMP-7 may play a role in future biologic therapies for meniscus healing in tandem or even in lieu of surgical repairs.

Cellular Therapy

Given the regenerative potential of stem cells, many investigations have assessed whether there is a role for stem cell-based adjuvant therapy in the management of meniscal tears and defects. Many stem cell populations can be used for new tissue generation, but depending on their tissue origin, certain populations have a tendency to differentiate into specific pathways [31, 133]. To enhance meniscus defect repair, MSCs from a variety of different sources have also been studied [17]. The mechanism by which MSCs may contribute to meniscus defect healing likely has to do with the activation of Indian hedgehog cell signaling pathways, which stimulates the deposition of collagen type II [134]. BMSCs are readily available in abundant quantities in autologous grafts, possess a versatile differentiation capacity, and have been used in various therapeutic modalities [135]. However, in the setting of meniscus tissue formation, BMSCs have a tendency to undergo detrimental hypertrophy during chondrogenesis, interfering with their ability to form adequate fibrocartilaginous tissue necessary for meniscus development [136]. Studies have attempted to circumvent this characteristic by exposing BMSCs to native MDCs during culture in vitro; however, this limitation persists [6, 59, 136–138]. Nonetheless, investigations with BMSCs have yielded some positive results in the context of meniscus regeneration. Vangsness et al. conducted a 55-patient randomized clinical trial assessing the efficacy and safety of allogeneic BMSC intra-articular injections after partial medial meniscectomy [139]. The study demonstrated that patients receiving the stem cell injection, versus the saline control, had new meniscus tissue within the meniscectomy defect at 12 months post-injection. However, the quantity of cells injected did not correlate with amount of new meniscus generated. Additionally, the BMSC-injected groups had better clinical outcomes with respect to pain scores at follow-up [139]. BMSCs have also been shown in equine meniscus defect models to possess significant regenerative capability after 12 months in conjunction with a scaffold for tissue repair [140].

ADSCs have also been investigated in the setting of meniscus repair given their relative accessibility and potential for clinical translation [141–143]. Similar to BMSCs, ADSCs possess multilineage differentiation capacities, including chondrogenesis, which allows for the formation of the fibrocartilage needed for meniscus generation [142]. Animal studies demonstrate that ADSCs are able to engraft within defects, form new meniscus tissue, and remain viable cells for a substantial amount of time in meniscus tissue. Further, ADSCs are apparently adequate supplements to suture-based meniscus tear repairs, as demonstrated in murine models [141, 142]. In a rabbit model on total meniscectomy, Qi et al. studied treatment with ADSCs labeled with superparamagnetic iron oxide (SPIO) that allowed for in vivo orientation through the use of magnets. The animals were subsequently followed via imaging and histology at 12 weeks. New tissue resembling native meniscus both macro- and microscopically had formed in the experimental group. This not only provides evidence in support of ADSCs, but also further justifies the need to investigate SPIO-based delivery methods as potential therapeutic biologics in the treatment of osteoarthritis of the knee [142].

While BMSCs and ADSCs are readily and conveniently available, synovial stem cell populations appear to be superior at meniscus regeneration and healing [11]. When comparing rabbit BMSCs to MMSCs, MMSCs have a greater propensity for healing meniscus defects, while still possessing universal stem cell properties of clonicity, self-renewal, and multilineage potential. However, MMSCs tend to grow slower and form smaller colonies in vitro [17]. Synovial stem cell investigations have yielded promising results with single intra-articular injections into murine meniscal-deficient knees, showing significant healing as compared with saline controls at 6 months post-injection [12]. Allogeneic synovial MSCs have also been shown to regenerate new meniscus tissue in the setting of implantation after total meniscectomy models in rabbits. Allogeneic synovial MSCs demonstrated cell engraftment and differentiation into fibrochondrocytes at 12 weeks post-implantation [144]. Interestingly, these cells not only engraft well into meniscus tissue, but also remain localized to the region of implantation, as demonstrated by Horie et al. using gene labeling studies [11]. Kondo et al. were the first to describe autologous synovial MSC implantation in primates. After meniscectomy, primates received either MSC aggregates or nothing in order to assess efficacy, and at 16 weeks, the MSC group had healthier femoral articular cartilage and new healed meniscus tissue, as assessed by imaging and histology [145]. Baboolal et al. developed a technique stimulating mobilization of synovial MSCs intraoperatively that increased MSC mobilization up to 105-fold [63]. Chondroprogenitor MSCs have also been described as appropriate cell populations for meniscus regeneration. Similarly to synovial MSCs, chondroprogenitor MSCs also possess reduced expression of cellular hypertrophy marker collagen X, making them a desirable cell source for meniscus regeneration. Further, the stromal cell–derived factor 1/chemokine receptor type 4 (SDF-1/CXCR4) cell signal pathway appears to be critical in allowing this cell lineage to migrate into and heal meniscus defects in rats [146]. Similarly, injecting human MMSCs to rat meniscus defects also yielded meniscus defect healing, mediated through the SDF-1/CXCR4 signaling pathway. These cells expressed lower-than-normal levels of cell hypertrophy osteoarthritis markers, such as collagen X [147].

Gene Therapy

The relevance of growth factor and cytokine regulation [21, 98, 148] in meniscal tears and defects affecting repair and regeneration has provided insight into the potential role of gene therapy in managing this condition, especially given that genetic expression profiles after a meniscus tear are altered depending on the subject's age, sex, and comorbid injury patterns [149]. Groups have had success investigating the manipulation of meniscus genetic profiles using nonviral and viral vector-based alterations [64, 150–153]. Transduction of meniscus tissue with vectors capable of enhancing meniscus vascularity [152] and ECM synthesis [151] offers a new avenue to supplement traditional surgical repairs. Using gene-based therapy, there is potential for a more durable repair than with scaffolds [64, 150, 153]. A major limitation of gene therapy in clinical use is the need for ex vivo manipulation of the tissue for transduction purposes prior to reimplantation [64, 120, 154]. The use of recombinant adeno-associated virus (rAAV) vectors circumvents this by allowing in situ transduction of meniscus tissue, as demonstrated in human cells [64, 120, 154]. These vectors are especially applicable in meniscus cells as they can integrate successfully into replicating and nonreplicating cells [120, 154]. The rAAV has been used to upregulate FGF-2 expression as well as TFG-beta expression in vitro and in situ in intact and meniscal injury models, with resultant increased regenerative meniscus cell activity, as evidenced by alpha-smooth muscle actin expression [120, 154]. Genetic engineering efforts have also been combined with scaffold designs to create biologically augmented meniscus implants [155]. Seeding MSCs and meniscus cells previously transduced with TGF beta-1 into a collagen–GAG scaffold has proven beneficial in avascular meniscus tear repair in vitro, with notable increases in ECM formation 3 weeks after implantation [155]. Additional growth factor upregulation has also been investigated; upregulation of human insulin-like growth factor-1 using transfected BMSCs in calcium alginate gel has demonstrated increased proteoglycan formation in the transfected cells in vivo as compared with nontransfected controls. However, the level of ECM expression did not reach that of native meniscal cells [156]. MicroRNA manipulation has also been pivotal in gene therapy for many pathological conditions, given the role of these molecules in cell cycle regulatory processes [157]. Kawanishi et al. designed a synthetic microRNA (miR-210) to modulate meniscus cell metabolism, given the known effects of miR-210 on mitochondrial function, angiogenesis, and cell survival [158]. After intra-articular injection in a rat avascular meniscus tear model, miR-210 was shown to stimulate healing, with increased expression of itself, collagen type 2 alpha 1, VEGF, and FGF-2 in both meniscal cells and synovial cells compared with controls [158]. Given the minimally invasive approach, permanence of genetic integration, and lack of need for exogenous cell implantation, microRNA-based technology may certainly play a role in the future management of meniscus tears.

Drug Therapy

Small molecule-based regenerative modalities are also being explored for use in meniscus tissue repair. Zhang et al. found that adding simvastatin to hydrogel-based implants in meniscectomy rabbit models provided a more robust healing response than in controls [159]. The simvastatin group demonstrated more collagen I deposition, higher levels of BMP-2, BMP-7 on histological analysis, and stronger biomechanical profiles at 12 weeks post-implantation. The mechanism may involve modulation of BMP and genes COL1 and COL2 [159]. Qu et al. designed a nanofibrous scaffold that gradually degrades, releasing calculated amounts of collagenase and subsequent PDGF-AB to facilitate meniscus healing [66]. In a murine meniscal defect model, the collagenase allows for cell-permeable pore formation in the ECM. PDGF-AB acts as a chemoattractant, stimulating endogenous meniscus progenitor cell migration to facilitate healing of the defect [66]. This particular scaffold could be used to elute any desired combination of small molecules, including drugs, enzymes, cytokines, and ECM components.

Conclusion

Symptomatic meniscus tears and post-meniscectomy tissue defects remain a challenging scenario for clinicians to treat. Traditional management of these lesions has consisted of nonoperative therapy, resection, repair, and meniscal allograft transplantation. Outcomes of resection have been conclusively shown to be poor in the long term. Meniscal repair outcomes, while continually improving, remain suboptimal, and meniscal allograft transplantation is limited by graft availability, cost, and relatively short-term follow-up. Efforts to improve the treatment of meniscal defects are multi-faceted. Scaffolds have been partially successful in facilitating neomeniscal formation, tissue ingrowth, and arthroprotection, although long-term durability and sustained clinical benefits have been an issue. Biological augmentation of such implants is actively being investigated. Cell and growth factor-incorporating implants have the potential to improve upon the limitations of current designs. Advancements in gene therapy and small molecule-based applications will also likely play a role. Eventually, a combination of these strategies, incorporating the use of scaffolds, cell populations, biologics, and pharmacologics, will equip clinicians with the capacity to optimize native knee longevity.

References

1. Thompson WO, Thaete FL, Fu FH, Dye SF. Tibial meniscal dynamics using three-dimensional reconstruction of magnetic resonance images. Am J Sports Med. 1991;19(3):210–5; discussion 5-6.
2. Clark CR, Ogden JA. Development of the menisci of the human knee joint. Morphological changes and their potential role in childhood meniscal injury. J Bone Joint Surg Am. 1983;65(4):538–47.

3. Bursac P, Arnoczky S, York A. Dynamic compressive behavior of human meniscus correlates with its extra-cellular matrix composition. Biorheology. 2009;46(3):227–37.
4. Durselen L, Hebisch A, Claes LE, Bauer G. Gapping phenomenon of longitudinal meniscal tears. Clin Biomech (Bristol, Avon). 2003;18(6):505–10.
5. Ghadially FN, Lalonde JM, Wedge JH. Ultrastructure of normal and torn menisci of the human knee joint. J Anat. 1983;136(Pt 4):773–91.
6. Cui X, Hasegawa A, Lotz M, D'Lima D. Structured three-dimensional co-culture of mesenchymal stem cells with meniscus cells promotes meniscal phenotype without hypertrophy. Biotechnol Bioeng. 2012;109(9):2369–80.
7. Mueller SM, Shortkroff S, Schneider TO, Breinan HA, Yannas IV, Spector M. Meniscus cells seeded in type I and type II collagen-GAG matrices in vitro. Biomaterials. 1999;20(8):701–9.
8. Mueller SM, Schneider TO, Shortkroff S, Breinan HA, Spector M. Alpha-smooth muscle actin and contractile behavior of bovine meniscus cells seeded in type I and type II collagen-GAG matrices. J Biomed Mater Res. 1999;45(3):157–66.
9. Verdonk PC, Forsyth RG, Wang J, Almqvist KF, Verdonk R, Veys EM, et al. Characterisation of human knee meniscus cell phenotype. Osteoarthr Cartil. 2005;13(7):548–60.
10. Hiyama K, Muneta T, Koga H, Sekiya I, Tsuji K. Meniscal regeneration after resection of the anterior half of the medial meniscus in mice. J Orthop Res. 2017;35(9):1958–65.
11. Horie M, Sekiya I, Muneta T, Ichinose S, Matsumoto K, Saito H, et al. Intra-articular injected synovial stem cells differentiate into meniscal cells directly and promote meniscal regeneration without mobilization to distant organs in rat massive meniscal defect. Stem Cells. 2009;27(4):878–87.
12. Hatsushika D, Muneta T, Horie M, Koga H, Tsuji K, Sekiya I. Intraarticular injection of synovial stem cells promotes meniscal regeneration in a rabbit massive meniscal defect model. J Orthop Res. 2013;31(9):1354–9.
13. Ozeki N, Muneta T, Matsuta S, Koga H, Nakagawa Y, Mizuno M, et al. Synovial mesenchymal stem cells promote meniscus regeneration augmented by an autologous Achilles tendon graft in a rat partial meniscus defect model. Stem Cells. 2015;33(6):1927–38.
14. Matsukura Y, Muneta T, Tsuji K, Koga H, Sekiya I. Mesenchymal stem cells in synovial fluid increase after meniscus injury. Clin Orthop Relat Res. 2014;472(5):1357–64.
15. Mauck RL, Martinez-Diaz GJ, Yuan X, Tuan RS. Regional multilineage differentiation potential of meniscal fibrochondrocytes: implications for meniscus repair. Anat Rec (Hoboken). 2007;290(1):48–58.
16. Grogan SP, Pauli C, Lotz MK, D'Lima DD. Relevance of meniscal cell regional phenotype to tissue engineering. Connect Tissue Res. 2017;58(3–4):259–70.
17. Ding Z, Huang H. Mesenchymal stem cells in rabbit meniscus and bone marrow exhibit a similar feature but a heterogeneous multi-differentiation potential: superiority of meniscus as a cell source for meniscus repair. BMC Musculoskelet Disord. 2015;16:65.
18. Huang H, Wang S, Gui J, Shen H. A study to identify and characterize the stem/progenitor cell in rabbit meniscus. Cytotechnology. 2016;68(5):2083–103.
19. Freymann U, Endres M, Neumann K, Scholman HJ, Morawietz L, Kaps C. Expanded human meniscus-derived cells in 3-D polymer-hyaluronan scaffolds for meniscus repair. Acta Biomater. 2012;8(2):677–85.
20. Seol D, Zhou C, Brouillette MJ, Song I, Yu Y, Choe HH, et al. Characteristics of meniscus progenitor cells migrated from injured meniscus. J Orthop Res. 2017;35(9):1966–72.
21. Tarafder S, Gulko J, Sim KH, Yang J, Cook JL, Lee CH. Engineered healing of avascular meniscus tears by stem cell recruitment. Sci Rep. 2018;8(1):8150.
22. Gershuni DH, Hargens AR, Danzig LA. Regional nutrition and cellularity of the meniscus. Implications for tear and repair. Sports Med. 1988;5(5):322–7.
23. Hennerbichler A, Moutos FT, Hennerbichler D, Weinberg JB, Guilak F. Repair response of the inner and outer regions of the porcine meniscus in vitro. Am J Sports Med. 2007;35(5):754–62.
24. Makris EA, Hadidi P, Athanasiou KA. The knee meniscus: structure-function, pathophysiology, current repair techniques, and prospects for regeneration. Biomaterials. 2011;32(30):7411–31.

25. Travascio F, Jackson AR. The nutrition of the human meniscus: a computational analysis investigating the effect of vascular recession on tissue homeostasis. J Biomech. 2017;61:151–9.
26. Adesida AB, Mulet-Sierra A, Laouar L, Jomha NM. Oxygen tension is a determinant of the matrix-forming phenotype of cultured human meniscal fibrochondrocytes. PLoS One. 2012;7(6):e39339.
27. Bhargava MM, Attia ET, Murrell GA, Dolan MM, Warren RF, Hannafin JA. The effect of cytokines on the proliferation and migration of bovine meniscal cells. Am J Sports Med. 1999;27(5):636–43.
28. Bhargava MM, Hidaka C, Hannafin JA, Doty S, Warren RF. Effects of hepatocyte growth factor and platelet-derived growth factor on the repair of meniscal defects in vitro. In Vitro Cell Dev Biol Anim. 2005;41(8–9):305–10.
29. Lu Z, Furumatsu T, Fujii M, Maehara A, Ozaki T. The distribution of vascular endothelial growth factor in human meniscus and a meniscal injury model. J Orthop Sci. 2017;22(4):715–21.
30. Yuan X, Eng GM, Arkonac DE, Chao PH, Vunjak-Novakovic G. Endothelial cells enhance the migration of bovine meniscus cells. Arthritis Rheumatol. 2015;67(1):182–92.
31. Osawa A, Harner CD, Gharaibeh B, Matsumoto T, Mifune Y, Kopf S, et al. The use of blood vessel-derived stem cells for meniscal regeneration and repair. Med Sci Sports Exerc. 2013;45(5):813–23.
32. Zheng B, Cao B, Crisan M, Sun B, Li G, Logar A, et al. Prospective identification of myogenic endothelial cells in human skeletal muscle. Nat Biotechnol. 2007;25(9):1025–34.
33. Crisan M, Yap S, Casteilla L, Chen CW, Corselli M, Park TS, et al. A perivascular origin for mesenchymal stem cells in multiple human organs. Cell Stem Cell. 2008;3(3):301–13.
34. Aspden RM, Yarker YE, Hukins DWL. Collagen orientations in the meniscus of the knee-joint. J Anat. 1985;140(May):371–80.
35. Baek J, Chen X, Sovani S, Jin S, Grogan SP, D'Lima DD. Meniscus tissue engineering using a novel combination of electrospun scaffolds and human meniscus cells embedded within an extracellular matrix hydrogel. J Orthop Res. 2015;33(4):572–83.
36. Chatain F, Adeleine P, Chambat P, Neyret P. Societe Francaise dA. A comparative study of medial versus lateral arthroscopic partial meniscectomy on stable knees: 10-year minimum follow-up. Arthroscopy. 2003;19(8):842–9.
37. van de Graaf VA, Noorduyn JCA, Willigenburg NW, Butter IK, de Gast A, Mol BW, et al. Effect of early surgery vs physical therapy on knee function among patients with nonobstructive meniscal tears: the ESCAPE randomized clinical trial. JAMA. 2018;320(13):1328–37.
38. Holzer LA, Leithner A, Holzer G. Surgery versus physical therapy for meniscal tear and osteoarthritis. N Engl J Med. 2013;369(7):677.
39. Siemieniuk RAC, Harris IA, Agoritsas T, Poolman RW, Brignardello-Petersen R, Van de Velde S, et al. Arthroscopic surgery for degenerative knee arthritis and meniscal tears: a clinical practice guideline. BMJ. 2017;357:j1982.
40. Yim JH, Seon JK, Song EK, Choi JI, Kim MC, Lee KB, et al. A comparative study of meniscectomy and nonoperative treatment for degenerative horizontal tears of the medial meniscus. Am J Sports Med. 2013;41(7):1565–70.
41. Beaufils P, Becker R, Kopf S, Englund M, Verdonk R, Ollivier M, et al. Surgical management of degenerative meniscus lesions: the 2016 ESSKA meniscus consensus. Joints. 2017;5(2):59–69.
42. Rubman MH, Noyes FR, Barber-Westin SD. Arthroscopic repair of meniscal tears that extend into the avascular zone. A review of 198 single and complex tears. Am J Sports Med. 1998;26(1):87–95.
43. Kimura M, Shirakura K, Hasegawa A, Kobuna Y, Niijima M. Second look arthroscopy after meniscal repair. Factors affecting the healing rate. Clin Orthop Relat Res. 1995;314:185–91.
44. Noyes FR, Barber-Westin SD. Arthroscopic repair of meniscal tears extending into the avascular zone in patients younger than twenty years of age. Am J Sports Med. 2002;30(4):589–600.

45. Noyes FR, Barber-Westin SD. Arthroscopic repair of meniscus tears extending into the avascular zone with or without anterior cruciate ligament reconstruction in patients 40 years of age and older. Arthroscopy. 2000;16(8):822–9.
46. Driscoll MD, Robin BN, Horie M, Hubert ZT, Sampson HW, Jupiter DC, et al. Marrow stimulation improves meniscal healing at early endpoints in a rabbit meniscal injury model. Arthroscopy. 2013;29(1):113–21.
47. Kurzweil PR, Lynch NM, Coleman S, Kearney B. Repair of horizontal meniscus tears: a systematic review. Arthroscopy. 2014;30(11):1513–9.
48. Ahn JH, Kwon OJ, Nam TS. Arthroscopic repair of horizontal meniscal cleavage tears with marrow-stimulating technique. Arthroscopy. 2015;31(1):92–8.
49. Spahn G. Arthroscopic revisions in failed meniscal surgery. Int Orthop. 2003;27(6):378–81.
50. Tsujii A, Nakamura N, Horibe S. Age-related changes in the knee meniscus. Knee. 2017;24(6):1262–70.
51. Pauli C, Grogan SP, Patil S, Otsuki S, Hasegawa A, Koziol J, et al. Macroscopic and histopathologic analysis of human knee menisci in aging and osteoarthritis. Osteoarthr Cartil. 2011;19(9):1132–41.
52. Englund M, Guermazi A, Gale D, Hunter DJ, Aliabadi P, Clancy M, et al. Incidental meniscal findings on knee MRI in middle-aged and elderly persons. N Engl J Med. 2008;359(11):1108–15.
53. Frank RM, Cole BJ. Meniscus transplantation. Curr Rev Musculoskelet Med. 2015;8(4):443–50.
54. Zellner J, Taeger CD, Schaffer M, Roldan JC, Loibl M, Mueller MB, et al. Are applied growth factors able to mimic the positive effects of mesenchymal stem cells on the regeneration of meniscus in the avascular zone? Biomed Res Int. 2014;2014:537686.
55. Myers KR, Sgaglione NA, Goodwillie AD. Meniscal scaffolds. J Knee Surg. 2014;27(6):435–42.
56. Ozeki N, Muneta T, Koga H, Katagiri H, Otabe K, Okuno M, et al. Transplantation of Achilles tendon treated with bone morphogenetic protein 7 promotes meniscus regeneration in a rat model of massive meniscal defect. Arthritis Rheum. 2013;65(11):2876–86.
57. Zhang ZZ, Jiang D, Wang SJ, Qi YS, Zhang JY, Yu JK. Potential of centrifugal seeding method in improving cells distribution and proliferation on demineralized cancellous bone scaffolds for tissue-engineered meniscus. ACS Appl Mater Interfaces. 2015;7(28):15294–302.
58. Rothrauff BB, Shimomura K, Gottardi R, Alexander PG, Tuan RS. Anatomical region-dependent enhancement of 3-dimensional chondrogenic differentiation of human mesenchymal stem cells by soluble meniscus extracellular matrix. Acta Biomater. 2017;49:140–51.
59. McCorry MC, Bonassar LJ. Fiber development and matrix production in tissue-engineered menisci using bovine mesenchymal stem cells and fibrochondrocytes. Connect Tissue Res. 2017;58(3–4):329–41.
60. Shimomura K, Rothrauff BB, Hart DA, Hamamoto S, Kobayashi M, Yoshikawa H, et al. Enhanced repair of meniscal hoop structure injuries using an aligned electrospun nanofibrous scaffold combined with a mesenchymal stem cell-derived tissue engineered construct. Biomaterials. 2018;192:346–54.
61. Freymann U, Metzlaff S, Kruger JP, Hirsh G, Endres M, Petersen W, et al. Effect of human serum and 2 different types of platelet concentrates on human meniscus cell migration, proliferation, and matrix formation. Arthroscopy. 2016;32(6):1106–16.
62. Freymann U, Degrassi L, Kruger JP, Metzlaff S, Endres M, Petersen W. Effect of serum and platelet-rich plasma on human early or advanced degenerative meniscus cells. Connect Tissue Res. 2017;58(6):509–19.
63. Baboolal TG, Khalil-Khan A, Theodorides AA, Wall O, Jones E, McGonagle D. A novel arthroscopic technique for intraoperative mobilization of synovial mesenchymal stem cells. Am J Sports Med. 2018;46(14):3532–40.
64. Madry H, Cucchiarini M, Kaul G, Kohn D, Terwilliger EF, Trippel SB. Menisci are efficiently transduced by recombinant adeno-associated virus vectors in vitro and in vivo. Am J Sports Med. 2004;32(8):1860–5.

65. Lee KI, Olmer M, Baek J, D'Lima DD, Lotz MK. Platelet-derived growth factor-coated decellularized meniscus scaffold for integrative healing of meniscus tears. Acta Biomater. 2018;76:126–34.
66. Qu F, Holloway JL, Esterhai JL, Burdick JA, Mauck RL. Programmed biomolecule delivery to enable and direct cell migration for connective tissue repair. Nat Commun. 2017;8(1):1780.
67. Monllau JC, Gelber PE, Abat F, Pelfort X, Abad R, Hinarejos P, et al. Outcome after partial medial meniscus substitution with the collagen meniscal implant at a minimum of 10 years' follow-up. Arthroscopy. 2011;27(7):933–43.
68. Rodkey WG, Steadman JR, Li ST. A clinical study of collagen meniscus implants to restore the injured meniscus. Clin Orthop Relat Res. 1999;(367 Suppl):S281–92.
69. Bulgheroni P, Murena L, Ratti C, Bulgheroni E, Ronga M, Cherubino P. Follow-up of collagen meniscus implant patients: clinical, radiological, and magnetic resonance imaging results at 5 years. Knee. 2010;17(3):224–9.
70. Bulgheroni E, Grassi A, Campagnolo M, Bulgheroni P, Mudhigere A, Gobbi A. Comparative study of collagen versus synthetic-based meniscal scaffolds in treating meniscal deficiency in young active population. Cartilage. 2016;7(1):29–38.
71. Rodkey WG, DeHaven KE, Montgomery WH 3rd, Baker CL Jr, Beck CL Jr, Hormel SE, et al. Comparison of the collagen meniscus implant with partial meniscectomy. A prospective randomized trial. J Bone Joint Surg Am. 2008;90(7):1413–26.
72. Zaffagnini S, Giordano G, Vascellari A, Bruni D, Neri MP, Iacono F, et al. Arthroscopic collagen meniscus implant results at 6 to 8 years follow up. Knee Surg Sports Traumatol Arthrosc. 2007;15(2):175–83.
73. Zaffagnini S, Marcheggiani Muccioli GM, Lopomo N, Bruni D, Giordano G, Ravazzolo G, et al. Prospective long-term outcomes of the medial collagen meniscus implant versus partial medial meniscectomy: a minimum 10-year follow-up study. Am J Sports Med. 2011;39(5):977–85.
74. Verdonk R, Verdonk P, Huysse W, Forsyth R, Heinrichs EL. Tissue ingrowth after implantation of a novel, biodegradable polyurethane scaffold for treatment of partial meniscal lesions. Am J Sports Med. 2011;39(4):774–82.
75. Peters G, Wirth CJ. The current state of meniscal allograft transplantation and replacement. Knee. 2003;10(1):19–31.
76. de Groot JH, Zijlstra FM, Kuipers HW, Pennings AJ, Klompmaker J, Veth RP, et al. Meniscal tissue regeneration in porous 50/50 copoly(L-lactide/epsilon-caprolactone) implants. Biomaterials. 1997;18(8):613–22.
77. Tienen TG, Heijkants RG, de Groot JH, Pennings AJ, Schouten AJ, Veth RP, et al. Replacement of the knee meniscus by a porous polymer implant: a study in dogs. Am J Sports Med. 2006;34(1):64–71.
78. Zuidema J, van Minnen B, Span MM, Hissink CE, van Kooten TG, Bos RR. In vitro degradation of a biodegradable polyurethane foam, based on 1,4-butanediisocyanate: a three-year study at physiological and elevated temperature. J Biomed Mater Res A. 2009;90(3):920–30.
79. van Minnen B, van Leeuwen MB, Kors G, Zuidema J, van Kooten TG, Bos RR. In vivo resorption of a biodegradable polyurethane foam, based on 1,4-butanediisocyanate: a three-year subcutaneous implantation study. J Biomed Mater Res A. 2008;85(4):972–82.
80. de Groot JH. Polyurethane scaffolds for meniscal tissue regeneration. Med Device Technol. 2005;16(7):18–20.
81. Efe T, Getgood A, Schofer MD, Fuchs-Winkelmann S, Mann D, Paletta JR, et al. The safety and short-term efficacy of a novel polyurethane meniscal scaffold for the treatment of segmental medial meniscus deficiency. Knee Surg Sports Traumatol Arthrosc. 2012;20(9):1822–30.
82. Verdonk P, Beaufils P, Bellemans J, Djian P, Heinrichs EL, Huysse W, et al. Successful treatment of painful irreparable partial meniscal defects with a polyurethane scaffold: two-year safety and clinical outcomes. Am J Sports Med. 2012;40(4):844–53.
83. Bouyarmane H, Beaufils P, Pujol N, Bellemans J, Roberts S, Spalding T, et al. Polyurethane scaffold in lateral meniscus segmental defects: clinical outcomes at 24 months follow-up. Orthop Traumatol Surg Res. 2014;100(1):153–7.

84. Dhollander A, Verdonk P, Verdonk R. Treatment of painful, irreparable partial meniscal defects with a polyurethane scaffold: midterm clinical outcomes and survival analysis. Am J Sports Med. 2016;44(10):2615–21.

85. Leroy A, Beaufils P, Faivre B, Steltzlen C, Boisrenoult P, Pujol N. Actifit((R)) polyurethane meniscal scaffold: MRI and functional outcomes after a minimum follow-up of 5 years. Orthop Traumatol Surg Res. 2017;103(4):609–14.

86. Monllau JC, Poggioli F, Erquicia J, Ramirez E, Pelfort X, Gelber P, et al. Magnetic resonance imaging and functional outcomes after a polyurethane meniscal scaffold implantation: minimum 5-year follow-up. Arthroscopy. 2018;34(5):1621–7.

87. Barber FA. Editorial commentary: polyurethane meniscal scaffold: a perfect fit or flop? Arthroscopy. 2018;34(5):1628–30.

88. Schuttler KF, Haberhauer F, Gesslein M, Heyse TJ, Figiel J, Lorbach O, et al. Midterm follow-up after implantation of a polyurethane meniscal scaffold for segmental medial meniscus loss: maintenance of good clinical and MRI outcome. Knee Surg Sports Traumatol Arthrosc. 2016;24(5):1478–84.

89. Shin YS, Lee HN, Sim HB, Kim HJ, Lee DH. Polyurethane meniscal scaffolds lead to better clinical outcomes but worse articular cartilage status and greater absolute meniscal extrusion. Knee Surg Sports Traumatol Arthrosc. 2018;26(8):2227–38.

90. Faivre B, Bouyarmane H, Lonjon G, Boisrenoult P, Pujol N, Beaufils P. Actifit(R) scaffold implantation: influence of preoperative meniscal extrusion on morphological and clinical outcomes. Orthop Traumatol Surg Res. 2015;101(6):703–8.

91. Houck DA, Kraeutler MJ, Belk JW, McCarty EC, Bravman JT. Similar clinical outcomes following collagen or polyurethane meniscal scaffold implantation: a systematic review. Knee Surg Sports Traumatol Arthrosc. 2018;26(8):2259–69.

92. Elsner JJ, Portnoy S, Zur G, Guilak F, Shterling A, Linder-Ganz E. Design of a free-floating polycarbonate-urethane meniscal implant using finite element modeling and experimental validation. J Biomech Eng. 2010;132(9):095001.

93. Shemesh M, Asher R, Zylberberg E, Guilak F, Linder-Ganz E, Elsner JJ. Viscoelastic properties of a synthetic meniscus implant. J Mech Behav Biomed Mater. 2014;29:42–55.

94. Merriam AR, Patel JM, Culp BM, Gatt CJ Jr, Dunn MG. Successful total meniscus reconstruction using a novel fiber-reinforced scaffold: a 16- and 32-week study in an Ovine Model. Am J Sports Med. 2015;43(10):2528–37.

95. Gruchenberg K, Ignatius A, Friemert B, von Lubken F, Skaer N, Gellynck K, et al. Correction to: in vivo performance of a novel silk fibroin scaffold for partial meniscal replacement in a sheep model. Knee Surg Sports Traumatol Arthrosc. 2018;26(7):2216.

96. Yan R, Chen Y, Gu Y, Tang C, Huang J, Hu Y, et al. A collagen-coated sponge silk scaffold for functional meniscus regeneration. J Tissue Eng Regen Med. 2018;13:156.

97. Yuan Z, Liu S, Hao C, Guo W, Gao S, Wang M, et al. AMECM/DCB scaffold prompts successful total meniscus reconstruction in a rabbit total meniscectomy model. Biomaterials. 2016;111:13–26.

98. Lee CH, Rodeo SA, Fortier LA, Lu C, Erisken C, Mao JJ. Protein-releasing polymeric scaffolds induce fibrochondrocytic differentiation of endogenous cells for knee meniscus regeneration in sheep. Sci Transl Med. 2014;6(266):266ra171.

99. Shimomura K, Bean AC, Lin H, Nakamura N, Tuan RS. In vitro repair of meniscal radial tear using aligned electrospun nanofibrous scaffold. Tissue Eng Part A. 2015;21(13–14):2066–75.

100. Hayes JC, Curley C, Tierney P, Kennedy JE. Biomechanical analysis of a salt-modified polyvinyl alcohol hydrogel for knee meniscus applications, including comparison with human donor samples. J Mech Behav Biomed Mater. 2016;56:156–64.

101. Kang SW, Son SM, Lee JS, Lee ES, Lee KY, Park SG, et al. Regeneration of whole meniscus using meniscal cells and polymer scaffolds in a rabbit total meniscectomy model. J Biomed Mater Res A. 2006;78(3):659–71.

102. Lu HD, Cai DZ, Wu G, Wang K, Shi DH. Whole meniscus regeneration using polymer scaffolds loaded with fibrochondrocytes. Chin J Traumatol. 2011;14(4):195–204.

103. Liang Y, Idrees E, Andrews SHJ, Labib K, Szojka A, Kunze M, et al. Plasticity of human meniscus fibrochondrocytes: a study on effects of mitotic divisions and oxygen tension. Sci Rep. 2017;7(1):12148.
104. Baek J, Sovani S, Glembotski NE, Du J, Jin S, Grogan SP, et al. Repair of avascular meniscus tears with electrospun collagen scaffolds seeded with human cells. Tissue Eng Part A. 2016;22(5–6):436–48.
105. Oda S, Otsuki S, Kurokawa Y, Hoshiyama Y, Nakajima M, Neo M. A new method for meniscus repair using type I collagen scaffold and infrapatellar fat pad. J Biomater Appl. 2015;29(10):1439–48.
106. Kwak HS, Nam J, Lee JH, Kim HJ, Yoo JJ. Meniscal repair in vivo using human chondrocyte-seeded PLGA mesh scaffold pretreated with platelet-rich plasma. J Tissue Eng Regen Med. 2017;11(2):471–80.
107. Koch M, Achatz FP, Lang S, Pfeifer CG, Pattappa G, Kujat R, et al. Tissue engineering of large full-size meniscus defects by a polyurethane scaffold: accelerated regeneration by mesenchymal stromal cells. Stem Cells Int. 2018;2018:8207071.
108. Moradi L, Vasei M, Dehghan MM, Majidi M, Farzad Mohajeri S, Bonakdar S. Regeneration of meniscus tissue using adipose mesenchymal stem cells-chondrocytes co-culture on a hybrid scaffold: in vivo study. Biomaterials. 2017;126:18–30.
109. DeLise AM, Fischer L, Tuan RS. Cellular interactions and signaling in cartilage development. Osteoarthr Cartil. 2000;8(5):309–34.
110. Hwang NS, Varghese S, Puleo C, Zhang Z, Elisseeff J. Morphogenetic signals from chondrocytes promote chondrogenic and osteogenic differentiation of mesenchymal stem cells. J Cell Physiol. 2007;212(2):281–4.
111. Zhang ZZ, Wang SJ, Zhang JY, Jiang WB, Huang AB, Qi YS, et al. 3D-printed poly(epsilon-caprolactone) scaffold augmented with mesenchymal stem cells for total meniscal substitution: a 12- and 24-week animal study in a Rabbit Model. Am J Sports Med. 2017;45(7):1497–511.
112. Pabbruwe MB, Kafienah W, Tarlton JF, Mistry S, Fox DJ, Hollander AP. Repair of meniscal cartilage white zone tears using a stem cell/collagen-scaffold implant. Biomaterials. 2010;31(9):2583–91.
113. Koh RH, Jin Y, Kang BJ, Hwang NS. Chondrogenically primed tonsil-derived mesenchymal stem cells encapsulated in riboflavin-induced photocrosslinking collagen-hyaluronic acid hydrogel for meniscus tissue repairs. Acta Biomater. 2017;53:318–28.
114. Sasaki H, Rothrauff BB, Alexander PG, Lin H, Gottardi R, Fu FH, et al. In vitro repair of meniscal radial tear with hydrogels seeded with adipose stem cells and TGF-beta3. Am J Sports Med. 2018;46(10):2402–13.
115. Yuan X, Wei Y, Villasante A, Ng JJD, Arkonac DE, Chao PG, et al. Stem cell delivery in tissue-specific hydrogel enabled meniscal repair in an orthotopic rat model. Biomaterials. 2017;132:59–71.
116. Whitehouse MR, Howells NR, Parry MC, Austin E, Kafienah W, Brady K, et al. Repair of torn avascular meniscal cartilage using undifferentiated autologous mesenchymal stem cells: from in vitro optimization to a first-in-human study. Stem Cells Transl Med. 2017;6(4):1237–48.
117. Hutchinson ID, Rodeo SA, Perrone GS, Murray MM. Can platelet-rich plasma enhance anterior cruciate ligament and meniscal repair? J Knee Surg. 2015;28(1):19–28.
118. Boesen AP, Hansen R, Boesen MI, Malliaras P, Langberg H. Effect of high-volume injection, platelet-rich plasma, and sham treatment in chronic midportion achilles tendinopathy: a randomized double-blinded prospective study. Am J Sports Med. 2017;45(9):2034–43.
119. de Vos RJ, Weir A, van Schie HT, Bierma-Zeinstra SM, Verhaar JA, Weinans H, et al. Platelet-rich plasma injection for chronic Achilles tendinopathy: a randomized controlled trial. JAMA. 2010;303(2):144–9.
120. Cucchiarini M, Schetting S, Terwilliger EF, Kohn D, Madry H. rAAV-mediated overexpression of FGF-2 promotes cell proliferation, survival, and alpha-SMA expression in human meniscal lesions. Gene Ther. 2009;16(11):1363–72.

121. Holmes HL, Wilson B, Goerger JP, Silverberg JL, Cohen I, Zipfel WR, et al. Facilitated recruitment of mesenchymal stromal cells by bone marrow concentrate and platelet rich plasma. PLoS One. 2018;13(3):e0194567.
122. Griffin JW, Hadeed MM, Werner BC, Diduch DR, Carson EW, Miller MD. Platelet-rich plasma in meniscal repair: does augmentation improve surgical outcomes? Clin Orthop Relat Res. 2015;473(5):1665–72.
123. Kemmochi M, Sasaki S, Takahashi M, Nishimura T, Aizawa C, Kikuchi J. The use of platelet-rich fibrin with platelet-rich plasma support meniscal repair surgery. J Orthop. 2018;15(2):711–20.
124. Kaminski R, Kulinski K, Kozar-Kaminska K, Wielgus M, Langner M, Wasko MK, et al. A prospective, randomized, double-blind, parallel-group, placebo-controlled study evaluating meniscal healing, clinical outcomes, and safety in patients undergoing meniscal repair of unstable, complete vertical meniscal tears (bucket handle) augmented with platelet-rich plasma. Biomed Res Int. 2018;2018:9315815.
125. Pujol N, Salle De Chou E, Boisrenoult P, Beaufils P. Platelet-rich plasma for open meniscal repair in young patients: any benefit? Knee Surg Sports Traumatol Arthrosc. 2015;23(1):51–8.
126. Jang SH, Ha JK, Lee DW, Kim JG. Fibrin clot delivery system for meniscal repair. Knee Surg Relat Res. 2011;23(3):180–3.
127. Port J, Simon TM, Jackson DW. Preparation of an exogenous fibrin clot. Arthroscopy. 1995;11(3):332–7.
128. Kamimura T, Kimura M. Meniscal repair of degenerative horizontal cleavage tears using fibrin clots: clinical and arthroscopic outcomes in 10 cases. Orthop J Sports Med. 2014;2(11):2325967114555678.
129. Kamimura T, Kimura M. Repair of horizontal meniscal cleavage tears with exogenous fibrin clots. Knee Surg Sports Traumatol Arthrosc. 2011;19(7):1154–7.
130. Ra HJ, Ha JK, Jang SH, Lee DW, Kim JG. Arthroscopic inside-out repair of complete radial tears of the meniscus with a fibrin clot. Knee Surg Sports Traumatol Arthrosc. 2013;21(9):2126–30.
131. Longo UG, Campi S, Romeo G, Spiezia F, Maffulli N, Denaro V. Biological strategies to enhance healing of the avascular area of the meniscus. Stem Cells Int. 2012;2012:528359.
132. Muhammad H, Schminke B, Bode C, Roth M, Albert J, von der Heyde S, et al. Human migratory meniscus progenitor cells are controlled via the TGF-beta pathway. Stem Cell Rep. 2014;3(5):789–803.
133. Blank U, Karlsson G, Karlsson S. Signaling pathways governing stem-cell fate. Blood. 2008;111(2):492–503.
134. Horie M, Choi H, Lee RH, Reger RL, Ylostalo J, Muneta T, et al. Intra-articular injection of human mesenchymal stem cells (MSCs) promote rat meniscal regeneration by being activated to express Indian hedgehog that enhances expression of type II collagen. Osteoarthr Cartil. 2012;20(10):1197–207.
135. Lu Y, Wang Y, Lin M, Zhou J, Wang Z, Jiang M, et al. A systematic review of randomised controlled trials examining the therapeutic effects of adult bone marrow-derived stem cells for non-ischaemic dilated cardiomyopathy. Stem Cell Res Ther. 2016;7(1):186.
136. Saliken DJ, Mulet-Sierra A, Jomha NM, Adesida AB. Decreased hypertrophic differentiation accompanies enhanced matrix formation in co-cultures of outer meniscus cells with bone marrow mesenchymal stromal cells. Arthritis Res Ther. 2012;14(3):R153.
137. Chowdhury A, Bezuidenhout LW, Mulet-Sierra A, Jomha NM, Adesida AB. Effect of interleukin-1beta treatment on co-cultures of human meniscus cells and bone marrow mesenchymal stromal cells. BMC Musculoskelet Disord. 2013;14:216.
138. Matthies NF, Mulet-Sierra A, Jomha NM, Adesida AB. Matrix formation is enhanced in co-cultures of human meniscus cells with bone marrow stromal cells. J Tissue Eng Regen Med. 2013;7(12):965–73.
139. Vangsness CT Jr, Farr J 2nd, Boyd J, Dellaero DT, Mills CR, LeRoux-Williams M. Adult human mesenchymal stem cells delivered via intra-articular injection to the knee following

partial medial meniscectomy: a randomized, double-blind, controlled study. J Bone Joint Surg Am. 2014;96(2):90–8.

140. Gonzalez-Fernandez ML, Perez-Castrillo S, Sanchez-Lazaro JA, Prieto-Fernandez JG, Lopez-Gonzalez ME, Lobato-Perez S, et al. Assessment of regeneration in meniscal lesions by use of mesenchymal stem cells derived from equine bone marrow and adipose tissue. Am J Vet Res. 2016;77(7):779–88.

141. Toratani T, Nakase J, Numata H, Oshima T, Takata Y, Nakayama K, et al. Scaffold-free tissue-engineered allogenic adipose-derived stem cells promote meniscus healing. Arthroscopy. 2017;33(2):346–54.

142. Ruiz-Iban MA, Diaz-Heredia J, Garcia-Gomez I, Gonzalez-Lizan F, Elias-Martin E, Abraira V. The effect of the addition of adipose-derived mesenchymal stem cells to a meniscal repair in the avascular zone: an experimental study in rabbits. Arthroscopy. 2011;27(12):1688–96.

143. Qi Y, Yang Z, Ding Q, Zhao T, Huang Z, Feng G. Targeted transplantation of iron oxide-labeled, adipose-derived mesenchymal stem cells in promoting meniscus regeneration following a rabbit massive meniscal defect. Exp Ther Med. 2016;11(2):458–66.

144. Horie M, Driscoll MD, Sampson HW, Sekiya I, Caroom CT, Prockop DJ, et al. Implantation of allogenic synovial stem cells promotes meniscal regeneration in a rabbit meniscal defect model. J Bone Joint Surg Am. 2012;94(8):701–12.

145. Kondo S, Muneta T, Nakagawa Y, Koga H, Watanabe T, Tsuji K, et al. Transplantation of autologous synovial mesenchymal stem cells promotes meniscus regeneration in aged primates. J Orthop Res. 2017;35(6):1274–82.

146. Jayasuriya CT, Twomey-Kozak J, Newberry J, Desai S, Feltman P, Franco JR, et al. Human cartilage-derived progenitors resist terminal differentiation and require CXCR4 activation to successfully bridge meniscus tissue tears. Stem Cells. 2018;37:102.

147. Shen W, Chen J, Zhu T, Chen L, Zhang W, Fang Z, et al. Intra-articular injection of human meniscus stem/progenitor cells promotes meniscus regeneration and ameliorates osteoarthritis through stromal cell-derived factor-1/CXCR4-mediated homing. Stem Cells Transl Med. 2014;3(3):387–94.

148. Stone AV, Loeser RF, Vanderman KS, Long DL, Clark SC, Ferguson CM. Pro-inflammatory stimulation of meniscus cells increases production of matrix metalloproteinases and additional catabolic factors involved in osteoarthritis pathogenesis. Osteoarthr Cartil. 2014;22(2):264–74.

149. Brophy RH, Rai MF, Zhang Z, Torgomyan A, Sandell LJ. Molecular analysis of age and sex-related gene expression in meniscal tears with and without a concomitant anterior cruciate ligament tear. J Bone Joint Surg Am. 2012;94(5):385–93.

150. Goto H, Shuler FD, Lamsam C, Moller HD, Niyibizi C, Fu FH, et al. Transfer of lacZ marker gene to the meniscus. J Bone Joint Surg Am. 1999;81(7):918–25.

151. Goto H, Shuler FD, Niyibizi C, Fu FH, Robbins PD, Evans CH. Gene therapy for meniscal injury: enhanced synthesis of proteoglycan and collagen by meniscal cells transduced with a TGFbeta(1)gene. Osteoarthr Cartil. 2000;8(4):266–71.

152. Hidaka C, Ibarra C, Hannafin JA, Torzilli PA, Quitoriano M, Jen SS, et al. Formation of vascularized meniscal tissue by combining gene therapy with tissue engineering. Tissue Eng. 2002;8(1):93–105.

153. Martinek V, Usas A, Pelinkovic D, Robbins P, Fu FH, Huard J. Genetic engineering of meniscal allografts. Tissue Eng. 2002;8(1):107–17.

154. Cucchiarini M, Schmidt K, Frisch J, Kohn D, Madry H. Overexpression of TGF-beta via rAAV-mediated gene transfer promotes the healing of human meniscal lesions ex vivo on explanted menisci. Am J Sports Med. 2015;43(5):1197–205.

155. Steinert AF, Palmer GD, Capito R, Hofstaetter JG, Pilapil C, Ghivizzani SC, et al. Genetically enhanced engineering of meniscus tissue using ex vivo delivery of transforming growth factor-beta 1 complementary deoxyribonucleic acid. Tissue Eng. 2007;13(9):2227–37.

156. Zhang H, Leng P, Zhang J. Enhanced meniscal repair by overexpression of hIGF-1 in a full-thickness model. Clin Orthop Relat Res. 2009;467(12):3165–74.

157. Bartel DP. MicroRNAs: genomics, biogenesis, mechanism, and function. Cell. 2004;116(2):281–97.
158. Kawanishi Y, Nakasa T, Shoji T, Hamanishi M, Shimizu R, Kamei N, et al. Intra-articular injection of synthetic microRNA-210 accelerates avascular meniscal healing in rat medial meniscal injured model. Arthritis Res Ther. 2014;16(6):488.
159. Zhang S, Matsushita T, Kuroda R, Nishida K, Matsuzaki T, Matsumoto T, et al. Local administration of Simvastatin stimulates healing of an avascular meniscus in a Rabbit Model of a meniscal defect. Am J Sports Med. 2016;44(7):1735–43.

Index

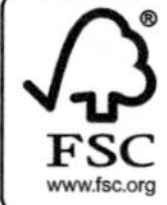